Genetics of Human Infertility

Monographs in Human Genetics

Vol. 21

Series Editor

Michael Schmid Würzburg

Genetics of Human Infertility

Volume Editor

Peter H. Vogt Heidelberg

24 figures, 16 in color, and 8 tables, 2017

KARGER

Basel · Freiburg · Paris · London · New York · Chennai · New Delhi · Bangkok · Beijing · Shanghai · Tokyo · Kuala Lumpur · Singapore · Sydney

Peter H. Vogt
Sektion für Reproduktionsgenetik
Abt. Gynäkologische
Endokrinologie u.
Fertilitätsstörungen
Universitätsklinikum Heidelberg
Im Neuenheimer Feld 440
D–69120 Heidelberg (Germany)

Library of Congress Cataloging-in-Publication Data

Names: Vogt, Peter, 1950- editor.
Title: Genetics of human infertility / volume editor, Peter Vogt.
Other titles: Monographs in human genetics ; v. 21. 0077-0876
Description: Basel ; New York : Karger, [2017] | Series: Monographs in human genetics, ISSN 0077-0876 ; vol. 21 | Includes bibliographical references and indexes.
Identifiers: LCCN 2017032899| ISBN 9783318060973 (hardcover : alk. paper) | ISBN 9783318060980 (ebook)
Subjects: | MESH: Infertility--genetics | Infertility--physiopathology
Classification: LCC RC889 | NLM WP 570 | DDC 616.6/92042--dc23 LC record available at https://lccn.loc.gov/2017032899

Bibliographic Indices. This publication is listed in bibliographic services, including Thomson Reuters indices.

www.karger.com
Printed on acid-free and non-aging paper (ISO 9706)
ISSN 0077–0876
e-ISSN 1662–3835
ISBN 978–3–318–06097–3
e-ISBN 978–3–318–06098–0

Contents

Editorial

It is my great pleasure to introduce volume 21 of the book series *Monographs in Human Genetics*, entitled "Genetics of Human Infertility." The concept of this book emerged in the summer of 2014 during a telephone call with my colleague of many years, Peter Vogt, from the University of Heidelberg. From a demographic point of view, it appears that in endlessly and exponentially growing world populations that can account for hunger crises, diseases, epidemics, and even war conflicts between nations, any concerns about possibly overcoming infertility or subfertility factors in the human genome are unnecessary. However, it is a well-established fact that many individual couples who have faced a personal battle with involuntary childlessness have journeyed through an immense burden in the form of social, emotional, and psychological strain. Fortunately, the past decades have been witness to remarkable advances in human infertility treatments that include assisted reproductive technologies. In parallel, genetic aetiologies of female and male infertility have been unravelled by a variety of genetic disciplines and different techniques. These landmark discoveries call for a timely and thorough overview of this area with the assistance of expert investigators.

The present volume has been organized in an exquisite way. I am very thankful to Peter Vogt for all the time he invested and the efforts he made in processing the 11 chapters of this captivating book. In addition to 9 chapters on the genetic aspects of human infertility, 2 chapters focus on germ cell development in mice and primates. Internationally renowned authors have contributed superb articles that are well prepared and flawlessly illustrated. Finally, I am grateful to Karger Publishers for their enduring support of this book series.

Michael Schmid, Würzburg

Preface

The cover picture of this volume is the first drawing of a severe human sperm pathology, termed teratozoospermia. It was prepared 340 years ago in 1677 by Antoni van Leeuwenhoek, who is considered to be the world's first microbiologist. He gazed through a tiny lens set into a brass holder, looked into the sun, and by this simple construction achieved the magnification of nearly 300 times normal vision. This picture was never published in an original paper or book, but came to light through his correspondence with the Royal Society of England in London, which published these letters in their *Philosophical Transactions* (vol. 12, pp. 1040–1046). It remains unclear whether such human sperm dysmorphologies have some genetic origin despite their high incidence in human males with distinct infertility problems.

Today we know that human male and female infertility affects nearly 15–20% of all couples worldwide and that this condition presents with highly heterogeneous pathologies. Sometimes they are only visible in the germ line, but often they are also affecting the common health condition. Their aetiology often, but not always, includes genetic factors besides anatomical defects, immunological interference, and environmental aspects. Nearly 30% of infertility cases are probably due primarily to only genetic defects. Experimental animal knockout models mainly performed with mouse and *Drosophila* convincingly show that male or female infertility can be caused by single or multiple gene defects. However, translating these findings into the practice of an infertility clinic is challenging because human is not an experimental species. Genetic causes for human infertility therefore often remain unexplained – also called "idiopathic" – for the vast majority of male or female infertility patients. Nevertheless, a large number of human candidate genes have been identified by sophisticated molecular methods. However, since also many structural polymorphism and polymorphic sequence variants have been identified in the human genome in different populations, it remains a major challenge to select those gene and genome mutations causing infertility unless one has the chance to also analyse the patient's genetic family background.

At present, there are therefore only a handful of genetic defects that have been shown to cause, or to be strongly associated with, primary male or female infertility. This situation may change in the near future since sophisticated molecular diagnostic test systems are now also becoming available in the infertility clinic, including tools like CGH (comparative genomic hybridization) array analyses and genomic sequencing with NGS (next-generation sequencing) machines.

With this background in mind, I would like to thank all of the authors of this volume who have contributed to an actual comprehensive overview on what is known today about the major genetic conditions causing male or female infertility in humans. All authors have focused their papers on finding answers to the basic question of how to translate their results into the clinical practice as soon as possible. The authors are also thanked for their willingness to incorporate some future insights into their chapters, including the presentation of diagnostic tools for the analysis of the epigenetic equipment required for fertility, and putative experimental systems for the imminent generation of male or female germ cells from pluripotent stem cells. I also highly appreciate the discussions concerning the heterogeneity of somatic pathologies, including infertility caused by distinct genetic defects due to chromosome aneuploidies like the Klinefelter syndrome (47,XXY) or single gene mutations in the *CFTR* and *AR* gene, respectively. Special thanks also go to my colleagues who critically compared the genetic and epigenetic control of male germ cell development in mice and primates with that in humans. A critical description of the putative functional and nonfunctional aspects of mutations in the azoospermia factor locus (AZF) located on the long arm of the human Y chromosome reveals the importance of chromosome studies and family studies in all sporadic cases of human infertility.

Peter H. Vogt
Heidelberg, March 2017

Vogt PH (ed): Genetics of Human Infertility. Monogr Hum Genet.
Basel, Karger, 2017, vol 21, pp 1–16 (DOI: 10.1159/000477275)

Genetic Basis of Male and Female Infertility

Rathika Mallepaly[b] · Peter R. Butler[a, b] · Amin S. Herati[a, b] · Dolores J. Lamb[a–c]

[a]Center for Reproductive Medicine, [b]Scott Department of Urology and [c]Department of Molecular and Cellular Biology, Baylor College of Medicine, Houston, TX, USA

Abstract

Male and female infertility affects close to 50 million couples worldwide according to a recent World Health Organization estimate. Many of the 25–30% of couples with idiopathic infertility likely have a genetic etiology for their condition. Next-generation sequencing has identified many new putative causes of infertility in recent years, which are discussed in this chapter. Genetic and genomic causes of infertility can be divided into cytogenetic anomalies, gene defects, and epigenetic aberrances. The discussion of male infertility focuses on genetic factors impairing spermatogenesis and includes numerical chromosomal anomalies such as Klinefelter syndrome, structural chromosomal anomalies such as Y-chromosome microdeletions, certain single gene mutations, syndromic diseases, and epigenetic mutations. The discussion of female infertility includes chromosomal anomalies like Turner syndrome, as well as genetic and epigenetic mutations identified as causes of hypogonadotropic hypogonadism, premature ovarian insufficiency, endometriosis, and polycystic ovarian syndrome. In conclusion, new genetic testing methods have significantly advanced our knowledge of the genetic basis of male and female infertility. However, the list of known candidate abnormalities is not exhaustive, and further research is required to understand how each candidate mutation influences fertility.

Infertility is a complex, heterogeneous disorder that is influenced by many biological factors, which can affect the male, female, or both partners. In 2010, the World Health Organization (WHO) estimated that 48.5 million couples worldwide were infertile, with a rising prevalence due to a growing world population [1]. According to the American Society for Reproductive Medicine, when a cause for infertility is identified among heterosexual couples of reproductive age, it is due to a male factor in a third of cases, due to a female factor in another third, and the remaining third are due to combined male and female factors [2]. However, in approximately 25–30% of couples, no cause is identified and the infertility is considered idiopathic [3].

R.M. and P.R.B. are co-first authors.

Many of these idiopathic infertility cases are likely genetic or genomic in nature. These defects may contribute to nearly 50% of male factor infertility causes [4, 5]. The 2 most common female factor conditions, ovulatory dysfunction (25%) and endometriosis (15%), have a demonstrable familial predisposition, also suggesting a genetic basis [6–8]. Our understanding of the genetic basis of male infertility has advanced beyond our understanding of female infertility as sperm are continuously undergoing meiotic division and are easier to obtain through ejaculation or surgical extraction. Moreover, male fecundity is less influenced by age and hormonal milieu.

With the advent of advanced genetic testing, such as next-generation sequencing (NGS), the medical community is identifying a genetic basis of reproductive disease with ever increasing frequency. Genetic and genomic abnormalities, such as chromosomal aneuploidy, chromosomal structural defects, genetic mutations, and epigenetic dysregulation, can cause infertility in both males and females through the disruption of spermatogenesis and oogenesis, respectively. Herein we present the known genetic causes and associations for both male and female infertility.

Male Infertility

Standard Work-Up

Evaluation of the infertile male consists of a medical history, physical examination, hormone measurement, and semen analysis (SA). Routine SA includes an evaluation of sperm density, motility, and morphology. Conditions of suboptimal SA parameters include absent sperm in the ejaculate (azoospermia), low sperm density (oligozoospermia; OS), abnormal sperm morphology (teratozoospermia), or impaired motility (asthenozoospermia). Although the SA allows for the assignment of infertile men into various categories based on their kind and degree of spermatogenic impairment, it often fails to detect the ultimate cause of male infertility. Semen parameters cannot define a man as fertile or infertile unless there are no sperm in the ejaculate. It is not a test of fertility.

Cytogenetic Anomalies in Male Infertility

The relationship between chromosomal anomalies and male infertility is fairly well studied. In a retrospective review of 668 subfertile males who underwent karyotype analysis, the rate of cytogenetic abnormality was found to be the highest among azoospermic men (13.3%), followed by those with severe OS (sOS; 10.9%), OS (4.2%), and mild OS (1.2%) [9]. The overall incidence of cytogenic abnormality in this study was 8.2%, which is more than 10 times the incidence among the normozoospermic (NS) population (0.6%) [10, 11]. Several other studies found similar incidences ranging from 4.3 to 10.3% among subfertile men and up to 15.4% among azoospermic men [12–18]. Furthermore, studies associating chromosomal abnormalities with categories of abnormal semen parameters have identified a higher likelihood of detecting a gonosomal abnormality in men with nonobstructive azoospermia (NOA) and an autosomal abnormality in men with a less severe phenotype, such as sOS, oligoasthenoteratozoospermia (OAT), oligoteratozoospermia, and isolated OS [9, 18]. Reciprocal and Robertsonian translocations have also been reported at a higher frequency in OS men compared to NOA men (1.7 vs. 0.6 and 0.9 vs. 0.3%, respectively) [19].

Chromosome Aneuploidy and Male Infertility

Infertile men have significantly increased rates of sperm aneuploidy relative to fertile men [20]. Most embryos conceived from aneuploid sperm will spontaneously abort [21], but sperm with aneuploidies of chromosomes 13, 18, 21, X, or Y can generate viable offspring. Patients with trisomy of either chromosome 13 (Patau syndrome) or 18 (Edwards syndrome) generally do not reach reproductive age [22]. While case reports of men with trisomy 21 (Down syndrome) with proven fertility exist, they are generally sterile [23–26]. Aneuploidy of the X chromosome is not lethal and is commonly implicated in the development of male infertility.

Aneuploidy of the X Chromosome
Klinefelter syndrome (KS) is the most common chromosomal disorder associated with male infertility, implicated in 10–26.7 and 1.4–5% of cases of NOA and OS, respectively [19, 27, 28]. The clinical presentation of KS entails hypergonadotropic hypogonadism, gynecomastia, small testes, and increased stature. Eighty percent of KS cases possess a 47XXY karyotype, whereas the remaining 20% are either mosaic (46XY/47XXY) or have higher-grade aneuploidy (48XXXY, 49XXXXY) [29]. The extra X chromosome may be either maternally or paternally inherited with an almost equal proportion [29–31].

Unassisted fertility among KS patients is uncommon, as 74.7% of mosaic KS patients and 90% of nonmosaic KS patients are azoospermic [32]. The testes of KS patients often undergo progressive atrophy and gradual depletion of germ cells, hastened at puberty [32–34]. Assisted reproductive technology can enable reproductive success in KS patients. Ramasamy et al. [35] reported that 45 of 68 (66.2%) nonmosaic KS patients underwent successful microscopic testicular sperm extraction for in vitro fertilization, and 45% of the sperm retrieved resulted in viable pregnancies.

Small Supranumerary Marker Chromosomes
The sensitivity and resolution of fluorescence in situ hybridization and array comparative genomic hybridization (aCGH) over traditional karyotype has increased the detection of small supranumerary marker chromosomes (sSMCs) among infertile males. Infertile males are approximately 5 times more likely to carry sSMCs than a general population of newborns [17]. Out of 149 infertile male patients in a recent systematic review, sSMCs were associated with OAT in 40 cases (26.8%), recurrent pregnancy loss in 32 cases (21.5%), and idiopathic infertility in 77 cases (51.7%) [36, 37]. The causative mechanism of sSMCs in male infertility has not been well characterized, but it may be that the presence of spermatogenesis-related genes on sSMCs could disrupt sperm development.

Chromosome Structural Anomalies and Male Infertility
Structural anomalies, including translocations and inversions, as well as deletions such as the Y-chromosome microdeletions, have been associated with male infertility. The type and severity of structural anomalies depends on the location and size of the anomaly as well as the presence of interchromosomal effects during meiotic recombination [38].

Translocations
Translocations account for 1.8–3.3% of autosomal abnormalities among infertile males [9]. Translocations can either be balanced (or reciprocal) or unbalanced depending on the conservation of genetic material, which is critically important for the development of normal spermatozoa and the embryos inheriting their genetic material. People with balanced translocations carry a full, diploid complement of the human genome and rarely manifest a phenotype like infertility. Deleterious phenotypes manifest if the translocation breakpoint occurs within a gene or its regulatory regions. Spermatozoa from men with balanced translocations have been reported to have a higher rate of meiotic errors (such as impaired synaptic complex pairing or recombination), resulting in disomy and/or unbalanced translocations in 29–81% of the spermatozoa [39, 40]. Consequently, these spermatozoa may produce embryos with unbalanced translocations or aneuploidies.

Rearrangement of chromosomal material between the gonosomes and autosomes is strongly associated with male infertility. Translocation of material between autosomes and the X chromosome is associated with sterility via disruption in spermatogenesis regardless of the position of the

X chromosome break [41]. Rearrangements between the Y chromosome and autosomes also result in sterility if the breakpoint occurs in a pseudoautosomal region of the Y chromosome, in the region of Yq11, or its boundaries. Both Yq11 and the Y chromosome pseudoautosomal region contain genes which play important roles in meiosis and fertility.

Robertsonian translocations occur among the acrocentric chromosomes (chromosomes 13, 14, 15, 21, and 22) and are 8.5-fold enriched in infertile males relative to unselected newborns [17]. Acrocentric chromosomes possess a single recombination focus in the q-arm of the chromosome. Dysfunction of that single focus can result in achiasmate bivalents (bivalents lacking recombination foci), leading to meiotic defects. Of sperm from men with Robertsonian translocations, 3–36% are genetically unbalanced [39]. Moreover, these translocations are more commonly associated with OS than NOA (1.6 vs. 0.09%) [17].

Inversions
Chromosomal inversions are 8 times more frequent in infertile males than in the general population (0.16 vs. 0.02%) [17]. Similar to other structural anomalies, unbalanced gametes are produced at higher frequencies (range 0.7–54.3%) depending on the size and location of the inversion [40]. Inversions of chromosome 1 carry the highest risk for male infertility, which is likely because chromosome 1 carries the most genetic material [17].

Y Chromosome Microdeletion
Three Yq11 bands (Yq11.21, Yq11.22, and Yq11.23) are of particular importance in evaluating the genetic causes of male infertility as it possesses genes essential for spermatogenesis and are error prone due to the abundance of palindromic sequences comprising a quarter of the q11 band [42, 43]. These sequences are prone to recombinational errors, such as microdeletions, leading to loss of Yq11 spermatogenesis-associated genes [44]. For further discussion on the genes lost in the Yq11 band, please read the chapter of Vogt et al. in this volume (pp. 57). Figure 1 describes subregions of the Yq11 band and candidate genes for the NOA phenotype associated with Y-chromosome microdeletions.

Gene Polymorphisms and Male Infertility
In addition to larger genomic anomalies spanning multiple genes or whole chromosomes, mutations of many single genes are associated with male infertility. Although hundreds of genes have been associated, the type and strength of supporting evidence for these candidate genes varies. In a 2008 review, Matzuk and Lamb [45] identified 464 genes for which mouse models supported a role in male infertility, and over 100 genes or genetic factors with human data implicating them in male infertility. These numbers have increased exponentially since that publication. Advances in high-throughput sequencing and molecular karyotyping have allowed for the identification of more candidate genes, although validation and corroboration of evidence for single genes playing a role is important.

Single Gene Mutations
A small number of genes are supported as infertility candidate genes by both human and rodent data. Spermatogenesis and oogenesis-specific basic helix-loop-helix 1 (*SOHLH1*) is a transcription factor necessary for spermatogonial proliferation and differentiation [46]. Synaptonemal complex protein 3 (*SYCP3*) encodes a protein that mediates meiotic homologous recombinations [47]. Nuclear receptor subfamily 5 group A member 1 (*NR5A1*) is associated with fetal gonadal development, and multiple missense mutations in this gene have been associated with NOA and sOS [48]. Heat shock transcription factor 2 (*HSF2*) promotes the transcription of heat-shock proteins to protect the cell against toxic stimuli like heat, and loss of function (LoF) of this gene in both humans and mice has been associated with maturation arrest and meiotic defects in spermatocytes

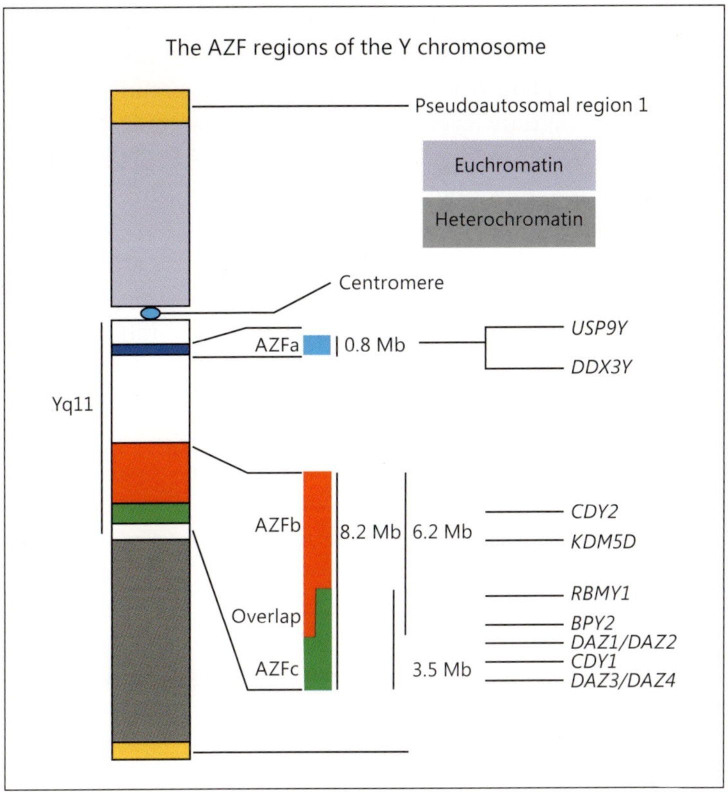

Fig. 1. The azoospermia factor (AZF) regions of the Y chromosome with spermatogenesis-relevant genes. For further information presenting the complete complexity of the AZF region gene content the reader is referred to the chapter of Vogt et al. in this volume (pp. 57).

[49]. The protamines, PRM1 and PRM2, are highly basic chromatin structure proteins which effect tight DNA compaction in mature spermatozoa, and mutations in these genes have been associated with infertility [50]. Testis-expressed gene 11 (*TEX11*) is associated with synaptonemal complex formation and DNA damage repair, and LoF results in maturation arrest in both humans and mice [51]. E2F transcription factor 1 (*E2F1*) is associated with the p53 cancer pathway and present in spermatogonial stem cells and spermatocytes. It has been associated with NOA in humans and subfertility in mice [52].

Syndromic Genetic Causes of Male Infertility

In addition to the previously discussed syndromes arising from chromosomal abnormalities, there are some genetic syndromes that include male infertility among their phenotypes. Some of the best studied of these are the mutations of the cystic fibrosis transmembrane conductance regulator (*CFTR*) gene, which causes infertility through spermatogenic impairment as well as congenital bilateral absence of the vas deferens [53]. Kallmann syndrome (KalS) is characterized by anosmia and infertility secondary to congenital gonadotropin-releasing hormone (GnRH) deficiency. The absence of GnRH precludes the release of follicle-stimulating hormone (FSH) and luteinizing hormone (LH) from the pituitary of both males and females, causing infertility in both genders. A number of genes have been associated with KalS, including anosmin-1 (*ANOS1*, also known as *KAL1*), semaphorin 3A (*SEMA3A*), fibroblast growth factor receptor 1 (*FGFR1*), kisspeptin 1 (*KISS1*), and kisspeptin receptor 1 (*KISS1R*) [54–57]. Myotonic dystrophy associated with mutations in myotonic dystrophy protein kinase (*DMPK*) also includes male infertility in a range of syndromic phenotypes [58].

Ciliopathies perturb flagellar function and result in male infertility. Primary ciliary dyskinesia (PCD) is characterized by defective ciliary function, which can range from completely immotile cilia to abnormal but motile cilia. Kartagener syndrome (PCD/KS) is one of the most prevalent instances of PCD associated with infertility, as well as the triad of bronchiectasis, situs inversus, and sinusitis. Autosomal recessive mutations of dynein axonemal intermediate chain 1 (*DNAI1*) and dynein axonemal heavy chain 5 (*DNAH5*) are reported in patients with PCD/KS [59, 60], and NGS has also implicated mutations of the HYDIN, axonemal central pair apparatus protein (*HYDIN*) gene in PCD/KS patients, including some with male infertility [61]. Moreover, axonemal defects can have more ominous consequences due to interactions of cilia and flagella in cell signaling pathways, affecting embryologic development and homeostasis [62]. This is particularly true for polycystin 1 (*PKD1*) mutations, which cause autosomal dominant polycystic kidney disease (ADPKD) and sterility in men, potentially through interactions with the transforming growth factor-β (TGF-β) or wingless-integrated (Wnt) signaling pathways [63].

Aberrant Epigenetic Regulation and Male Infertility

Gene expression during spermatogenesis is regulated by epigenetics, and thus epigenetic defects can lead to infertility. Epigenetic regulation includes posttranscriptional modulation with microRNA (miRNA) and transcriptional modulation via DNA methylation and modification of chromatin structure.

miRNAs are highly conserved, short (18–22 nucleotide long), noncoding RNAs that bind to the 3′ or 5′ untranslated regions of messenger RNA (mRNA) and interfere with translation of the tagged mRNA. Dysregulation of miRNA is associated with spermatogenic defects, including NOA [64, 65], asthenozoospermia [66], and OS [66]. Specifically, dysregulation of miR-449a and miR-34b/c is associated with impaired spermatogenesis in mice [67, 68]. Herati et al. [69] reported 35 miRNAs aberrantly expressed in the sperm of men with teratozoospermia. miRNA 449a displayed the largest reduction in expression compared to sperm from NS men, while hsa-let-7b-5p was the most overexpressed. The let7 family of miRNA may be involved in silencing certain genes involved in the self-renewing program of spermatogonial stem cells [70].

DNA methylation is the modification of cytosine nucleotides with a methyl group at the carbon 5 position, predominantly occurring in CpG (5′-cytosine-phosphate-guanine-3′) dinucleotides, which can be clustered at the promoter regions of genes. Hypermethylation is usually associated with the silencing of gene expression while hypomethylation is associated with an abnormally increased expression [71].

As a result of sex-specific methylation, certain genes are expressed during development in a monoallelic, parent-of-origin-specific manner, a phenomenon referred to as imprinting [72]. Imprinted genes are more often aberrantly methylated in men with OS and NOA compared to NS men [73–75]. In addition to imprinted genes, broad, genome-wide hypermethylation has been reported in sperm DNA from OAT men [76]. Hypermethylation of the methylenetetrahydrofolate reductase (*MTHFR*) and discoidin domain receptor 1 (*DDR1*) genes have been associated with NOA [77, 78]. Furthermore, hypermethylation of the genes deleted in azoospermia-like (*DAZL*) and cAMP responsive element modulator (*CREM*) are associated with OAT and OS, respectively [79, 80].

Spermatozoa are unique in that DNA is organized around protamines rather than histones. Tight DNA compaction is facilitated by protamines in the sperm nucleus. There is some evidence that in addition to compressing the DNA to facilitate transport to the ovum, this compaction also confers protection against DNA fragmentation [81]. In the process of protamination, histones are first replaced by 4 transition proteins, which are subsequently replaced by protamines [72]. This process never results in complete protamination, however. In sperm from NS men, approximately 10–15% of chromatin structural proteins are still histones, and most of those histones are associated with loci known to play important roles in embryonic development [82]. This suggests that the incomplete protamination of sperm DNA may be an intentional modulation of gene expression in the developing offspring.

Though little is known about the specific interactions between DNA and protamines, it is well established that the levels of PRM1 and PRM2 must be close to equal in order for sperm to function properly. Indeed, ratios of PRM1 to PRM2 (P1/P2) below 0.8 or greater than 1.2 have been associated with OS, oligoasthenozoospermia, and OAT [83]. In contrast, abnormal P1/P2 ratios have not been reported in NS men [72].

Female Infertility

Standard Work-Up

An evaluation for female factor infertility should be performed after 12 months of unprotected intercourse, though it may be initiated earlier for women ≥35 years of age or those with risk factors for female factor infertility (such as oligomenorrhea or amenorrhea) [3, 84]. The work-up begins with a history, physical, hormonal evaluation (including postovulatory serum progesterone levels and mid-cycle urinary LH levels), and imaging of the uterus and fallopian tubes to ensure patency with either transvaginal ultrasonography or hysterosalpingography [84]. Additional testing can be pursued with serum thyroid-stimulating hormone and prolactin levels for anovulatory women and serum FSH and estradiol (E2) levels for women with amenorrhea. The reproductive potential of an infertile female can be further assessed with a cycle-day 3 FSH and E2 measurement, clomiphene citrate challenge test, sonographic evaluation of early follicular phase antral follicle count, and assessment of anti-Müllerian hormone levels. More invasive examinations, such as diagnostic laparoscopy, are prompted by clinical suspicion of endometriosis and/or other tuboperitoneal disorders, such as pelvic adhesions, pelvic inflammatory disease, and peritoneal adhesions.

Cytogenetic Anomalies in Female Infertility

For unknown reasons, female gametes are more prone to meiotic recombination errors and a higher likelihood of aneuploidy [85]. These errors can occur during chromosomal pairing and/or recombination of meiosis I, or during the segregation of chromosomes with anaphase I and/or II. Identifying these cytogenetic errors in females can be challenging as errors in anaphase I and/or II manifest in select oocytes with each ovulatory cycle.

Chromosome Aneuploidy and Female Infertility

Monosomy – Turner Syndrome

Turner syndrome (TS) is characterized by short stature, a broad "shield" chest with widely set nipples, a webbed neck, and a low posterior hairline. TS represents the most common aneuploidy disorder causing female infertility, occurring in 1 of every 2,500 live female births. The aneuploidy occurs due to meiotic nondisjunction, varying from a partial to complete absence of the 46th X chromosome, and can be present in a nonmosaic or mosaic state. In a PCR-based genotyping study performed by Uematsu et al. [86], the solitary X chromosome was determined to be of maternal origin in 76.2% of patients. In TS patients with partial X chromosome deletions, the location of the deletion perturbs different genes resulting in variable somatic features. Deletions of the long arm of the X chromosome result in the loss of the diaphanous-related formin 2 (*DIAPH2*) gene; whereas deletions of the short arm of the X

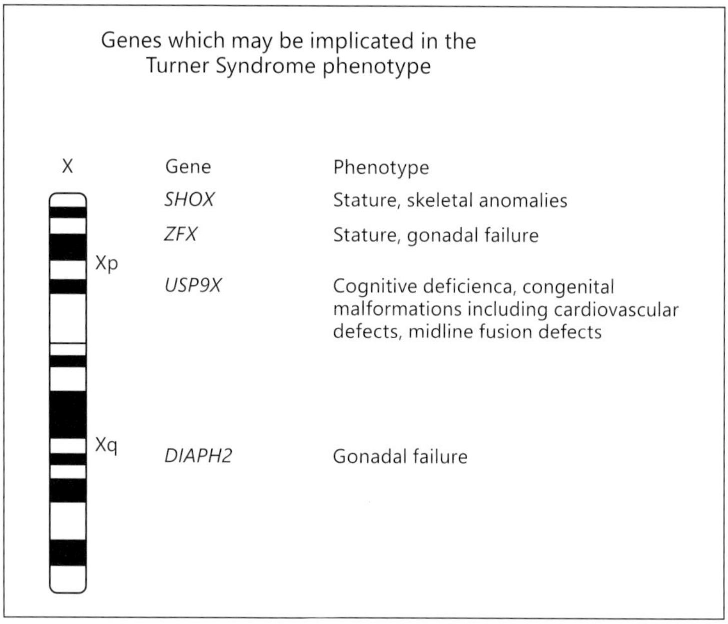

Fig. 2. Genes implicated in the phenotype of TS.

chromosome result in loss of the short stature homeobox (*SHOX*), zinc finger protein, X-linked (*ZFX*), ubiquitin-specific peptidase 9, X-linked (*USP9X*) genes (Fig. 2) [87].

Over 90% of TS patients possess gonadal dysgenesis, rendering them infertile. Analogous to the increased spermatogonial apoptosis rate of KS, ovarian dysfunction in TS is posited to occur due to accelerated follicular atresia rather than abnormal germ cell development [88]. Modi et al. [88] demonstrated a significantly higher rate of apoptosis in the oocytes of aborted 45X fetal ovaries using TUNEL (terminal deoxynucleotidyl transferase-mediated dUTP nick-end labeling) assays compared to the oocytes in the ovary of aborted fetuses with 46XX karyotypes, measured as 50–70% versus 3–7%, respectively. The mechanism for accelerated oocyte loss is believed to be due to meiotic pairing failure of homologous chromosomes [88]. Multiple karyotype abnormalities have been associated with TS and severe gonadal failure: 45X; 45X,i (Xq); 46X,idic (Xq), and 46X,idic (Xp) [89].

Mosaic TS manifests a less severe phenotype than monosomic TS with 5–6% of patients achieving spontaneous pregnancy [90]. Compared to the general population, mosaic TS women suffer markedly higher rates of miscarriages (30.8 vs. 15%) and are at a theoretically higher risk of primary ovarian insufficiency (POI); however, the risk of eventual POI in these patients is unknown [91]. Significant progress has been made in the last decade to harvest and cryopreserve viable oocytes with or without ovarian stimulation, as reviewed by Grynberg et al. [92]. Although further studies using in vitro maturation of immature oocytes are necessary, it appears to be a promising modality to preserve fertility in prepubertal TS patients.

Chromosome Structural Anomalies and Female Infertility

Translocations

Similar to males, females can also be phenotypically normal carriers of balanced reciprocal (X:A and A:A) and Robertsonian translocations. Balanced reciprocal X:A (chromosomes 1 [93], 2

[94], 3 [94], 4 [95], 6 [96], 7 [97], 9 [94], 11 [98], 15 [99], and 22 [100]) and A:A (ex. t[18:22] [101]) translocations have been identified using karyotypic analysis among infertile women. The location of the X chromosome translocation determines the severity of ovarian insufficiency. The proximal short arm of the X chromosome is of interest as it contains a region of critical importance in normal ovarian function, Xp11.1 to Xp21, that can result in POI. Similarly, Xq13–26 of the long arm of the X chromosome is another region critical in the maintenance of ovarian function as it contains the premature ovarian failure (POF)1 and POF2 loci, which when disrupted cause late (age 24–39 years) and early (age 16–21 years) onset POI, respectively [102, 103]. However, meiotic segregation patterns differ between male and female carriers with more frequent unbalanced gametes produced by female Robertsonian translocation carriers [104]. In a study comparing meiotic segregation patterns and preimplantation genetic diagnosis data from the embryos of male and female Robertsonian carriers to determine pregnancy outcomes, Ko et al. [105] showed higher rates of unbalanced, nonviable embryos from the female Robertsonian carriers (75.3 vs. 66.3%, $p < 0.005$).

Gene Defects

While a multitude of X-lined and autosomal candidate genes have been discovered that perturb gonadal and/or neuroendocrine function, challenges exist in proving causality with female infertility. We will focus on syndrome-associated gene mutations that disrupt the hypothalamic-pituitary-gonadal axis and nonsyndromic mutations that are associated with POI, endometriosis, and polycystic ovarian syndrome (PCOS).

Hypogonadotropic Hypogonadism

Females with congenital hypogonadotropic hypogonadism (HH) often present with symptoms of delayed menarche, thelarche, and infertility. HH can be divided into congenital and acquired causes. Congenital causes can be further divided into KalS (which was discussed in the male infertility section above) and normosmic isolated HH (or idiopathic hypergonadotropic hypogonadism; IHH). The most commonly mutated gene among female patients with KalS is the *ANOS1* gene, which is located at Xp23.3 and codes for an extracellular glycoprotein that functions in neuronal adhesion and axonal migration [106]. Other major genes linked with KalS include *FGFR1*, fibroblast growth factor 8 (*FGF8*), chromodomain helicase DNA binding protein 7 (*CHD7*), prokineticin 2 (*PROK2*), and prokineticin receptor 2 (*PROKR2*) [107]. While several gene mutations have been linked to KalS, the aforementioned mutations account for only 30% of all KalS cases [107].

Specific IHH-related gene mutations are more readily detected in the era of NGS. Despite its obvious candidacy to cause HH, it was not until 2009 that a homozygous frameshift mutation of the *GNRH1* gene was detected using whole-exome sequencing in a brother and sister with IHH [108]. Compound heterozygous mutations of the GnRH receptor gene (*GNRHR*) have also been identified in 2 families with IHH (reviewed by Layman [8]). Recently, LoF mutations of G-protein coupled receptor 54 (*GPR54*) have been suggested as the etiology for 1–2% of IHH cases and confirmed by in vitro studies and in vivo mouse models [109].

Premature Ovarian Insufficiency

Menopause is defined by hypergonadotropic hypoestrogenic amenorrhea for more than 12 months in women over 40 years of age and signifies the depletion of the ovulatory reserve [110]. While this pivotal event in a woman's lifetime varies according to individual genetic and environmental factors, the median age of menopause inception is 47.5 years [111]. Premature exhaustion of the primordial follicles before the age of 40 reduces the reproductive duration of the female and is called POI. It is estimated in developed countries that 1% of women under the age 40 and 0.1% of women under the age of 30 will develop POI [112]. Idiopathic POI accounts for 25% and identifiable genetic etiologies account for another 20% of all patients with POI. The proportion of identifiable genetic causes increases in the cohort of POI women under the age of 20 years, with almost half expected to have a genetic basis [112]. While menopause signals irreversible infertility, women with POI may have intermittent ovarian function and reproductive potential.

The presence of trinucleotide repeat expansion of the 5′-untranslated region of the fragile X mental retardation 1 gene (*FMR1*) is a well-established risk factor for POI. Expansion of CGG beyond the normal 55 but less than 200 copies is classified as "premutation" and puts female carriers at risk of POI; however, >200 copies, which causes fragile X syndrome in males, does not confer an increased risk of POI in female carriers. Approximately 20–28% of female carriers of the permutated *FMR1* gene develop POI, whereas only 2% of women with POI carry the mutation [113]. Trinucleotide expansion is believed to cause follicular atresia due to the accumulation of mutated *FMR1* mRNA (reviewed by Bilgin and Kovanci [114]).

Multiple candidate genes have been investigated based on their physiologic roles, extrapolation from animal models, and/or associations with a syndrome that possesses POI phenotype. Linkage studies investigating reproductive physiology genes have yielded candidates for POI; however, validation studies have produced inconsistent results. These candidates include progesterone receptor membrane component 1 (*PGRMC1*), estrogen receptor α (*ESR*), aromatase (*ARO*), inhibin gene family, and FSH receptor (*FSHR*) [114]. Among candidate genes derived from animal models of POI, overlapping human data have been shown for NOBOX oogenesis homeobox (*NOBOX*), growth differentiation factor 9 (*GDF9*), bone morphogenetic protein 15 (*BMP15*), and steroidogenic factor 1 (*SF1*). Moreover, syndromic gene mutations associated with POI include the gene candidates forkhead box L2 (*FOXL2*), galactose-1-phosphate uridylyltransferase (*GALT*), autoimmune regulator (*AIRE*), eukaryotic translation initiation factor 2B subunit epsilon (*EIF2B*), noggin (*NOG*), and DNA polymerase gamma, catalytic subunit (*POLG*) [115, 114].

Array CGH and genome-wide association studies have identified a number of candidate gene SNP associations with POI (reviewed by Simpson [116]). Maguire et al. [117] used high-resolution aCGH with probe spacing of 2.2 kb to assay for candidate copy-number variations (CNVs) in 89 women with POI. Seven of the 89 POI women possessed novel hemizygous mutations of 8p24.13, 10p15-p14, 10q26.3, 15q25.2, and 18q21.32, which involved the genes synaptonemal complex central element protein 1 (*SYCE1*) and cytoplasmic polyadenylation element binding protein 1 (*CPEB1*). Knockout mouse models of these 2 genes recapitulated the ovarian failure phenotype. More recently, Tsuiko et al. [118] compared 301 women with POI to 3,188 control individuals using high-resolution aCGH. Eleven novel microdeletions and microduplications were identified encompassing 8 POI relevant genes, formin 2 (*FMN2*), shugoshin-like 2 (*SGOL2*), TATA box binding protein (*TBP*), scavenger receptor class b, member 1 (*SCARB1*), *BNC1*, ADP-ribosylation factor GTPase-activating protein 3 (*ARFGAP3*), *SYCE1*, and *CPEB1*. Functional enrichment analysis using web-based software (g:Profiler) determined a notable number of POI candidate genes that possessed the dual function of immune cell development and germ and granulosa cell differentiation and maturation. Interestingly, Tsuiko et al. [118] found a negative relationship between the number of CNVs and the age of menopause in the POI cohort, and a larger cumulative size of all CNVs was also associated with later first pregnancy (each year of delay was associated with an 80-kb larger size of cumulative CNV load).

Pu et al. [119] performed a meta-analysis of 59 genetic association studies evaluating polymorphisms and POI. Ten common SNPs of 5 genes (*BMP15*, estrogen receptor 1 [*ESR1*], *FMR1*, *FSHR*, and inhibin alpha subunit [*INHA*]) and 2 less prevalent SNPs of BMP15 (538G>A) and INHA (769G>A) were assessed for their strength of association with POI. While BMP15 (538G>A) was present significantly more often in POI patients compared to control patients, none of the other SNPs reached statistical significance.

Genetics of Endometriosis and Polycystic Ovarian Syndrome

Endometriosis is defined as ectopic estrogen-dependent endometrial glands and/or stroma located outside the uterus and is present in 30–40% of women with pelvic pain and infertility (reviewed by Barnhart et al. [120]). Ectopic endometrial tissue implant on peritoneal cavity sites, such as the ovaries, peritoneum, bowel, and bladder. Although the most widely accepted mechanism for endometriosis remains the retrograde menstruation theory, 22.4% of respondents to a 1971 questionnaire study reported either a first- or second-degree relative with endometriosis, supporting a role for genetics in the pathophysiology [121]. An important family of genes associated with endometriosis are the *HOX* genes, namely homeobox A10 (*HOXA10*) and *HOXA11*, which are important for uterine implantation. In a comparison of 40 patients with endometriosis to 40 women with normal ovulatory cycles, endometriosis patients failed to show the expected mid-luteal rise of *HOX* gene expression in eutopic endometrial tissue using Northern blot analysis, suggesting a uterine-based mechanism for the lower reproductive potential of females with endometriosis [122]. In a study examining methylation patterns of various gynecologic disorders, Kulp et al. [123] found hypomethylation of CpG sites within the *HOXA10* gene in women with endometriosis compared to controls as a proposed mechanism for the altered midluteal *HOX* transcript levels. Candidate genes have also been identified from gene polymorphism association studies and can be classified into 4 broad categories: xenobiotic metabolism genes, hormone receptor or hormone metabolism, inflammation/angiogenesis genes, and "other" process genes [124]. Candidate genes from each of these categories with the most number of positive to negative association studies include glutathione M-transferase 1 (*GSTM1*), *ESR1*, interleukin-10 (*IL-10*), and HLA class II histocompatibility antigen, DRB1–9 β-chain (*HLA-DRB1*).

Meta-analyses of multiple published genome-wide association studies on women with endometriosis have identified SNPs of an additional set of candidate genes, including Wnt family member 4 (*WNT4*), growth regulation by estrogen in breast cancer 1 (*GREB1*), inhibitor of DNA binding 4 (*ID4*), CDKN2B antisense RNA 1 (*CDKN2BAS*), vezatin (*VEZT*), fibronectin 1 (*FN1*), and interleukin 1α (*IL1A*) [125]. It is important to note that causation has not been confirmed with these gene mutations.

PCOS is a complex endocrine disorder characterized by irregular menstruation or amenorrhea, hyperandrogenism, and polycystic ovaries. PCOS is believed to be a multifactorial condition, reflecting the influences of genetic, environmental, metabolic, and endocrine abnormalities [126]. Ovarian theca cells produce androgens, so mutations modulating androgen synthesis, transport, and regulation are obvious candidates. Despite these targets, few genes have been identified in PCOS women. Mutations of fibrillin-3 (*FBN3*) and LH receptor (*LHR*) have been detected in PCOS women of Chinese and European descent (reviewed by De Leo et al. [126]). The *FBN3* gene encodes for extracellular fibrillin protein, which interacts with TGF-β binding proteins [127]. In the absence of fibrillin from *FBN3*, unregulated TGF-β signaling stimulates ovarian fibroblast and collagen production in the ovarian cortex. Variants of the *LHR* also predispose to PCOS through activating mutations to enhance the effects of pituitary LH on ovarian thecal cells [126].

Epigenetics and Female Infertility

Epigenetics guides gene expression during oogenesis just as it does with spermatogenesis. Altered regulation of DNA methylation, histone function, and small coding RNAs can all contribute to female infertility. In addition to meiotic recombinational failure, epigenetic aberrances accumulate with age and may impede fertility. DNA methyltransferases are enzymes responsible for maintaining methylation patterns following DNA replication and help guide oogenesis. Lower gene expression of *Dnmt1*, *Dnmt3a*, *Dnmt3b*, and *Dnmt3L* were observed in the oocytes of aged mice compared to younger mice [128]. Not surprisingly, these aged oocytes had genome-wide hypomethylation, lower cleavage and blastocyst formation rates, lower pregnancy rates, and more stillbirths and fetal malformations.

Dysfunctional histone modification with aberrant methylation, acetylation, and/or ubiquitination also contribute to abnormal oogenesis and impaired fertility. During meiosis, histones are deacetylated during meiosis I and II by HDAC (histone deacetylase). With advancing age, preovulatory oocyte *HDAC* mRNA levels decrease, which prevents proper histone deacetylation and results in embryo death if the oocyte is fertilized. Similar changes in histone methylation are also present in the di- and trimethylated histone H3 lysine 4 (H3K4), which is aberrantly methylated in older mouse germinal vesicle stage oocytes [129].

While the oocyte genome is transcriptionally silent, miRNA are enriched in meiosis II (MII) oocytes and may play essential roles in follicular development [130]. Assou et al. [130] used RNA-seq technology to analyze the RNAome of pooled MII oocytes and found 3 miRNA that were abundantly expressed, including miR184, miR100, and miR10A. These miRNAs were predicted by in silico prediction algorithms to regulate transcription and cell cycle genes.

Conclusion

With the advent of NGS, it is now possible to understand the genetic underpinnings of male and female infertility at a higher resolution. Despite these advances, significant work remains to validate and determine the mechanisms by which candidate gene mutations and epigenetic modifications influence fertility potential.

Acknowledgements

A.S.H. is a National Institutes of Health (NIH) K12 Scholar supported by a Male Reproductive Health Research (MHRH) Career Development Physician-Scientist Award (HD073917-01) from the Eunice Kennedy Shriver National Institute of Child Health and Human Development (NICHD) Program (to Dolores J. Lamb).

References

1 Mascarenhas MN, Flaxman SR, Boerma T, Vanderpoel S, Stevens GA: National, regional, and global trends in infertility prevalence since 1990: a systematic analysis of 277 health surveys. PLoS Med 2012;9:e1001356.

2 ASRM: Causes of infertility. 2016. http://www.reproductivefacts.org/infographic_causes_of_infertility/ (accessed June 6, 2016)

3 Smith S, Pfeifer SM, Collins JA: Diagnosis and management of female infertility. JAMA 2003;290:1767–1770.

4 Hwang K, Yatsenko AN, Jorgez CJ, et al: Mendelian genetics of male infertility. Ann NY Acad Sci 2010;1214:E1–E17.

5 Dohle GR, Colpi GM, Hargreave TB, et al: EAU guidelines on male infertility. Eur Urol 2005;48:703–711.

6 Unuane D, Tournaye H, Velkeniers B, Poppe K: Endocrine disorders and female infertility. Best Pract Res Clin Endocrinol Metab 2011;25:861–873.
7 Beck-Peccoz P, Persani L: Premature ovarian failure. Orphanet J Rare Dis 2006;1:9.
8 Layman LC: The genetic basis of female reproductive disorders: etiology and clinical testing. Mol Cell Endocrinol 2013;370:138–148.
9 Yatsenko AN, Yatsenko SA, Weedin JW, et al: Comprehensive 5-year study of cytogenetic aberrations in 668 infertile men. J Urol 2010;183:1636–1642.
10 Berger R: The incidence of constitutional chromosome aberrations (in French). J Genet Hum 1975;23(suppl):42–49.
11 Baer RJ, Flessel MC, Jelliffe-Pawlowski LL, et al: Detection rates for aneuploidy by first-trimester and sequential screening. Obstet Gynecol 2015;126:753–759.
12 Retief AE, van Zyl JA, Menkveld R, Fox MF, Kotze GM, Brusnicky J: Chromosome studies in 496 infertile males with a sperm count below 10 million/mL. Hum Genet 1984;66:162–164.
13 Bourrouillou G, Dastugue N, Colombies P: Chromosome studies in 952 infertile males with a sperm count below 10 million/ml. Hum Genet 1985;71:366–367.
14 Chandley AC: The chromosomal basis of human infertility. Br Med Bull 1979;35: 181–186.
15 Kosar PA, Ozcelik N, Kosar A: Cytogenetic abnormalities detected in patients with non-obstructive azoospermia and severe oligozoospermia. J Assist Reprod Genet 2010;27:17–21.
16 Abramsson L, Beckman G, Duchek M, Nordenson I: Chromosomal aberrations and male infertility. J Urol 1982;128: 52–53.
17 van Assche E, Bonduelle M, Tournaye H, et al: Cytogenetics of infertile men. Hum Reprod 1996;11(suppl 4):1–24, discussion 25–26.
18 Elghezal H, Hidar S, Braham R, Denguezli W, Ajina M, Saad A: Chromosome abnormalities in one thousand infertile males with nonobstructive sperm disorders. Fertil Steril 2006;86:1792–1795.
19 Ceylan GG, Ceylan C, Elyas H: Genetic anomalies in patients with severe oligozoospermia and azoospermia in eastern Turkey: a prospective study. Genet Mol Res 2009;8:915–922.
20 Moosani N, Pattinson HA, Carter MD, Cox DM, Rademaker AW, Martin RH: Chromosomal analysis of sperm from men with idiopathic infertility using sperm karyotyping and fluorescence in situ hybridization. Fertil Steril 1995;64: 811–817.
21 Hassold T, Hunt PA, Sherman S: Trisomy in humans: incidence, origin and etiology. Curr Opin Genet Dev 1993;3: 398–403.
22 Jedraszak G, Copin H, Demailly M, et al: Azoospermia and trisomy 18p syndrome: a fortuitous association? A patient report and a review of the literature. Mol Cytogenet 2015;8:34.
23 Bobrow M, Barby T, Hajianpour A, Maxwell D, Yau SC: Fertility in a male with trisomy 21. J Med Genet 1992;29: 141.
24 Sheridan R, Llerena J Jr, Matkins S, Debenham P, Cawood A, Bobrow M: Fertility in a male with trisomy 21. J Med Genet 1989;26:294–298.
25 Pradhan M, Dalal A, Khan F, Agrawal S: Fertility in men with Down syndrome: a case report. Fertil Steril 2006;86:1765 e1–e3.
26 Johannisson R, Gropp A, Winking H, Coerdt W, Rehder H, Schwinger E: Down's syndrome in the male: reproductive pathology and meiotic studies. Hum Genet 1983;63:132–138.
27 Gekas J, Thepot F, Turleau C, et al: Chromosomal factors of infertility in candidate couples for ICSI: an equal risk of constitutional aberrations in women and men. Hum Reprod 2001;16:82–90.
28 Ferlin A, Arredi B, Foresta C: Genetic causes of male infertility. Reprod Toxicol 2006;22:133–141.
29 Thomas NS, Hassold TJ: Aberrant recombination and the origin of Klinefelter syndrome. Hum Reprod Update 2003;9:309–317.
30 Hassold TJ, Sherman SL, Pettay D, Page DC, Jacobs PA: XY chromosome nondisjunction in man is associated with diminished recombination in the pseudoautosomal region. Am J Hum Genet 1991;49:253–260.
31 Vallabhajosyula R, Rajangam S, C L: Association of parental origin with clinical profile in Klinefelter syndrome. J Clin Diagn Res 2015;9:GC01–GC03.
32 Rives N, Milazzo JP, Perdrix A, et al: The feasibility of fertility preservation in adolescents with Klinefelter syndrome. Hum Reprod 2013;28:1468–1479.
33 Aksglaede L, Wikstrom AM, Rajpert-De Meyts E, Dunkel L, Skakkebaek NE, Juul A: Natural history of seminiferous tubule degeneration in Klinefelter syndrome. Hum Reprod Update 2006;12: 39–48.
34 Mau-Holzmann UA: Somatic chromosomal abnormalities in infertile men and women. Cytogenet Genome Res 2005;111:317–336.
35 Ramasamy R, Ricci JA, Palermo GD, Gosden LV, Rosenwaks Z, Schlegel PN: Successful fertility treatment for Klinefelter's syndrome. J Urol 2009;182: 1108–1113.
36 Liehr T, Weise A: Frequency of small supernumerary marker chromosomes in prenatal, newborn, developmentally retarded and infertility diagnostics. Int J Mol Med 2007;19:719–31.
37 Armanet N, Tosca L, Brisset S, Liehr T, Tachdjian G: Small supernumerary marker chromosomes in human infertility. Cytogenet Genome Res 2015;146: 100–108.
38 Tempest HG, Cheng SY, Gillott DJ, Handyside AH, Thornhill AR, Griffin DK: Scoring of sperm chromosomal abnormalities by manual and automated approaches: qualitative and quantitative comparisons. Asian J Androl 2010;12: 257–262.
39 Tempest HG: Meiotic recombination errors, the origin of sperm aneuploidy and clinical recommendations. Syst Biol Reprod Med 2011;57:93–101.
40 Sarrate Z, Blanco J, Anton E, Egozcue S, Egozcue J, Vidal F: FISH studies of chromosome abnormalities in germ cells and its relevance in reproductive counseling. Asian J Androl 2005;7:227–236.
41 Madan K: Balanced structural changes involving the human X: effect on sexual phenotype. Hum Genet 1983;63:216–21.
42 Rives N: Y chromosome microdeletions and alterations of spermatogenesis, patient approach and genetic counseling. Ann Endocrinol (Paris) 2014;75:112–114.
43 Vogt PH: Azoospermia factor (AZF) in Yq11: towards a molecular understanding of its function for human male fertility and spermatogenesis. Reprod Biomed Online 2005;10:81–93.
44 Lange J, Skaletsky H, van Daalen SK, et al: Isodicentric Y chromosomes and sex disorders as byproducts of homologous recombination that maintains palindromes. Cell 2009;138:855–869.

45 Matzuk MM, Lamb DJ: The biology of infertility: research advances and clinical challenges. Nat Med 2008;14:1197–1213.
46 Choi Y, Jeon S, Choi M, et al: Mutations in SOHLH1 gene associate with nonobstructive azoospermia. Hum Mutat 2010;31:788–793.
47 Miyamoto T, Hasuike S, Yogev L, et al: Azoospermia in patients heterozygous for a mutation in SYCP3. Lancet 2003; 362:1714–1719.
48 Ropke A, Tewes AC, Gromoll J, Kliesch S, Wieacker P, Tuttelmann F: Comprehensive sequence analysis of the NR5A1 gene encoding steroidogenic factor 1 in a large group of infertile males. Eur J Hum Genet 2013;21:1012–1015.
49 Mou L, Wang Y, Li H, et al: A dominant-negative mutation of HSF2 associated with idiopathic azoospermia. Hum Genet 2013;132:159–165.
50 Imken L, Rouba H, El Houate B, et al: Mutations in the protamine locus: association with spermatogenic failure? Mol Hum Reprod 2009;15:733–738.
51 Yatsenko AN, Georgiadis AP, Ropke A, et al: X-linked TEX11 mutations, meiotic arrest, and azoospermia in infertile men. N Engl J Med 2015;372:2097–2107.
52 Jorgez CJ, Wilken N, Addai JB, et al: Genomic and genetic variation in E2F transcription factor-1 in men with nonobstructive azoospermia. Fertil Steril 2015; 103:44–52.e1.
53 Kaplan E, Shwachman H, Perlmutter AD, Rule A, Khaw KT, Holsclaw DS: Reproductive failure in males with cystic fibrosis. N Engl J Med 1968;279:65–69.
54 Franco B, Guioli S, Pragliola A, et al: A gene deleted in Kallmann's syndrome shares homology with neural cell adhesion and axonal path-finding molecules. Nature 1991;353:529–536.
55 Young J, Metay C, Bouligand J, et al: SEMA3A deletion in a family with Kallmann syndrome validates the role of semaphorin 3A in human puberty and olfactory system development. Hum Reprod 2012;27:1460–1465.
56 Dode C, Levilliers J, Dupont JM, et al: Loss-of-function mutations in FGFR1 cause autosomal dominant Kallmann syndrome. Nat Genet 2003;33:463–465.
57 Seminara SB, Messager S, Chatzidaki EE, et al: The *GPR54* gene as a regulator of puberty. N Engl J Med 2003;349: 1614–1627.
58 Jansen G, Groenen PJ, Bachner D, et al: Abnormal myotonic dystrophy protein kinase levels produce only mild myopathy in mice. Nat Genet 1996;13:316–324.
59 Afzelius BA, Eliasson R, Johnsen O, Lindholmer C: Lack of dynein arms in immotile human spermatozoa. J Cell Biol 1975;66:225–232.
60 Sha YW, Ding L, Li P: Management of primary ciliary dyskinesia/Kartagener's syndrome in infertile male patients and current progress in defining the underlying genetic mechanism. Asian J Androl 2014;16:101–106.
61 Olbrich H, Schmidts M, Werner C, et al: Recessive HYDIN mutations cause primary ciliary dyskinesia without randomization of left-right body asymmetry. Am J Hum Genet 2012;91:672–684.
62 Fliegauf M, Benzing T, Omran H: When cilia go bad: cilia defects and ciliopathies. Nat Rev Mol Cell Biol 2007;8:880–893.
63 Linck RW, Chemes H, Albertini DF: The axoneme: the propulsive engine of spermatozoa and cilia and associated ciliopathies leading to infertility. J Assist Reprod Genet 2016;33:141–156.
64 Lian J, Zhang X, Tian H, et al: Altered microRNA expression in patients with non-obstructive azoospermia. Reprod Biol Endocrinol 2009;7:13.
65 Abu-Halima M, Backes C, Leidinger P, et al: MicroRNA expression profiles in human testicular tissues of infertile men with different histopathologic patterns. Fertil Steril 2014;101:78–86.e2.
66 Abu-Halima M, Hammadeh M, Schmitt J, et al: Altered microRNA expression profiles of human spermatozoa in patients with different spermatogenic impairments. Fertil Steril 2013;99:1249–1255.e16.
67 Comazzetto S, Di Giacomo M, Rasmussen KD, et al: Oligoasthenoteratozoospermia and infertility in mice deficient for miR-34b/c and miR-449 loci. PLoS Genet 2014;10:e1004597.
68 Bao J, Li D, Wang L, et al: MicroRNA-449 and microRNA-34b/c function redundantly in murine testes by targeting E2F transcription factor-retinoblastoma protein (E2F-pRb) pathway. J Biol Chem 2012;287:21686–21698.
69 Herati A, Mielnik A, Schlegel P, Paduch D: MP76–20 human sperm miRNA profile in patients with normozoospermia and teratozoospermia. J Urol 2015; 193:e991.
70 Tong MH, Mitchell D, Evanoff R, Griswold MD: Expression of *Mirlet7* family microRNAs in response to retinoic acid-induced spermatogonial differentiation in mice. Biol Reprod 2011;85:189–197.
71 Deaton AM, Bird A: CpG islands and the regulation of transcription. Genes Dev 2011;25:1010–1022.
72 Rajender S, Avery K, Agarwal A: Epigenetics, spermatogenesis and male infertility. Mutat Res 2011;727:62–71.
73 Kobayashi H, Sato A, Otsu E, et al: Aberrant DNA methylation of imprinted loci in sperm from oligospermic patients. Hum Mol Genet 2007;16:2542–2551.
74 Marques CJ, Francisco T, Sousa S, Carvalho F, Barros A, Sousa M: Methylation defects of imprinted genes in human testicular spermatozoa. Fertil Steril 2010;94:585–594.
75 Minor A, Chow V, Ma S: Aberrant DNA methylation at imprinted genes in testicular sperm retrieved from men with obstructive azoospermia and undergoing vasectomy reversal. Reproduction 2011;141:749–757.
76 Houshdaran S, Cortessis VK, Siegmund K, Yang A, Laird PW, Sokol RZ: Widespread epigenetic abnormalities suggest a broad DNA methylation erasure defect in abnormal human sperm. PLoS One 2007;2:e1289.
77 Ramasamy R, Ridgeway A, Lipshultz LI, Lamb DJ: Integrative DNA methylation and gene expression analysis identifies discoidin domain receptor 1 association with idiopathic nonobstructive azoospermia. Fertil Steril 2014;102:968–973.e3.
78 Khazamipour N, Noruzinia M, Fatehmanesh P, Keyhanee M, Pujol P: MTHFR promoter hypermethylation in testicular biopsies of patients with non-obstructive azoospermia: the role of epigenetics in male infertility. Hum Reprod 2009; 24:2361–2364.
79 Navarro-Costa P, Nogueira P, Carvalho M, et al: Incorrect DNA methylation of the DAZL promoter CpG island associates with defective human sperm. Hum Reprod 2010;25:2647–2654.
80 Nanassy L, Carrell DT: Abnormal methylation of the promoter of CREM is broadly associated with male factor infertility and poor sperm quality but is improved in sperm selected by density gradient centrifugation. Fertil Steril 2011;95:2310–2314.

81 Boissonnas CC, Jouannet P, Jammes H: Epigenetic disorders and male subfertility. Fertil Steril 2013;99:624–631.
82 Hammoud SS, Nix DA, Zhang H, Purwar J, Carrell DT, Cairns BR: Distinctive chromatin in human sperm packages genes for embryo development. Nature 2009;460:473–478.
83 Aoki VW, Liu L, Carrell DT: Identification and evaluation of a novel sperm protamine abnormality in a population of infertile males. Hum Reprod 2005;20:1298–1306.
84 Practice Committee of the American Society for Reproductive Medicine: Diagnostic evaluation of the infertile female: a committee opinion. Fertil Steril 2015;103:e44–e50.
85 Hulten M, Smith E, Delhanty J: Errors in chromosome segregation during oogenesis and early embryogenesis; in Carrell DT, Peterson CM (eds): Reproductive Endocrinology and Infertility: Integrating Modern Clinical and Laboratory Practice, ed 1. Berlin, Springer, 2010, pp 1602–1675.
86 Uematsu A, Yorifuji T, Muroi J, et al: Parental origin of normal X chromosomes in Turner syndrome patients with various karyotypes: implications for the mechanism leading to generation of a 45,X karyotype. Am J Med Genet 2002;111:134–139.
87 Ranke MB, Saenger P: Turner's syndrome. Lancet 2001;358:309–314.
88 Modi DN, Sane S, Bhartiya D: Accelerated germ cell apoptosis in sex chromosome aneuploid fetal human gonads. Mol Hum Reprod 2003;9:219–225.
89 Ogata T, Matsuo N: Turner syndrome and female sex chromosome aberrations: deduction of the principal factors involved in the development of clinical features. Hum Genet 1995;95:607–629.
90 Bernard V, Donadille B, Zenaty D, et al: Spontaneous fertility and pregnancy outcomes amongst 480 women with Turner syndrome. Hum Reprod 2016;31:782–788.
91 Santoro N: Mechanisms of premature ovarian failure. Ann Endocrinol (Paris) 2003;64:87–92.
92 Grynberg M, Bidet M, Benard J, et al: Fertility preservation in Turner syndrome. Fertil Steril 2016;105:13–19.
93 Venkateshwari A, Srilekha A, Veena K, Sujatha M, Jyothy A: A rare de novo balanced X; 1 translocation in an Indian female with primary amenorrhea. J Reprod Infertil 2015;16:171–173.
94 Moysés-Oliveira M, Guilherme Rdos S, Dantas AG, et al: Genetic mechanisms leading to primary amenorrhea in balanced X-autosome translocations. Fertil Steril 2015;103:1289–1296.e2.
95 Phelan JP, Upton RT, Summitt RL: Balanced reciprocal X-4 translocation in a female patient with early secondary amenorrhea. Am J Obstet Gynecol 1977;129:607–613.
96 Sills ES, Cotter PD, Marron KD, Shkrobot LV, Walsh HM, Salem RD: Ovarian dysgenesis associated with an unbalanced X;6 translocation: first characterisation of reproductive anatomy and cytogenetic evaluation in partial trisomy 6 with breakpoints at Xq22 and 6p23. Mol Med Rep 2012;5:29–31.
97 Vasu VR, Chandra N, Santhiya ST: X;7 translocation in an Indian woman with hypergonadotropic amenorrhea – a case report. Genet Test Mol Biomarkers 2009;13:533–536.
98 Dorus E, Amarose AP, Tredway DR, Reale FR, Hatch R, Serrano LF: A reciprocal translocation (X;11) in a female with gonadal dysgenesis. Clin Genet 1979;16:263–269.
99 Ji XW, Chen XY, Tan J, Liang H: Balanced X;15 translocation 46,X,t(X;15)(q21;q23) associated with primary amenorrhea. Am J Med Genet 1988;31:783–786.
100 Grzesiuk JD, Pereira CS, Grangeiro CH, et al: Familial chromosomal translocation X; 22 associated with infertility and recurrent X mosaicism. Mol Cytogenet 2016;9:45.
101 Dutta UR, Ponnala R, Dalal A: A novel de novo balanced reciprocal translocation t(18;22) associated with recurrent miscarriages: a case report. J Reprod Infertil 2014;15:113–116.
102 Krauss CM, Turksoy RN, Atkins L, McLaughlin C, Brown LG, Page DC: Familial premature ovarian failure due to an interstitial deletion of the long arm of the X chromosome. N Engl J Med 1987;317:125–131.
103 Marozzi A, Vegetti W, Manfredini E, et al: Association between idiopathic premature ovarian failure and fragile X premutation. Hum Reprod 2000;15:197–202.
104 Munne S, Escudero T, Sandalinas M, Sable D, Cohen J: Gamete segregation in female carriers of Robertsonian translocations. Cytogenet Cell Genet 2000;90:303–308.
105 Ko DS, Cho JW, Lee HS, et al: Preimplantation genetic diagnosis outcomes and meiotic segregation analysis of robertsonian translocation carriers. Fertil Steril 2013;99:1369–1376.
106 Ahmadzadeh A, Ghods E, Mojarrad M, et al: Study on KAL1 gene mutations in idiopathic hypogonadotropic hypogonadism patients with X-linked recessive inheritance. Int J Mol Cell Med 2015;4:152–159.
107 Hardelin JP, Dode C: The complex genetics of Kallmann syndrome: KAL1, FGFR1, FGF8, PROKR2, PROK2, et al. Sex Dev 2008;2:181–193.
108 Bouligand J, Ghervan C, Tello JA, et al: Isolated familial hypogonadotropic hypogonadism and a *GNRH1* mutation. N Engl J Med 2009;360:2742–2748.
109 Karges B, de Roux N: Molecular genetics of isolated hypogonadotropic hypogonadism and Kallmann syndrome. Endocr Dev 2005;8:67–80.
110 Butler L, Santoro N: The reproductive endocrinology of the menopausal transition. Steroids 2011;76:627–635.
111 McKinlay SM, Brambilla DJ, Posner JG: The normal menopause transition. Maturitas 2008;61:4–16.
112 Fenton AJ: Premature ovarian insufficiency: pathogenesis and management. J Midlife Health 2015;6:147–153.
113 Murray A, Schoemaker MJ, Bennett CE, et al: Population-based estimates of the prevalence of *FMR1* expansion mutations in women with early menopause and primary ovarian insufficiency. Genet Med 2014;16:19–24.
114 Bilgin EM, Kovanci E: Genetics of premature ovarian failure. Curr Opin Obstet Gynecol 2015;27:167–174.
115 Vujovic S, Ivovic M, Tancic-Gajic M, et al: Premature ovarian failure. Srp Arh Celok Lek 2012;140:806–811.
116 Simpson JL: Genetics of female infertility due to anomalies of the ovary and mullerian ducts. Methods Mol Biol 2014;1154:39–73.
117 McGuire MM, Bowden W, Engel NJ, Ahn HW, Kovanci E, Rajkovic A: Genomic analysis using high-resolution single-nucleotide polymorphism arrays reveals novel microdeletions associated with premature ovarian failure. Fertil Steril 2011;95:1595–1600.

118 Tsuiko O, Noukas M, Zilina O, et al: Copy number variation analysis detects novel candidate genes involved in follicular growth and oocyte maturation in a cohort of premature ovarian failure cases. Hum Reprod 2016;31: 1913–1925.

119 Pu D, Xing Y, Gao Y, Gu L, Wu J: Gene variation and premature ovarian failure: a meta-analysis. Eur J Obstet Gynecol Reprod Biol 2014;182:226–237.

120 Barnhart K, Dunsmoor-Su R, Coutifaris C: Effect of endometriosis on in vitro fertilization. Fertil Steril 2002;77: 1148–1155.

121 Ranney B: Endometriosis. IV. Hereditary tendency. Obstet Gynecol 1971;37: 734–737.

122 Taylor HS, Bagot C, Kardana A, Olive D, Arici A: HOX gene expression is altered in the endometrium of women with endometriosis. Hum Reprod 1999;14:1328–1331.

123 Kulp JL, Mamillapalli R, Taylor HS: Aberrant HOXA10 Methylation in Patients With Common Gynecologic Disorders: Implications for Reproductive Outcomes. Reprod Sci 2016;23:455–463.

124 Dun EC, Taylor RN, Wieser F: Advances in the genetics of endometriosis. Genome Med 2010;2:75.

125 Fung JN, Rogers PA, Montgomery GW: Identifying the biological basis of GWAS hits for endometriosis. Biol Reprod 2015;92:87.

126 De Leo V, Musacchio MC, Cappelli V, Massaro MG, Morgante G, Petraglia F: Genetic, hormonal and metabolic aspects of PCOS: an update. Reprod Biol Endocrinol 2016;14:38.

127 Prodoehl MJ, Hatzirodos N, Irving-Rodgers HF, et al: Genetic and gene expression analyses of the polycystic ovary syndrome candidate gene fibrillin-3 and other fibrillin family members in human ovaries. Mol Hum Reprod 2009;15:829–841.

128 Yue MX, Fu XW, Zhou GB, et al: Abnormal DNA methylation in oocytes could be associated with a decrease in reproductive potential in old mice. J Assist Reprod Genet 2012;29:643–650.

129 Shao GB, Wang J, Zhang LP, et al: Aging alters histone H3 lysine 4 methylation in mouse germinal vesicle stage oocytes. Reprod Fertil Dev 2015;27: 419–426.

130 Assou S, Al-edani T, Haouzi D, et al: MicroRNAs: new candidates for the regulation of the human cumulus-oocyte complex. Hum Reprod 2013;28: 3038–3049.

Dolores J. Lamb, PhD
Center for Reproductive Medicine
Scott Department of Urology, Baylor College of Medicine
1 Baylor Plaza Suite N730, Houston, TX 77030 (USA)
E-Mail dlamb@bcm.edu

Vogt PH (ed): Genetics of Human Infertility. Monogr Hum Genet.
Basel, Karger, 2017, vol 21, pp 17–39 (DOI: 10.1159/000477276)

Genetics of Premature Ovarian Failure: New Developments in Etiology

Yinying Qin[a–d] · Joe Leigh Simpson[g, h] · Zi-Jiang Chen[a–f]

[a]Center for Reproductive Medicine, Shandong Provincial Hospital, Shandong University, [b]National Research Center for Assisted Reproductive Technology and Reproductive Genetics, [c]The Key Laboratory for Reproductive Endocrinology of the Ministry of Education, and [d]Shandong Provincial Key Laboratory of Reproductive Medicine, Jinan, and [e]Center for Reproductive Medicine, Ren Ji Hospital, School of Medicine, Shanghai Jiao Tong University, and [f]Shanghai Key Laboratory for Assisted Reproduction and Reproductive Genetics, Shanghai, China; [g]The March of Dimes Foundation, White Plains, NY, and [h]Herbert Wertheim College of Medicine, Florida International University, Miami, FL, USA

Abstract

Premature ovarian failure (POF), also termed primary ovarian insufficiency, is a common disorder in women of reproductive age. This discussion focuses predominately on single genes whose perturbations are associated with POF. Perturbations known to have deleterious effects were initially derived from hypothesis-driven candidate gene interrogations. Genes on the X chromosome considered causative for isolated POF include *FMR1*, *PGRMCI*, and *BMP15*. Genes identified on autosomes include *FSHR*, *GDF9*, *NR5A1*, *NOBOX*, *FIGLA*, *STAG3*, *FOXL2*, *HFM1*, *SOHLH1*, *MCM8*, *MCM9*, and *MSH5*. The most common single nuclear causative gene in syndromic POF is a premutation of *FMR1*, but other examples of proven syndromic POF include the blepharophimosis-ptosis-epicanthus inversus syndrome due to *FOXL2*, and proximal symphalangism (*SYM1*) and multiple synostosis syndrome (*SYNS1*) due to NOG perturbations. Mitochondrial DNA mutations or nuclear DNA mutations disrupting mitochondrial function can also be causative for syndromic POF, as illustrated by Perrault syndrome (several genes) and progressive external ophthalmoplegia due to DNA polymerase γ. Genome-wide association studies are also revealing regions potentially associated with POF, some of which are plausible, but often without obvious causative genes.

In premature ovarian failure (POF), menstruation ceases before the expected age of menopause. Diagnosis is traditionally confirmed by elevated serum FSH levels (>40 IU/L) prior to the age of 40 years. More recently a threshold of >25IU/L has been proposed [1].

Approximately 1% of the women are affected with POF before the age of 40 years, and perhaps 0.1% before the age of 30 years. The spectrum of causes includes genetic, autoimmune, metabolic, infectious, and iatrogenic etiologies. However, the etiology remains to be elucidated in most cases. The importance of genetic causation is evident as 10–15% of cases have an affected first-degree relative [2].

Table 1. Autosomal genes causing POF that are codified in OMIM

OMIM nomenclature	Gene name	Chromosomal location
Location		
POF1	*FMR1*	Xq27.3
POF2	*DIAPH2 (POF2A)* *POF1B (POF2B)*	Xq13.3-q21.1
POF3	*FOXL2*	3q23
POF4	*BMP15*	Xp11.2
POF5	*NOBOX*	7q35
POF6	*FIGLA*	2p13.3
POF7	*NR5A1*	9q33
POF8	*STAG3*	7q22.1
POF9	*HFM1*	1p22.2
POF10	*MCM8*	20p12.3
POF11	*ERCC6 (PGBD3)*	10q11.23

Nomenclature

In addition to POF, the designations primary ovarian insufficiency (POI) and premature menopause are also used and nearly synonymous. The latter is preferred by ESHRE [1]. However, in our view, POI better designates the broader spectrum of disorders with diminished ovarian reserve, regardless of any etiology, thus covering a larger cohort, including occult, biochemical, and overt stages. POF can therefore be considered the final stage of POI. The authoritative Online Mendelian Inheritance in Man (OMIM) has long applied the appellation POF to proven causative genes (Table 1). POF is then the appropriate term for of this genetic report.

Chromosomal Anomalies in Premature Ovarian Failure

Chromosomal abnormalities were initially the only way to verify a genetic etiology of POF. Long-known karyotypic abnormalities include numerical defects (monosomy X), X-chromosome deletions, X-autosome translocations, and isochromosomes. Prevalences range widely, with selection and ascertainment biases presumably accounting for differences in diverse cohorts [3].

Monosomy and Trisomy

The X chromosome plays an essential role in the maintenance of ovarian development and function. Females lacking an X chromosome are well known to display ovarian failure.

X monosomy (Turner syndrome) is characterized by ovarian dysgenesis due to accelerated follicular atresia, typically resulting in primary amenorrhea. However, in 1975, Simpson [4] reported that 3% (5/178) of 45,X patients menstruated. That is, 45,X women may present with POF and secondary amenorrhea as well as the more typical primary amenorrhea. Mosaicism may also result in POF with secondary amenorrhea.

X trisomy is also associated with ovarian dysfunction, 47,XXX women may sometimes experience oligomenorrhea, secondary amenorrhea, and early menopause. Goswami et al. [5] found 2 of 52 47,XXX cases to have POF (3.8%), and in a Chinese population, Jiao et al. [6] reported a prevalence of 1.5% (8/531). The association of 47,XXX with autoimmune diseases is a potential confounding explanation [5, 7]. Overexpression of genes that escape X inactivation could also explain POF in 47,XXX. However, the responsible genes remain to be defined [8]. Finally, the association of 3 X chromosomes could also result in a meiotic disturbance that might secondarily induce ovarian failure.

Structural Chromosomal Abnormalities
Many X chromosome deletions and X-autosome balanced translocations have frequently been reported in patients with POF. These cases have been studied to identify and localize causative genes. Thus, phenotypic-karyotypic correlations have revealed that almost all terminal deletions originating at the proximal X short arm (Xp13) are associated with primary amenorrhea, lack of breast development, and complete ovarian failure. The most proximal region of the X-short arm can be presumed to contain pivotal loci for ovarian maintenance [9, 10].

The X long arm likewise contains pivotal genes, independent of those on Xp. Of particular note are 2 loci on the X chromosome that appear critical for the POF phenotype and have been defined as critical regions (CR): CRI Xq13-Xq21 or POF2, and CRII Xq23-q27 or POF1. Given that XIST is in CRII, it has been reasonably proposed that epigenetic mechanisms downregulate the oocyte-expressed autosomal genes translocated to CRI [11–13]. By contrast, with CRII in terminal deletions arising at Xq25 or Xq26, the more common phenotype is not primary amenorrhea but POF. Similarly, the most distal deletions arising at Xq27 or Xq28 exert a less severe effect on stature than proximal deletions.

Autosomal rearrangements not involving the X chromosomes are also associated with premature or complete ovarian failure. Robertsonian or reciprocal autosomal translocations have been surveyed in Belgian, American, Japanese, and Chinese women [6, 14–16]. No autosome appears to be preferentially involved. Perturbations presumably confer cryptic haploinsufficiency or interrupt pivotal genes in these regions. Nonspecific defective meiotic pairing or a position effect on contiguous genes are also possible explanations [9, 17].

X-autosomal translocations are another way to detect genes causing the POF phenotype. X-autosome translocations frequently involve Xq21, but protein-coding genes have still not been identified with certainty. Other putative POF genes on the X chromosome identified in this fashion include *DIAPH2* on Xq22, *XPNPEP2* on Xq25, *DACH2* on Xq21.3, *POF1B* on Xq21.1, *CHM* on Xq21.1, *PGRMC1* on Xq24, *COL4A6* on Xq22.3, and *NXF5* on Xq22.1 [18–24]. Several of these are discussed below, but for others robust functional evidence is lacking.

Genes on the X Chromosome

Bone Morphogenetic Protein 15, BMP15, POF4 (Xp11.2)

BMP15 is located on chromosome Xp11.2. A role for *BMP15* in human POF pathogenesis was first supported by evidence from various animal models. *Bmp15* knockout female mice are subfertile, showing decreased ovulation rates, reduced litter sizes, and a decreased number of litters per lifetime [25]. Primary ovarian failure occurs in homozygous ewes [26].

In humans, BMP15 was first implicated in POF by Di Pasquale et al. [27], who reported a heterozygous p.Y235C missense mutation in each of 2 sisters with ovarian failure. In vitro evidence highlighted a dominant negative effect. BMP15 is a member of the TGFB (transforming growth factor beta) family; the gene products of family members dimerize, which is consistent with a dominant negative effect. Other BMP15 variants have been identified in Caucasian, Indian, and Chinese women with POF effects of varying frequencies, ranging from 1.5 to 15% [28–35]. Most reports have found variants occurring in the region corresponding to the propeptide of the protein, an essential component for dimerization and subsequent posttranslational processing to generate a biologically active protein. Other variants have been associated with a marked reduction of mature protein production [34].

Androgen Receptor, AR (Xq12)

Located on Xq12, *AR* encodes the nuclear AR and is pivotal for sex differentiation and reproduction. In the ovary, *AR* is expressed in the developing follicles, in particular granulosa cells. *AR* deficiency in female mice results in a POF-like phenotype, accompanied by the dysregulation of major genes critical for folliculogenesis [36]. Thus, normal folliculogenesis requires AR-mediated androgen action. Missense mutations p.T650A and p.O658K were found in Indian women with POF [37].

A different molecular mechanism involving *AR* has been proposed to explain POF. This considers whether aberrations in CAG repeat length in exon 1 of the *AR* gene result in POF [37–40].

Forkhead Box O4, FOXO4 (Xq13.1)
FOXO4 plays a functional role during ovarian physiology. The gene encodes a member of the O class of the winged helix/forkhead transcription factor family (FOXO). *FOXO4* is expressed in granulosa cells in mice and humans, and is involved in the PI3K/Akt/Cdkn1b molecular pathway. Mutation screening in Tunisian patients identified an intronic variant IVS2+41T>G [41].

Dachshund Family Transcription Factor 2, DACH2, POF2 (Xq21.3)
DACH2 is located on Xq21.3. It was first identified by the fine mapping of genes disrupted in an X-autosome translocation in POF patients. Two novel missense mutations, p.R37L and p.F316S, were detected in an Italian cohort of POF patients [20]. However, more recent studies do not appear to exist.

Premature Ovarian Failure 1B, POF1B, POF2 (Xq21.2)
POF1B (Xq21.2) is the designation of a gene region accepted in the genome community as being proven for POF. This gene was initially found when interrupted by a translocation breakpoint in an X-autosome translocation in a woman with secondary amenorrhea (POF). Mutation analysis in an Italian POF cohort revealed a rare variant in 2 patients [20]. Lacombe et al. [42] studied a Lebanese family with 5 affected sisters; linkage to Xq21 was shown by whole-genome SNP typing and homozygosity-by-descent mapping. A homozygous R329Q mutation in exon 10 impaired the capacity to bind nonmuscle actin filaments, and plausibly could lead to exaggerated germ-cell apoptosis and POF.

Progesterone Receptor Membrane Component-1, PGRMC1 (Xq22–24)
Located at Xq22–24, the *PGRMC1* progesterone-binding membrane receptor is expressed in a variety of tissues, including the liver, kidneys, adrenal glands, uterus, and leukocytes [22, 43, 44]. As the name implies, this gene is involved in progesterone signaling in the reproductive system.

In 2008, Mansouri et al. [22] reported POF in a mother and daughter, both of whom carried an X-autosome translocation [t(X;11)(q24;q13)]. The RNA expression was reduced for *PGRMC1*. Mutation screening of 67 females with idiopathic POF then identified a third patient with a missense mutation (p.H165R) located in the cytochrome b5 domain. This mutation abolished the binding of cytochrome P450 7A1 (CYP7A1) to PGRMC1 and attenuated the ability of PGRMC1 to mediate the antiapoptotic action of progesterone in ovarian cells. Reduced levels of PGRMC1 might cause POF through impaired activation of the microsomal cytochrome P450 and increased apoptosis of ovarian cells. Wang et al. [45] identified a novel missense mutation (C.556C>T, p.Pro186Ser) in a Chinese POF case, but no functional studies were performed.

Genes on Autosomes

Autosomal genes count for the great majority of genes that, in our opinion, can be considered causative or strong candidates for POF in at least certain ethnic groups. These are discussed in order of their chromosomal location.

ATP-Dependent DNA Helicase Homolog, HFM1, POF9 (1p22.2)
Wang et al. [45] identified a compound heterozygous mutation in the *HFM1* gene in 2 affected sis-

ters. More broadly, this suggests that mutations in genes encoding proteins that regulate meiosis could result in autosomal recessive primary ovarian insufficiency in humans. This section will allude to several other genes in which meiosis is disturbed in POF.

Mismatch Homology 4 and 5, MSH4 and MSH5 (1p31; 6p21.3)

MSH4 and MSH5 belong to the DNA mismatch repair gene family, which plays an important role in meiotic recombination. MSH4 and MSH5 proteins form a heterodimeric complex and facilitate chromosome synapsis during the zygotene stage. Disruption of *Msh4* or *Msh5* in female mice results in sterility, degenerated ovaries, and loss of oocytes progressively due to meiotic failure [46, 47]. In Caucasians sequenced for *MSH4* and *MSH5*, a heterozygous mutation p.Pro29Ser (c.2547C>T) in *MSH5* was found in 2 of 41 cases (4.88%). This variant was located in the Hmsh4-binding domain of MSH5 and could disrupt the integrity of the interaction between MSH5 and MSH4 proteins [48]. A novel homozygous missense mutation (c.1459G>T, p.D487Y) in the *MSH5* gene in 2 Chinese sisters with POI was identified. The homologous mutation in mice resulted in atrophic ovaries without oocytes, and an in vitro functional study revealed that mutant MSH5 impaired DNA homologous recombination repair [49].

Transforming Growth Factor Beta Receptor III, TGFBR3 (1p33-p32)

Human *TGFBR3* encodes the TGF-β type III receptor. This receptor is a membrane proteoglycan that can function as a coreceptor with other TGF-β receptor superfamily members (e.g., BMP15 and GDF9). Two missense variants (p.E458G and p.P825L) were found by Qin et al. [50] in Chinese women with idiopathic POF. Each was predicted to have functional and structural impacts on the TGFBR3 protein. Another missense mutation (p.P775S) was found in an Indian POF case [51].

G Protein-Coupled Receptor 3, GPR3 (1p36.1-p35)

GPR3 is located on 1p36.1-p35. A 2-exon gene, GRP3 is a member of the G protein-coupled receptor family and is predominantly expressed in oocytes. GPR3 maintains meiotic arrest in antral follicles until the luteinizing hormone surge, exerting action through pathways involving cAMP and cGMP. In *Gpr3*$^{-/-}$ mice, most oocytes in antral follicles spontaneously undergo the premature resumption of meiosis [52]. A single synonymous variant (c.135G>A, p.Val45Val) in a Chinese patient was identified [53]. Another study also failed to find any potential disease-associated changes in 82 North-American Caucasian women with POF [54].

Wingless-Type MMTV Integration Site Family Member 4, WNT4 (1p36.23-p35.1)

WNT4 encodes a secreted extracellular signaling protein and is expressed in human ovaries from early embryonic development [55]. *Wnt4* plays a critical role in female sex determination and differentiation. In the ovaries of *Wnt4* mutant mice, the rate of apoptosis is similar to that of wild-type mice at birth, but apoptotic cells then progressively increase during follicular development [55]. Sequencing the coding region of *WNT4* in 55 Tunisian women with POF identified 1 synonymous variant in exon 2 (c.99G>A, p.Ser33Ser) [56]. In 145 Chinese women with POF, no causative variants were found [57].

Factor in the Germline Alpha, FIGLA, POF6 (2p13.3)

FIGLA is a germ cell-specific, basic helix-loop-helix (HLH) transcription factor that plays a crucial role in the formation of the primordial follicle and coordinates the expression of zona pellucida genes. Zhao et al. [58] screened 100 Chinese women with POF, identifying 3 variants in 4 women. Missense mutation p.A4E was found in 2 women. A truncated protein (p.G6fsX66) was found in a third woman, caused by a frameshift that led to haploinsufficiency. In the fourth, deletion p.140delN was shown by the yeast 2-hybrid assay to have disrupted FIGLA binding to the TCF3 HLH domain. A nonsynonymous variant, p.Arg83Cys, was recently found in Indian POF cases, which lies in the bHLH domain of the *FIGLA* gene [59].

Follicle-Stimulating Hormone Receptor, FSHR (2p21-p16)

Follicle-stimulating hormone (FSH)/FSHR signaling plays a well-known role in regulating follicular growth, estrogen production, and oocyte maturation. Perturbation of this important G protein receptor is a common cause of ovarian failure in Finland. The initial *FSHR* mutation (c.566C>T, p.Ala189Val) associated with POF was found in 6 Finnish families in each of which multiple siblings had hypergonadotropic ovarian dysgenesis [60, 61]. Population studies revealed a segregation coefficient of 0.23, confirming autosomal recessive inheritance. *FSHR* mutations have proven to be a common cause of XX gonadal dysgenesis in Finland, but cohort screening studies subsequently failed to find mutations in most other ethnicities [33, 62–70].

Inhibins: INHA (2q35), INHBA (7p15-p13), INHBB (2cen-q13)

Inhibins are dimeric glycoprotein hormones that belong to the superfamily of TGF-β and exert negative regulation on FSH. Several genes exist in the inhibin family, including INHA, INHBB, and INHBA.

In *INHA*, 1 missense coding variant (p.G769A) and 2 promoter alleles (–16T, –124T) of the *INHA* gene have been associated with POF. The p. G769A mutation was first found in a New Zealand and Slovenian cohort by Shelling et al. [71], who believed interference with receptor binding adversely influenced the subsequent signal transduction pathway. This was proposed to result in increased FSH and, hence, accelerated the number of follicles recruited per cycle. Variants were also reported in Italian and Indian POF samples [72–74]. No disease-causing variants were revealed in Korean, Argentinean, and Italian samples [75–77].

Dixit et al. [73] later expanded his Indian sample, finding 2 additional missense variants, p.Ser92Asn, p.His175Gln. The mother of 1 POF patient also had the same (p.His175Gln) variant; she underwent premature menopause at 36 years of age.

INHBB encodes for the inhibin *βB* subunit expressed exclusively in granulosa cells. Low serum inhibin in POF cases is consistent with a role in the pathogenesis of POF. Plausible causative mutations have been found in POF patients in India, New Zealand, and Slovenia [71, 72].

INHBA encodes for the inhibin βA subunit. A silent mutation c.1032C>T was detected in 1 of 12 New Zealand POF patients [71]. Gene association studies in an Indian cohort showed a missense mutation c.896A>C (p.Gln299Pro) in a woman with primary amenorrhea [72]. However, mutations in *INHBA* have not shown an association with secondary amenorrhea (POF).

Eukaryotic Initiation Factor 2B, EIF2B: EIF2B2 (14q24.3), EIF2B4 (2p23.3), EIF2B5 (3q27.1)

EIF2B genes encode 5 subunits (α–ε) of eIF2B protein and play critical roles in the initial steps of protein synthesis. Three of the 5 *EIF2B* genes (*EIF2B2, 4,* and *5*) were found perturbed in 7 women with ovarioleukodystrophy (POF; white matter abnormalities as shown on MRI) [78]. However, no novel variants were then identified in an aggregate totaling 93 isolated POF patients [79].

Growth Differentiation Factor 9, GDF9 (5q31.1)

Expressed in oocytes, GDF is, like BMP15, a member of the TGF family. Dimerization can occur, setting the stage for dominant negative mechanisms of action. Heterozygous mutations have been detected in European, Caucasian, and Asian patients, but less so, if at all, in Japanese and New Zealand subjects [30, 80–84]. Variants include a hydrophobic to hydrophilic amino acid change, which could plausibly account causally for a proportion of the 1–4% of *GDF9* variants in POF cohorts. On the other hand, variants found in POF cases are rarely novel but rather just more frequent than in controls.

POU Class 5 Homeobox 1, POU5F1 (6p21.31)
This transcription factor gene is significantly downregulated in *Nobox* knockout mice. On this basis, *POU5F1* becomes a potential candidate gene for POF, i.e., a downstream target of *NOBOX*. Wang et al. [85] sequenced 175 Chinese POF cases and found 1 nonsynonymous variant (p.P13T), a heterozygous hydrophobic to hydrophilic substitution.

Forkhead Box O3, FOXO3 (6q21)
Forkhead transcription factor *FOXO3*, located on 6q21, encodes a master regulator and potent suppressor of primordial follicle activation. Loss of *Foxo3* in mice leads to POF, likely due to premature global follicle activation. Variants in POF cohorts range from 1.3 to 13.2% in different ethnic groups, the wide range suggesting many reported variants are not pathogenic [86–88].

Minichromosome Maintenance Complex Component 8 and 9: MCM8 (20p12.3), MCM9 (6q22.31)
These genes are implicated in homologous recombination and repair of double-stranded DNA breaks. *Mcm8*- and *Mcm9*-deficient mice are infertile and have small gonads due to germ cell depletion [89]. Rajkovic and colleagues discovered homozygous mutations in *MCM8* and *MCM9* genes in consanguineous families, using whole-exome sequencing [90, 91]. The homozygous mutant c.446C>G (p.P149R) found in MCM8 inhibited recruitment of *MCM8* to sites of DNA damage and led to genomic instability. One of the 2 mutations found in *MCM9* – c.1732t2T>C – resulted in abnormal alternative splicing, and truncated forms of *MCM9* are also unable to be recruited to sites of DNA damage. The other mutation [c.394C>T (p.Arg132*)] results in loss of function of *MCM9*. It is suspected that preferential sensitivity of germline meiosis to *MCM9* functional deficiency and compromised DNA repair in the somatic component most likely accounts for ovarian failure and also the short stature observed. The MCM8/MCM9 complex is likely required for the resolution of dsDNA breaks that occur during homologous recombination in the pachytene of meiosis I. Failure to resolve breaks likely leads to oocyte death and small or absent ovaries.

Cbp/p300-Interacting Transactivator with Glu/Asp-Rich Carboxy-Terminal Domain 2, CITED2 (6q23.3)
CITED2 is essential for early embryonic development. This is evidenced by the delayed differentiation of gonads in *Cited2*$^{-/-}$ mice [92]. Fonseca et al. [93] reported 1 novel missense mutation c.604C>A (p.Pro202Thr) in 116 Tunisian POF cases.

Stromal Antigen 3, STAG3 (7q22.1)
STAG3 encodes a subunit of cohesion essential for assembly of the meiotic cohesin ring and the synaptonemal complex during meiosis. Female mice deficient of Stag3 are sterile, with early oocyte depletion. In a highly consanguineous Palestinian pedigree characterized by subjects with primary amenorrhea and gonadoblastoma, Caburet et al. [94] found a homozygous mutation (c.968delC, p.F187fs*7) in *STAG3*. Recently, another homozygous duplication (c.1947_48dupCT, Y650Sfs*22) was identified in a Lebanese POI family, confirming its causative role in POI [42].

Newborn Ovary Homeobox Gene, NOBOX, POF5 (7q35)
NOBOX is an oocyte-specific homeobox gene that plays a critical role in early folliculogenesis. Rajkovic et al. [95] showed that deficiency of *Nobox* disrupted early folliculogenesis and

oocyte-specific gene expression in mice. Lack of *Nobox* accelerated postnatal oocyte loss and abolished the transition from primordial to growing follicles. Follicles were replaced by fibrous tissue in female mice lacking *Nobox*, analogous to histological features observed in nonsyndromic ovarian failure in women. Several other genes expressed in oocytes (*Oct4* and *Gdf9*) are downregulated in *Nobox*$^{-/-}$ mice, demonstrating downstream regulation. Lechowska et al. [96] later showed that POF in *Nobox*-deficient mice resulted from faulty signaling between somatic and germ line components during embryonic development. In addition, the extremely unusual and abnormal presence of adherens junctions between unseparated oocytes within syncytial follicles indicates that faulty communication between somatic and germ cells is involved in, or leads to, abnormalities in the programmed cell adhesion. Qin et al. [97] demonstrated that the heterozygous mutation p.R355H disrupted NOBOX homeodomain binding to NOBOX DNA-binding element, thus exerting a dominant negative effect. This perturbation was found in 1 of 96 Caucasian women; no perturbations were found in 200 Chinese POF women [98]. In other ovarian insufficiency cohorts, Bouilly et al. [99, 100] reported novel *NOBOX* loss-of-function variants in 6.2 and 5.6%, respectively. Functional studies have demonstrated that haploinsufficiency is the likely genetic mechanism responsible for human POF.

Nuclear Receptor Subfamily 5, Group A, Member 1, NR5A1; Steroidogenic Factor-1, SF-1, POF7 (9q33)

NR5A1 encodes an orphan nuclear receptor that regulates the transcription of several genes involved in reproduction, steroidogenesis, or male sexual differentiation. These genes include *AMH*, *DAX1*, *CYP11A*, steroidogenic acute regulatory protein, and genes encoding steroid hydroxylases, gonadotropins, and aromatase. Inactivation of *Nr5a1*, specifically in mouse granulosa cells, causes infertility associated with hypoplastic ovaries [101].

Philibert et al. [102] identified *NR5A1* mutations as a frequent cause of primary amenorrhea in 46,XY females with low testosterone concentrations. Sequencing identified *NR5A1* mutations in: (a) 4 kindreds, each unusually having within the single kindred both 1 family member with a 46,XY disorder of sex development and another family member with 46,XX primary ovarian insufficiency, and (b) 25 other sporadic subjects having just a single family member with 46,XX ovarian failure. Mutations impaired the transactivational activity of *NR5A1* [103]. Janse et al. [104] later sequenced the coding regions of *NR5A1* in a well-phenotyped cohort of 356 Dutch women with POF; 9 different mutations were identified in 10 patients. Functional prediction showed low to intermediate pathogenicity for all the nonconservative mutations. More recently, the mutation p.Y5D, located in a novel nondomain region, was presumed to result in haploinsufficiency in Chinese patients with POF [105].

Spermatogenesis- and Oogenesis-Specific Basic Helix-Loop-Helix Transcription Factor 1 and 2, SOHLH1/2 (9q34.3; 13q13.3)

The germ cell-specific master-master transcription factors SOHLH1 and SOHLH2 orchestrate different oocyte-specific gene transcription essential for early folliculogenesis. *Sohlh1/2*-deficient mice exhibit atrophied ovaries devoid of follicles, the result of defective primordial-to-primary follicle transition. Novel heterozygous variants have been identified in *SOHLH1* and *SOHLH2* in women of Han Chinese and Serbian origin [106, 107]. A plausible pathogenesis includes disturbing the expression, transactivation, or homo-/hetero-dimerization of SOHLH1/2 proteins. Bayram et al. [108] performed whole-exome sequencing in 2 families in each of which 2 siblings had primary amenorrhea rather than POF. The siblings in one family showed a frameshift [SHOLH1 c.705delT (p.Pro235fs*4)], while protein was truncated in the other [SOHLH1 c.27C>G 9p.Tyr9stop).

Tubulin Beta 8 Class VIII, TUBB8 (10p15.3)
TUBB8 is expressed exclusively in the oocyte and early embryo, where it accounts for almost all of the expressed β-tubulin. In affected women from 7 Chinese families with infertility due to oocyte meiosis 1 arrest, heterozygous missense mutations in the *TUBB8*, paternally inherited or de novo, were identified [109]. Mutations disrupt microtubule behavior on expression in cultured cells and alter microtubule dynamics in vivo. This causes catastrophic spindle-assembly defects and maturation arrest on expression in mouse and human oocytes.

PiggyBac Transposable Element Derived 3, PGBD3 (10q11)
In 1 Chinese nonconsanguineous POF kindred and 432 sporadic POF patients, 3 novel *CSB-PGBD3* heterozygous mutation were found. Functional studies suggested that all 3 mutants might impair oocyte DNA damage repair [110].

Phosphatase and Tensin Homolog, PTEN (10q23.3)
PTEN plays a causative role in early activation of primordial follicles by negatively regulating the *PI3K* (phosphoinositide 3-kinase) pathway [111]. Primordial follicles become depleted in *Pten* null mice in early adulthood, thus mimicking the phenotype of human POF. However, no causative mutation was detected in the coding regions of *PTEN* in Japanese and Chinese women with POF [112, 113].

Nanos Homolog 1, 2, 3 (Drosophila), NANOS1 (10q26.11), NANOS2 (19q13.32), NANOS3 (19p13.13)
NANOS is required for primordial germ cell (PGC) development and maintenance. There are 3 homologs: NANOS1, NANOS2, and NANOS3. In mice, disruption of *Nanos1* does not adversely affect germ cell development, but knockout of either *Nanos2* or *Nanos3* resulted in infertility with decreased gonad size due to loss of PGCs. *Nanos2* deficiency results in loss of spermatogonia, while *Nanos3* deficiency impairs PGC maintenance in both males and females [114]. Mutations in human *NANOS3* were first investigated in 80 Chinese and 88 Caucasian women with POF by Qin et al. [115]. No mutations were found in coding exons, but there was 1 known SNP (rs2016163) in exon 1. A potentially relevant heterozygous mutation (c.457C>T; p.R153W) was identified in a subsequent sample of 100 Chinese POF patients. In this mutation the stability of NANOS3 was decreased (hypomorph). Taken together, *NANOS3* is considered causative for POF [116].

Wilms Tumor 1, WT1 (11p13)
The Wilms' tumor gene *WT1* encodes an essential transcription factor, which functions in mammalian urogenital development [117]. In adult ovaries, WT1 is expressed in granulosa cells of ovarian follicles. $Wt1^{+/R394W}$ mice were found to be subfertile due to defects in follicle development [118]. In 384 Chinese patients with POF, 2 novel missense mutations (p.Pro126Ser in exon1 and p.Arg370His in exon7) were found. In vitro experiments showed that both mutants repressed the expression of *Amh* and *Cdh1*, induced the expression of *Fshr* and *Cyp19* in mRNA and protein levels, and potentially impaired GC differentiation and oocyte-GC interaction. This cascade should result in the loss of follicles prematurely [119].

Cyclin-Dependent Kinase Inhibitor 1B, CDKN1B (12p13.1-p12)
CDKN1B, also known as P27 or KIP1, is a cyclin-dependent kinase inhibitor that regulates proliferation and differentiation in many tissues. In ovaries, it suppresses ovarian follicle endowment and activation, and promotes follicle atresia. In mice, premature follicle depletion occurred due to accelerated activation in *Cdkn1b* knockouts [120]. Sequence analysis of *CDKN1B* revealed 1 novel heterozygous mutation, c.356T>C (p.Ile-119Thr), in 87 Tunisian POF patients [121].

However, no variants were identified in Chinese cohorts, suggesting that mutations in *CDKN1B* might not be common in POF [122, 123].

Anti-Müllerian Hormone Receptor Type II, AMHR2 (12q13)
AMHR2, located on 12q13, encodes a receptor in the well-known AMH pathway that plays a crucial role in the development and maintenance of various reproductive organs (uterus, ovary). The –482 A>G polymorphism (rs2002555) in *AMHR2* was found to be associated with age at menopause in Dutch women [124]. However, no variants in *AMHR2* were detected in 16 Japanese women with POF [125].

KIT Ligand, KITLG (12q22)
KITLG is located on 12q22, encoding the ligand of tyrosine-kinase receptor. KIT/KITLG plays a critical role during oogenesis and folliculogenesis. Mice with deficiency in *Kitlg* manifested with impaired PGCs. No perturbations were reported in the coding region of *KITLG* in 40 Caucasian women with POF [126].

Forkhead Box 1, FOXO1 (13q14.1)
FOXO1, another member of the forkhead family of transcription factors, is important in granulosa cell function and follicle maturation. Watkins et al. [127] identified one 5′UTR mutation (c.–30C>T) and 1 missense mutation (p.P84L) in *FOXO1A* in a New Zealand and Slovenian POF cohort.

Spalt-Like Transcription Factor 4, SALL4 (20q13.2)
Sall4 is a zinc finger transcription factor that is expressed in murine oocytes and capable of binding to Pou5fl to regulate its expression. Both *Sall4* and *Pou5fl* are downregulated in Nobox$^{-/-}$ newborn ovaries [128, 129]. Wang et al. [130] screened the coding regions of *SALL4* in 100 Han Chinese females with nonsyndromic POF, identifying 2 heterozygous missense mutations (p.V181M and p.T817A) in the evolutionarily conserved region. Thus, these might be POF-associated gene variants; however, functional studies are necessary.

Meiotic Protein Covalently Bound to Double-Strand Breaks, SPO11 (20q13.31)
SPO11 is implicated in meiosis by forming the double-strand breaks that initiate meiotic recombination. *Spo11*$^{-/-}$ mice were infertile, showing a premature depletion of oocytes as a result of defective meiosis. However, no novel variants were found in 41 women with nonsyndromic POF [48]. The role of *SPO11* mutations in human POF is not yet clear.

DNA Meiotic Recombinase 1, DMC1 (22q13.1)
DMC1 encodes a member of the superfamily of recombinases, which is important for repairing double-strand DNA breaks during mitosis and meiosis. Any gene perturbing meiosis is a logical candidate for nonsyndromic POF [9, 131]. Indeed, Mandon-Pepin et al. [48] found the homozygous mutation p.M200V in *DMC1* in 1 of 41 women with POF.

Genes Causing Syndromic Premature Ovarian Failure

Apart from nonsyndromic POF, Mendelian disorders exist in which POF is a major component of a pleiotropic phenotypic spectrum (varied expressivity). In fact, the most common single cause of POF, fragile X syndrome, falls into this category. The role of arguably the most important ovarian differentiation gene, *FOXL2*, was also identified through a syndrome – blepharophimosis-ptosis-epicanthus syndrome (BPES).

Familial Mental Retardation 1, FMR1, Fragile × Syndrome (Xq27.3)
In fragile X syndrome, pathogenesis involves >200 CGG repeats at a specific site on the X chromosome. The normal number of CGG repeats is 30–

32. Mental retardation, facial features, and large testes are characteristic. Affected women (>200 CGG) do not have POF, but paradoxically women with above the normal number but fewer than 200 repeats do [132]. This range is 54–200 CGG repeats, and is termed "premutation." Premutation *FMR1* explains at least 5% of sporadic cases of POF and 10–15% of familial cases. From the perspective of clinical presentation, 15–20% of women with an FMR1 premutation develop POF [133]. It is not known why the number of CGG repeats correlates with risk of POF only within this selected ("subclinical") range (54–200 CGG repeats). Still, the likelihood of POF increases from 40–54, to its maximum of 80–99 repeats; the risk then plateaus with no further increase between 100 and 200 repeats. One possible explanation is that selected genes are suppressed and, hence, generate POF only at 54–200 repeats; however, suppression of additional genes beyond 200 repeats must reverse the phenotype.

Given the approximate 5% frequency of the *FMR1* premutation in POF women, *FMR1* testing is recommended for women with POF by ESHRE [1]. This may or may not be applicable in all venues [134, 135]. In Chinese subjects, only 2 premutation carriers were found among 379 sporadic POF cases; none were found in 402 controls (0.49%) [136]. This rate is lower than that in Caucasians. Rates measured among other populations include 1.56% in Japanese and 4.8% in Slovenians [137, 138].

Forkhead Box L2, FOXL2 (3q23)

FOXL2 appears to be the pivotal player in ovarian development. Initial realization of the importance of FOXL2 and other forkhead DNA-binding proteins in humans came from studying BPES, an autosomal dominant disorder in which POF occurs along with the somatic features that describe the syndrome [139]. More than 100 unique *FOXL2* mutations have been described in BPES in multiple populations [140].

In contrast to the high frequency in BPES, few *FOXL2* mutations have been described in nonsyndromic (isolated) POF [141]. No mutations were found by Chatterjee et al. [142], Ni et al. [143], or De Baere et al. [144].

Symphalangism, SYM1, and Multiple Synostosis Syndrome, SYNS1, NOG (17q22)

The polypeptide of *NOG* is expressed in various reproductive tissues and organs. NOG binds to and inactivates members of the TGF-β superfamily (i.e., BMP2, 4, 7, 14, and GDF5). *NOG* mutations are found in the proximal symphalangism (SYM1) and multiple synostoses (SYNS1) syndromes [145]. Kosaki et al. [146] described a heterozygous mutation (p.E48K) in *NOG* in a female presenting with SYM1 and POF. Laissue et al. [147] screened 100 nonsyndromic sporadic POF patients and identified only 1 heterozygous mutation (p.G92E).

Other Syndromic Premature Ovarian Failure Genes

Other syndromic forms of POF involving nuclear genes exist. *EIF2B*, which is causative for ovarioleukodystrophy (*EIF2B*), has been discussed previously. Others include *GALT*-associated galactosemia and *AIRE; AIRE* causes autoimmune polyendocrinopathy candidiasis ectodermal dystrophy syndrome. Overall, these syndromes in aggregate explain at best 0.5% of cases with POF. Nonetheless, clinicians caring for female adolescents with these or other syndromes should consider the above genes if menstrual irregularities arise. Scientifically, syndrome-related POF can also point to new genetic mechanisms that, if perturbed, cause isolated POF.

Mitochondrial Dysfunction Resulting in Syndromic Premature Ovarian Failure

A mature oocyte during oogenesis has the most mitochondria of any human cell. Thus, mitochondrial biogenesis plays an essential role in oocyte maturation, fertilization, and embryo development. Dysregulation of mitochondrial dynamics (bioenergetics) leads to excessive oxidative stress and apoptosis initiation, thus accelerating follicle depletion. Decreased mitochondrial DNA (mtDNA) in oocytes and peripheral blood cells has been observed in women with ovarian insufficiency [148, 149]. The causes could be mutations in mtDNA itself, or mutations in nuclear genes responsible for mitochondrial function.

Progressive External Opthalmoplegia: Polymerase γ, POLG (15q25)
Mutations have been identified in DNA polymerase γ (*POLG*), a mitochondrial gene that encodes the catalytic subunit of mtDNA polymerase responsible for mtDNA replication and repair. The resulting syndrome – progressive external ophthalmoplegia – includes proximal myopathy, sensory ataxia, and parkinsonism. Screening for *POLG* mutations in isolated POF revealed a single p.R953C mutation isolated in 201 cases of POF (0.5%) [148, 150, 151].

Perrault Syndrome: HAS2 (5qB1.3), LARS2 (3p21.3), CLPP (19p13.3), C10orf2 (10q.24)
Perrault syndrome is a recognized syndrome characterized by sensorineural deafness and POF. The genetic etiology involves mitochondrial perturbations and several genes – *HARS2, LARS2, CLPP,* and *C10orf2* – each of which encodes nuclear genes capable of mitochondrial tRNA synthetase and chambered protease. Mutations are responsible for POF in Perrault syndrome [152–154].

Genome-Wide Association Studies and Copy Number Variants in Premature Ovarian Failure

Whole genome-wide association studies (GWAS), whole-exome sequencing, and whole-genome sequencing are increasingly being conducted. In GWAS, 6 studies have been performed to identify POF-associated variants. The first showed association with the PTH-responsive B1 gene (*PTHB1*) in a small discovery set of 24 women and 24 controls [155]. Knauff et al. [156] identified an association for an intron SNP in *ADAMTS19* in a discovery set of 99 Dutch women and 181 controls, but not in the replication set. *LAMC1* was reported to be significantly associated with POF in a Korean study of 122 cases and 242 controls [157]. Using a genome-wide linkage scan, 5q14.1-q15 was found to be a susceptibility region in a single Dutch POF family subjected to secondary amenorrhea [158]. Caburet et al. [159] reported a genome-wide linkage and homozygosity analysis in a large consanguineous Middle-Eastern POF-affected family presenting with an autosomal recessive pattern of inheritance. Two syntenic regions on chromosome 7, 7p21-p15.3 and 7q21.3-q22.2, were identified and proposed as candidate regions on the basis of homozygosity mapping. However, the 3 candidate genes sequenced from this region, *DLX5*, *DLX6*, and *DSS1*, showed no causative mutations.

Ours is the only study conducted in Chinese Han women with idiopathic POF that is even modestly close to adequate size. The initial discovery by Qin et al. [160] consisted of 391 cases and 895 controls, followed by an independently replicated set of 400 cases and 800 controls. Significant associations were observed at 8q22.3, but no attractive candidate genes exist in this region. Existence of an as yet undefined long-distance regulatory region affecting ovarian differentiation and oogenesis might exist, analogous to the role played by SOX9 in male differentiation.

In addition to linkage analysis and GWAS based on SNPs, there is increasing interest in the association of copy number variants (CNVs) with complex traits like POF. As of our 2015 review, 6 array CGH genomic hybridization studies had been published associating CNVs associated with

POF [3]. Aboura et al. [161] identified 8 known CNVs in 99 French patients with POF. Among these were 5 potential candidate genes, *DNAH5*, *NAIP*, *DUSP22*, *NUPR1*, and *AKT1*. Quilter et al. [162] found 15 novel discrete X chromosome intervals in a total of 20 out of 42 UK women with POF. However, Dudding et al. [163] detected only 2 microduplications (Xp22.33 and Xq13.3) at a low frequency of 4% in a New Zealand sample. Another array CGH involved 74 German cases with POF/ovarian dysgenesis: 44 losses or gains were believed to be potentially causative for POF [164]. Knauff et al. [165] found CNVs in Xq21.3 to be associated with POF in a region where *PCHCHIIX* and *TGHF2LX* are located. McGuire et al. [166] identified 17 novel microduplications and 7 novel microdeletions among 89 POF patients. Two novel microdeletions caused haploinsufficiency for *SYCE1* and *CPEB1*, genes known to generate ovarian failure in knockout mouse models. On the other hand, no CNVs have been found in regions considered to be pivotal on the basis of cytogenetic studies (see the section entitled Chromosomal Anomalies in Premature Ovarian Failure, above) [10].

There are logical explanations for these apparent inconsistencies. First, there are no studies in which the sample size is truly adequate. No GWAS study has ever exceeded 1,000, the universally accepted minimum sample size given evaluation involving hundreds of thousands of SNPs and necessity to correct for multiple comparisons. Second, POF is rare compared to common disorders like even polycystic ovary syndrome or endometriosis, for which sample sizes of thousands can be readily recruited for GWAS studies [167–169]. Third, POF is a disorder adversely affected by reproductive fitness, a further impediment for identifying genes.

Interrogating for CNVs (array CGH) is likely to be superseded by whole-exome or whole-genome sequencing. Low prevalence and impaired fecundity result in relatively few pedigrees, with multiple family members having isolated POF. Family-based whole-exome or genome sequencing may be the most fruitful approach for detecting POF genes given this heterogeneity.

Conclusions

Several general principles are already apparent in identifying nuclear and mitochondrial genes causing POF.

(1) Several genes have already emerged as unassailably causative for nonsyndromic POF. X-linked genes include *BMP15*, *PGRMC1*, and premutation *FMR1* (54–200 CGG repeats). Autosomal genes include FSHR, *GDF9*, *NR5A1*, *NOBOX*, *FIGLA*, *STAG3*, *FOXL2*, *HFM1*, *SOHLH1*, *MCM8*, *MCM9*, and *MSH5*. For all these genes, there exists plausibility, functional studies, robust differences between comparator controls and cases, or presence of multiple affected family members.

(2) Several other autosomal genes are strong candidates but data are more limited. Novel variants have been reported but there are few associated cases and functional studies are lacking.

(3) These autosomal genes include *HFM1*, *TGFBR3*, *INA*, *CITED2*, *SOHLH2*, *PGBD3*, *WT1*, *FOX01*, *NOG*, and *SALL4* (Table 2).

(4) Genetic causes of syndromic POF include X-linked fragile X syndrome (*FMR1*), BPES due to *FOXL2*, ovarioleukodystrophy due to eIF2B mutations and NOG, which when perturbed causes proximal symphalangism (SYM1) and multiple synostosis syndrome (SYNS1).

(5) Mutations of nuclear genes disrupting mitochondrial function can cause POF. This is illustrated by syndromic POF occurring in progressive external ophthalmoplegia due to mtDNA polymerase γ (*POLG*), and by Perrault syndrome, due to several genes.

(6) A mild surprise is that many POF genes differ in function from those logically predicted on the basis of having known reproductive endocrine roles. Recurring themes include genes that

Table 2. Autosomal genes that can be considered causative for isolated POF

Gene	Location	Ethnicity	Mutation prevalence (%)	Sequence variation	Amino acid change	Reference
HFM1	1p22.2	Chinese	1/69 (1.5)	c.2206G>A/ c.3929_3930 delinsG	p.G736S/ p.P1310R fs*41	Wang et al. [45], 2014
TGFBR3	1p33-p32	Chinese	2/112 (1.8)	c.1370A>G c.2467C>T	p.E458G p.P824L	Qin et al. [160], 2012; Qin et al. [50], 2011
		Indian	1/133 (0.8)	c.2323C>T	p.P775S	Dixit et al. [51], 2006
FIGLA	2p13.3	Chinese	2/100 (2.0)	c.15-36del c.419-421del	p.G6fsX66 p.140delN	Zhao et al. [58], 2008
		Indian	2/219 (0.9)	c.649+8A>G		Tosh et al. [59], 2015
FSHR	2p21-p16	Swiss	1/1162 (0.9)	c.566C>T	p.A189V	Jiang et al. [170], 1998
		Finnish	19/1976 (0.96)	c.566C>T	p.A189V	Aittomäki et al. [60], 1995
		Finnish	22/52 (42.3)	c.566C>T	p.A189V	Aittomäki et al. [60], 1995 Aittomäki et al. [171], 1996
INHA	2q33-q36	Indian	2/133 (1.5)	c.275G>A c.525C>G	p.S92N p.H175O	Dixit et al. [73], 2006
		Indian	9/80 (11.2)	c.769G>A	p.A257T	Dixit et al. [72], 2004
FOXL2	3q23	New Zealand/ Slovenian	2/70 (2.9)	c.898-927del c.1009T>A	p.A221_A23 p.Y258N	Harris et al. [141], 2002
GDF9	5q31.1	Chinese	1/100 (1.0)	c.712A>G	p.T238A	Zhao et al. [82], 2007
		American	1/61 (1.6)	c.307C>T	p.P103S	Kovanci et al. [81], 2007
		Caucasian, African, Asian	1/203 (0.5)	c.557C>A	p.S186Y	Laissue et al. [30], 2006
		Indian	6/127 (4.7)	c.199A>C c.646G>A	p.K67E p.V216M	Dixit et al. [80], 2005
POU5F1	6p21.31	Chinese	1/115 (0.9)	c.37C>A	p.P13T	Wang et al. [85], 2011
MSH5	6p21.3	Caucasian Senegalese	2/41 (4.9)	g.2547C>T	p.P29S	Mandon-Pepin et al. [48], 2008
FOXO3	6q21	Chinese	15/114 (13.2)	c.71C>A c.140C>T c.184G>A c.1652C>T c.1697C>G	p.P24H p.P47L p.D62N p.S551F p.G566A	Wang et al. [88], 2010
		(Mixed Italian, North American, French German, South Korean)	4/302 (1.3)	c.280C>T c.1021G>A c.1156C>T	p.L94F p.A341T p.L386F	Gallardo et al. [86], 2008

Table 2. Continued

Gene	Location	Ethnicity	Mutation prevalence (%)	Sequence variation	Amino acid change	Reference
		French	3/50 (6.0)	c.1778A>C	p.Y593S	Vinci et al. [87], 2008
		New Zealand, Slovenian	2/90 (2.2)	c.1262C>T c.1517G>A	p.S421L p.R506H	Watkins et al. [127], 2006
MCM9	6q22.31	European, Hispanic, Indian, African American	1/109 (0.9)	c.1533C>A	p.Tyr511*	Wood-Trageser et al. [91], 2014
CITED2	6q23.3	Tunisian, Australian	1/116 (0.9)	c.604C>A	p.P202T	Fonseca et al. [93], 2012
NOBOX	7q35	Caucasian or African	12/213 (5.6)	c.271G>T c.331G>A c.349C>T c.1112A>C c.1856C>T	p.G91T, p.G111R p.R117W p.K371T p.P619L	Bouilly et al. [100], 2014
		Caucasian, Senegalese, Ban-tu	12/178 (6.2)	c.271G>T c.349C>T c.1025G>C c.1048G>T c.907C>T	p.G91W p.R117W p.S342T p.V350L p.R303X	Bouilly et al. [99], 2011
		Caucasian	1/96(1.0)	c.1064G>A	p.R355H	Qin et al. [97], 2007
NR5A1	9q33	French	3/180 (1.7)	c.162C>A c.593C>T	p.S54R p.P198L	Voican et al. [172], 2013
		Tunisian	1/26 (1.8)	c.763C>T	p.R255C	Philibert et al. [173], 2013
		Chinese	1/384 (0.26)	c.13T>G	p.Y5D	Jiao et al. [105], 2013
		Asian, Caucasian, Mediterranean	5/356 (1.4)	c.407C>T c.574G>T+ c.575C>T c.593C>T c.938G>A	p.P136L p.A192F/ S+A192V p.P198L p.R313H	Janse et al. [104], 2012
		Roman, Indian, Senegalese, Afri-can	2/28 (2.3)	c.691-699del c.368G>C/ c.386C>T	p.L231_ L233del p.G123A/ P129L	Lourenco et al. [103], 2009
SOHLH1	9q34.3	Chinese Serbian	2/561 (0.36)	c.950C>T c.1126G>A	p.S317F p.E376K	Zhao et al. [107], 2015
PGBD3	10q11	Chinese	1/432 (0.2)	c.3166G>A	p.V1056I	Qin et al. [110], 2015
WT1	11p13	Chinese	2/384 (0.5)	c.376C>T c.1109G>A	p. P126S p.R370H	Wang et al. [119], 2015

Table 2. (continued)

Gene	Location	Ethnicity	Mutation prevalence (%)	Sequence variation	Amino acid change	Reference
CDKN1B	12p13.1-p12	Tunisian Colombian	1/87 (1.5)	c.356T>C	p.I119T	Ojeda et al. [121], 2011
SOHLH2	13q13.3	Chinese Serbian	8/56 (1.4)	c.235G>A c.314A>G c.360A>T c.610C>T c.961A>C	p.E79K p.E105G p.L120F p.L204F p.T321P	Qin et al. [106], 2014
FOXO1	13q14.1	New Zealand, Slovenian	1/90 (1.1)	c.251C>T	p.P84L	Watkins et al. [127], 2006
POLG	15q25	Caucasian, African, Hispanic, Asian	1/201 (0.5)	c.2857C>T	p.R953C	Tong et al. [150], 2010
NOG	17q22	French	1/100 (1.0)	c.275G>A	p.G92E	Laissue, et al. [147], 2007
NANOS3	19p13.13	Chinese	1/100 (1)	c.457C>T	p.R153W	Wu, et al. [116], 2013
SALL4	20q13.2	Chinese	2/100 (2)	c.541G>A c.2449A>G	p.V181M p.T817A	Wang, et al. [130], 2009

Causation is considered to exist for a novel missense mutation that is not found in controls, a nonsense mutation, or protein truncation. See Qin et al. [3] for expanded data, including negative studies.

are major regulators of pathways involved in cell proliferation, survival, migration, and metabolism. A further example is genes deleteriously affecting meiosis. The latter have increased the spectrum of genes – *MCM8*, *MCM9*, and *MSH5*.

Overall, a reasonable estimate is that 25% of POF cases can already be explained by a single gene mutation. Future studies need to involve multiple ethnic groups for each putative candidate.

Acknowledgements

This work was supported in part by the National Basic Research Program of China (973 program 2012CB944700), the National Natural Science Foundation of China (81270662), the Foundation for the Author of National Excellent Doctoral Dissertation of China (201078), and the Independent Innovation Foundation of Shandong University, IIFSDU (2012TS130).

References

1 ESHRE: Guideline on the management of premature ovarian insufficiency. https://wwweshreeu/Guidelines-and-Legal/Guidelines/Management-of-premature-ovarian-insufficiencyaspx 2015.

2 Van Kastern YM, Shoemaker J: Premature ovarian failure: a systematic review on therapeutic interventions to restore ovarian function and achieve pregnancy. Hum Repro Update 1999;5:483–492.

3 Qin Y, Jiao X, Simpson JL and Chen ZJ: Genetics of primary ovarian insufficiency: new developments and opportunities. Hum Reprod Update 2015;21;787–808.

4 Simpson JL: Gonadal dysgenesis and abnormalities of the human sex chromosomes: current status of phenotypic-karyotypic correlations. Birth Defects Orig Artic Ser 1975;11:23–59.

5 Goswami R, Goswami D, Kabra M, Gupta N, Dubey S, Dadhwal V: Prevalence of the triple X syndrome in phenotypically normal women with premature ovarian failure and its association with autoimmune thyroid disorders. Fertil Steril 2003;80:1052–1054.

6 Jiao X, Qin C, Li J, Qin Y, Gao X, Zhang B, Zhen X, Feng Y, Simpson JL, Chen ZJ: Cytogenetic analysis of 531 Chinese women with premature ovarian failure. Hum Reprod 2012;27:2201–2207.

7 Holland CM: 47,XXX in an adolescent with premature ovarian failure and autoimmune disease. J Pediatr Adolesc Gynecol 2001;14:77–80.

8 Tartaglia NR, Howell S, Sutherland A, Wilson R and Wilson L: A review of trisomy X (47,XXX). Orphanet J Rare Dis 2010;5:8.

9 Simpson JL: Genetic and phenotypic heterogeneity in ovarian failure: overview of selected candidate genes. Ann NY Acad Sci 2008;1135:146–154.

10 Simpson JL, Rajkovic A: Ovarian differentiation and gonadal failure. Am J Med Genet 1999;1135:186–200.

11 Rizzolio F, Bione S, Sala C, Goegan M, Gentile M, Gregato G, Rossi E, Pramparo T, Zuffardi O, Toniolo D: Chromosomal rearrangements in Xq and premature ovarian failure: mapping of 25 new cases and review of the literature. Hum Reprod 2006;21:1477–1483.

12 Rizzolio F, Sala C, Alboresi S, Bione S, Gilli S, Goegan M, Pramparo T, Zuffardi O, Toniolo D: Epigenetic control of the critical region for premature ovarian failure on autosomal genes translocated to the X chromosome: a hypothesis. Hum Genet 2007;121:441–450.

13 Rizzolio F, Pramparo T, Sala C, Zuffardi O, De Santis L, Rabellotti E, Calzi F, Fusi F, Bellazzi R, Toniolo D: Epigenetic analysis of the critical region I for premature ovarian failure: demonstration of a highly heterochromatic domain on the long arm of the mammalian X chromosome. J Med Genet 2009;46:585–592.

14 Hens L, Devroey P, Van Waesberghe L, Bonduelle M, Van Steirteghem AC, Liebaers I: Chromosome studies and fertility treatment in women with ovarian failure. Clin Genet 1989;2:81–91.

15 Kawano Y, Narahara H, Matsui N, Miyakawa I: Premature ovarian failure associated with a Robertsonian translocation. Acta Obstet Gynecol Scand 1998; 77:467–469.

16 Orczyk GP, Pehrson J, Leventhal JM: Premature ovarian failure in a 35-year-old woman with a Robertsonian translocation. Int J Fertil 1989;34:184–187.

17 Persani L, Rossetti R, Cacciatore C, Bonomi M: Primary ovarian insufficiency: X chromosome defects and autoimmunity. J Autoimmun 2009;33: 35–41.

18 Bione S, Sala C, Manzini C, Arrigo G, Zuffardi O, Banfi S, Borsani G, Jonveaux P, Philippe C, Zuccotti M, et al: A human homologue of the *Drosophila* melanogaster diaphanous gene is disrupted in a patient with premature ovarian failure: evidence for conserved function in oogenesis and implications for human sterility. Am J Hum Genet 1998;62:533–541.

19 Prueitt RL, Ross JL, Zinn AR: Physical mapping of nine Xq translocation breakpoints and identification of XPNPEP2 as a premature ovarian failure candidate gene. Cytogenet Cell Genet 2000;89:44–50.

20 Bione S, Rizzolio F, Sala C, Ricotti R, Goegan M, Manzini MC, Battaglia R, Marozzi A, Vegetti W, Dalpra L, et al: Mutation analysis of two candidate genes for premature ovarian failure, DACH2 and POF1B. Hum Reprod 2004; 19:2759–2766.

21 Lorda-Sanchez IJ, Ibanez AJ, Sanz RJ, Trujillo MJ, Anabitarte ME, Querejeta ME, Rodriguez de Alba M, Gimenez A, Infantes F, Ramos C, et al: Choroideremia, sensorineural deafness, and primary ovarian failure in a woman with a balanced X-4 translocation. Ophthalmic Genet 2000;21:185–189.

22 Mansouri MR, Schuster J, Badhai J, Stattin EL, Losel R, Wehling M, Carlsson B, Hovatta O, Karlstrom PO, Golovleva I, et al: Alterations in the expression, structure and function of progesterone receptor membrane component-1 (*PGRMC1*) in premature ovarian failure. Hum Mol Genet 2008;17:3776–3783.

23 Nishimura-Tadaki A, Wada T, Bano G, Gough K, Warner J, Kosho T, Ando N, Hamanoue H, Sakakibara H, Nishimura G, et al: Breakpoint determination of X;autosome balanced translocations in four patients with premature ovarian failure. J Hum Genet 2011;56:156–160.

24 Bertini V, Ghirri P, Bicocchi MP, Simi P, Valetto A: Molecular cytogenetic definition of a translocation t(X;15) associated with premature ovarian failure. Fertil Steril 2010;94:1097.e5–8.

25 Yan C, Wang P, DeMayo J, DeMayo FJ, Elvin JA, Carino C, Prasad SV, Skinner SS, Dunbar BS, Dube JL, et al: Synergistic roles of bone morphogenetic protein 15 and growth differentiation factor 9 in ovarian function. Mol Endocrinol 2001; 15:854–866.

26 Galloway SM, McNatty KP, Cambridge LM, Laitinen MP, Juengel JL, Jokiranta TS, McLaren RJ, Luiro K, Dodds KG, Montgomery GW, et al: Mutations in an oocyte-derived growth factor gene (*BMP15*) cause increased ovulation rate and infertility in a dosage-sensitive manner. Nat Genet 2000;25:279–283.

27 Di Pasquale E, Beck-Peccoz P, Persani L: Hypergonadotropic ovarian failure associated with an inherited mutation of human bone morphogenetic protein-15 (*BMP15*) gene. Am J Hum Genet 2004; 75:106–111.

28 Di Pasquale E, Rossetti R, Marozzi A, Bodega B, Borgato S, Cavallo L, Einaudi S, Radetti G, Russo G, Sacco M, et al: Identification of new variants of human *BMP15* gene in a large cohort of women with premature ovarian failure. J Clin Endocrinol Metab 2006;91:1976–1979.

29 Dixit H, Rao LK, Padmalatha VV, Kanakavalli M, Deenadayal M, Gupta N, Chakrabarty B, Singh L: Missense mutations in the *BMP15* gene are associated with ovarian failure. Hum Genet 2006; 119:408–415.
30 Laissue P, Christin-Maitre S, Touraine P, Kuttenn F, Ritvos O, Aittomäki K, Bourcigaux N, Jacquesson L, Bouchard P, Frydman R, et al: Mutations and sequence variants in GDF9 and BMP15 in patients with premature ovarian failure. Eur J Endocrinol 2006;154:739–744.
31 Lakhal B, Laissue P, Braham R, Elghezal H, Saad A, Fellous M, Veitia RA: A novel BMP15 variant, potentially affecting the signal peptide, in a familial case of premature ovarian failure. Clin Endocrinol 2009;71:752–753.
32 Lakhal B, Laissue P, Braham R, Elghezal H, Saad A, Fellous M, Veitia RA: BMP15 and premature ovarian failure: causal mutations, variants, polymorphisms? Clin Endocrinol 2010;72:425–426.
33 Ledig S, Ropke A, Haeusler G, Hinney B, Wieacker P: *BMP15* mutations in XX gonadal dysgenesis and premature ovarian failure. Am J Obstet Gynecol 2008; 198:84.e1–5.
34 Rossetti R, Di Pasquale E, Marozzi A, Bione S, Toniolo D, Grammatico P, Nelson LM, Beck-Peccoz P, Persani L: BMP15 mutations associated with primary ovarian insufficiency cause a defective production of bioactive protein. Hum Mutat 2009;30:804–810.
35 Wang B, Wen Q, Ni F, Zhou S, Wang J, Cao Y, Ma X: Analyses of growth differentiation factor 9 (GDF9) and bone morphogenetic protein 15 (BMP15) mutation in Chinese women with premature ovarian failure. Clin Endocrinol 2010;72:135–136.
36 Shiina H, Matsumoto T, Sato T, Igarashi K, Miyamoto J, Takemasa S, Sakari M, Takada I, Nakamura T, Metzger D, et al: Premature ovarian failure in androgen receptor-deficient mice. Proc Natl Acad Sci USA 2006;103:224–229.
37 Panda B, Rao L, Tosh D, Dixit H, Padmalatha V, Kanakavalli M, Raseswari T, Deenadayal M, Gupta N, Chakrabarty B, et al: Germline study of AR gene of Indian women with ovarian failure. Gynecol Endocrinol 2010;27:572–578.
38 Bretherick KL, Hanna CW, Currie LM, Fluker MR, Hammond GL, Robinson WP: Estrogen receptor alpha gene polymorphisms are associated with idiopathic premature ovarian failure. Fertil Steril 2008;89:318–324.
39 Chatterjee S, Singh R, Kadam S, Maitra A, Thangaraj K, Meherji P, Modi D: Longer CAG repeat length in the androgen receptor gene is associated with premature ovarian failure. Hum Reprod 2009;24:3230–3235.
40 Sugawa F, Wada Y, Maruyama T, Uchida H, Ishizuka B, Ogata T: Premature ovarian failure and androgen receptor gene CAG repeat lengths weighted by X chromosome inactivation patterns. Fertil Steril 2009;91:649–652.
41 Fonseca DJ, Garzon E, Lakhal B, Braham R, Ojeda D, Elghezal H, Saad A, Restrepo CM and Laissue P: Screening for mutations of the *FOXO4* gene in premature ovarian failure patients. Reprod Biomed Online 2012;24:339–341.
42 Lacombe A, Lee H, Zahed L, Choucair M, Muller JM, Nelson SF, Salameh W, Vilain E: Disruption of POF1B binding to nonmuscle actin filaments is associated with premature ovarian failure. Am J Hum Genet 2006;79:113–119.
43 Losel RM, Besong D, Peluso JJ, Wehling M: Progesterone receptor membrane component 1 – many tasks for a versatile protein. Steroids 2008;73:929–934.
44 Cahill MA: Progesterone receptor membrane component 1: an integrative review. J Steroid Biochem Mol Biol 2007; 105:16–36.
45 Wang JL, Li SL, Qin YY and Chen ZJ: Analysis of progesterone receptor membrane component 1 mutation in Han Chinese women with premature ovarian failure. Reprod Biomed Online 2014;29: 640–643.
46 de Vries SS, Baart EB, Dekker M, Siezen A, de Rooij DG, de Boer P, te Riele H: Mouse MutS-like protein Msh5 is required for proper chromosome synapsis in male and female meiosis. Genes Dev 1999;13:523–531.
47 Kneitz B, Cohen PE, Avdievich E, Zhu L, Kane MF, Hou H Jr, Kolodner RD, Kucherlapati R, Pollard JW, Edelmann W: MutS homolog 4 localization to meiotic chromosomes is required for chromosome pairing during meiosis in male and female mice. Genes Dev 2000;14: 1085–1097.
48 Mandon-Pepin B, Touraine P, Kuttenn F, Derbois C, Rouxel A, Matsuda F, Nicolas A, Cotinot C, Fellous M: Genetic investigation of four meiotic genes in women with premature ovarian failure. Eur J Endocrinol 2008;158:107–115.
49 Guo T, Zhao S, Zhao S, Chen M, Li G, Jiao X, Wang Z, Zhao Y, Qin Y, Gao F, et al: Mutations in *MSH5* in primary ovarian insufficiency. Hum Mol Genet 2017; 26:1452–1457.
50 Qin CR, Chen SL, Yao JL, Wu WQ, Xie JS: Identification of novel missense mutations of the *TGFBR3* gene in Chinese women with premature ovarian failure. Reprod Biomed Online 2011;23:697–703.
51 Dixit H, Rao KL, Padmalatha VV, Kanakavalli M, Deenadayal M, Gupta N, Chakrabarty BN, Singh L: Mutational analysis of the betaglycan gene-coding region in susceptibility for ovarian failure. Hum Reprod 2006;21:2041–2046.
52 Mehlmann LM, Saeki Y, Tanaka S, Brennan TJ, Evsikov AV, Pendola FL, Knowles BB, Eppig JJ, Jaffe LA: The Gs-linked receptor GPR3 maintains meiotic arrest in mammalian oocytes. Science 2004;306:1947–1950.
53 Zhou S, Wang B, Ni F, Wang J, Cao Y, Ma X: GPR3 may not be a potential candidate gene for premature ovarian failure. Reprod Biomed Online 2010;20: 53–55.
54 Kovanci E, Simpson JL, Amato P, Rohozinski J, Heard MJ, Bishop CE, Carson SA: Oocyte-specific G-protein-coupled receptor 3 (*GPR3*): no perturbations found in 82 women with premature ovarian failure (first report). Fertil Steril 2008;90:1269–1271.
55 Jaaskelainen M, Prunskaite-Hyyrylainen R, Naillat F, Parviainen H, Anttonen M, Heikinheimo M, Liakka A, Ola R, Vainio S, Vaskivuo TE, et al: WNT4 is expressed in human fetal and adult ovaries and its signaling contributes to ovarian cell survival. Mol Cell Endocrinol 2010; 317:106–111.
56 Lakhal B, Ben-Hadj-Khalifa S, Bouali N, Philipert P, Audran F, Braham R, Hatem E, Sultan C, Saad A: Mutational screening of SF1 and WNT4 in Tunisian women with premature ovarian failure. Gene 2012;509:298–301.

57 Chen B, Suo P, Wang B, Wang J, Yang L, Zhou S, Zhu Y, Ma X, Cao Y: Mutation analysis of the WNT4 gene in Han Chinese women with premature ovarian failure. Reprod Biol Endocrinol 2011;9:75.

58 Zhao H, Chen ZJ, Qin Y, Shi Y, Wang S, Choi Y, Simpson JL, Rajkovic A: Transcription factor FIGLA is mutated in patients with premature ovarian failure. Am J Hum Genet 2008;82:1342–1348.

59 Tosh D, Rani HS, Murty US, Deenadayal A, Grover P: Mutational analysis of the FIGLA gene in women with idiopathic premature ovarian failure. Menopause 2015;22:520–526.

60 Aittomäki K, Lucena JL, Pakarinen P, Sistonen P, Tapanainen J, Gromoll J, Kaskikari R, Sankila EM, Lehvaslaiho H, Engel AR, et al: Mutation in the follicle-stimulating hormone receptor gene causes hereditary hypergonadotropic ovarian failure. Cell 1995;82:959–968.

61 Aittomäki K: The genetics of XX gonadal dysgenesis. Am J Hum Genet 1994;54:844–851.

62 Chen XN, Chen GA, Li MZ: Follicular stimulating hormone receptor gene C566T mutation in premature ovarian failure (in Chinese). Zhonghua Fu Chan Ke Za Zhi 2006;5:315–318.

63 Conway GS, Conway E, Walker C, Hoppner W, Gromoll J, Simoni M: Mutation screening and isoform prevalence of the follicle stimulating hormone receptor gene in women with premature ovarian failure, resistant ovary syndrome and polycystic ovary syndrome. Clin Endocrinol 1999;51:97–99.

64 da Fonte Kohek MB, Batista MC, Russell AJ, Vass K, Giacaglia LR, Mendonca BB, Latronico AC: No evidence of the inactivating mutation (C566T) in the follicle-stimulating hormone receptor gene in Brazilian women with premature ovarian failure. Fertil Steril 1998;70:565–567.

65 Prakash GJ, Kanth VV, Shelling AN, Rozati R, Sujatha M: Absence of 566C>T mutation in exon 7 of the *FSHR* gene in Indian women with premature ovarian failure. Int J Gynaecol Obstet 2009;105:265–266.

66 Sundblad V, Chiauzzi VA, Escobar ME, Dain L, Charreau EH: Screening of FSH receptor gene in Argentine women with premature ovarian failure (POF). Mol Cell Endocrinol 2004;222:53–59.

67 Takakura K, Takebayashi K, Wang HQ, Kimura F, Kasahara K, Noda Y: Follicle-stimulating hormone receptor gene mutations are rare in Japanese women with premature ovarian failure and polycystic ovary syndrome. Fertil Steril 2001;71:207–209.

68 Tong Y, Liao WX, Roy AC, Ng SC: Absence of mutations in the coding regions of follicle-stimulating hormone receptor gene in Singapore Chinese women with premature ovarian failure and polycystic ovary syndrome. Horm Metab Res 2001;33:221–226.

69 Vilodre LC, Kohek MB, Spritzer PM: Screening of follicle-stimulating hormone receptor gene in women with premature ovarian failure in southern Brazil and associations with phenotype. J Endocrinol Invest 2008;31:552–557.

70 Woad KJ, Prendergast D, Winship IM, Shelling AN: FSH receptor gene variants are rarely associated with premature ovarian failure. Reprod Biomed Online 2013;26:396–399.

71 Shelling AN, Burton KA, Chand AL, van Ee CC, France JT, Farquhar CM, Milsom SR, Love DR, Gersak K, Aittomäki K, et al: Inhibin: a candidate gene for premature ovarian failure. Hum Reprod 2000;15:2644–2649.

72 Dixit H, Deendayal M, Singh L: Mutational analysis of the mature peptide region of inhibin genes in Indian women with ovarian failure. Hum Reprod 2004;19:1760–1764.

73 Dixit H, Rao KL, Padmalatha V, Kanakavalli M, Deenadayal M, Gupta N, Chakravarty BN, Singh L: Expansion of the germline analysis for the *INHA* gene in Indian women with ovarian failure. Hum Reprod 2006;21:1643–1644.

74 Marozzi A, Porta C, Vegetti W, Crosignani PG, Tibiletti MG, Dalpra L, Ginelli E: Mutation analysis of the inhibin alpha gene in a cohort of Italian women affected by ovarian failure. Hum Reprod 2002;17:1741–1745.

75 Corre T, Schuettler J, Bione S, Marozzi A, Persani L, Rossetti R, Torricelli F, Giotti I, Vogt P, Toniolo D: A large-scale association study to assess the impact of known variants of the human INHA gene on premature ovarian failure. Hum Reprod 2009;24:2023–2028.

76 Jeong HJ, Cho SW, Kim HA, Lee SH, Cho JH, Choi DH, Kwon H, Cha WT, Han JE, Cha KY: G769A variation of inhibin α-gene in Korean women with premature ovarian failure. Yonsei Med J 2004;45:479–482.

77 Sundblad V, Chiauzzi VA, Andreone L, Campo S, Charreau EH, Dain L: Controversial role of inhibin alpha-subunit gene in the aetiology of premature ovarian failure. Hum Reprod 2006;21:1154–1160.

78 Fogli A, Rodriguez D, Eymard-Pierre E, Bouhour F, Labauge P, Meaney BF, Zeesman S, Kaneski CR, Schiffmann R, Boespflug-Tanguy O: Ovarian failure related to eukaryotic initiation factor 2B mutations. Am J Hum Genet 2003;72:1544–1550.

79 Fogli A, Gauthier-Barichard F, Schiffmann R, Vanderhoof VH, Bakalov VK, Nelson LM, Boespflug-Tanguy O: Screening for known mutations in *EIF2B* genes in a large panel of patients with premature ovarian failure. BMC Womens Health 2004;4:8.

80 Dixit H, Rao LK, Padmalatha V, Kanakavalli M, Deenadayal M, Gupta N, Chakravarty B, Singh L: Mutational screening of the coding region of growth differentiation factor 9 gene in Indian women with ovarian failure. Menopause 2005;12:749–754.

81 Kovanci E, Rohozinski J, Simpson JL, Heard MJ, Bishop CE, Carson SA: Growth differentiating factor-9 mutations may be associated with premature ovarian failure. Fertil Steril 2007;87:143–146.

82 Zhao H, Qin Y, Kovanci E, Simpson JL, Chen ZJ, Rajkovic A: Analyses of GDF9 mutation in 100 Chinese women with premature ovarian failure. Fertil Steril 2007;88:1474–1476.

83 Takebayashi K, Takakura K, Wang HQ, Kimura F, Kasahara K, Noda Y: Mutation analysis of the growth differentiation factor-9 and -9B genes in patients with premature ovarian failure and polycystic ovary syndrome. Fertil Steril 2000;74:976–979.

84 Chand AL, Ponnampalam AP, Harris SE, Winship IM, Shelling AN: Mutational analysis of BMP15 and GDF9 as candidate genes for premature ovarian failure. Fertil Steril 2006;86:1009–1012.

85 Wang J, Wang B, Song J, Suo P, Ni F, Chen B, Ma X, Cao Y: New candidate gene *POU5F1* associated with premature ovarian failure in Chinese patients. Reprod Biomed Online 2011;22:312–316.
86 Gallardo TD, John GB, Bradshaw K, Welt C, Reijo-Pera R, Vogt PH, Touraine P, Bione S, Toniolo D, Nelson LM, et al: Sequence variation at the human *FOXO3* locus: a study of premature ovarian failure and primary amenorrhea. Hum Reprod 2008;23:216–221.
87 Vinci G, Christin-Maitre S, Pasquier M, Bouchard P, Fellous M, Veitia RA: *FOXO3a* variants in patients with premature ovarian failure. Clin Endocrinol 2008;68:495–497.
88 Wang B, Mu Y, Ni F, Zhou S, Wang J, Cao Y, Ma X: Analysis of *FOXO3* mutation in 114 Chinese women with premature ovarian failure. Reprod Biomed Online 2010;20:499–503.
89 Lutzmann M, Grey C, Traver S, Ganier O, Maya-Mendoza A, Ranisavljevic N, Bernex F, Nishiyama A, Montel N, Gavois E, et al: *MCM8*- and *MCM9*-deficient mice reveal gametogenesis defects and genome instability due to impaired homologous recombination. Mol Cell 2012;47:523–534.
90 AlAsiri S, Basit S, Wood-Trageser MA, Yatsenko SA, Jeffries EP, Surti U, Ketterer DM, Afzal S, Ramzan K, Faiyaz-Ul Haque M, et al: Exome sequencing reveals *MCM8* mutation underlies ovarian failure and chromosomal instability. J Clin Invest 2015;125:258–262.
91 Wood-Trageser MA, Gurbuz F, Yatsenko SA, Jeffries EP, Kotan LD, Surti U, Ketterer DM, Matic J, Chipkin J, Jiang H, et al: *MCM9* mutations are associated with ovarian failure, short stature, and chromosomal instability. Am J Hum Genet 2014;95:754–762.
92 Combes AN, Spiller CM, Harley VR, Sinclair AH, Dunwoodie SL, Wilhelm D, Koopman P: Gonadal defects in *Cited2*-mutant mice indicate a role for SF1 in both testis and ovary differentiation. Int J Dev Biol 2010;54:683–689.
93 Fonseca DJ, Ojeda D, Lakhal B, Braham R, Eggers S, Turbitt E, White S, Grover S, Warne G, Zacharin M, et al: *CITED2* mutations potentially cause idiopathic premature ovarian failure. Transl Res 2012;160:384–388.
94 Caburet S, Arboleda VA, Llano E, Overbeek PA, Barbero JL, Oka K, Harrison W, Vaiman D, Ben-Neriah Z, Garcia-Tunon I, et al: Mutant cohesin in premature ovarian failure. N Engl J Med 2014;370:943–949.
95 Rajkovic A, Pangas SA, Ballow D, Suzumori N, Matzuk MM: NOBOX deficiency disrupts early folliculogenesis and oocyte-specific gene expression. Science 2004;305:1157–1159.
96 Lechowska A, Bilinski S, Choi Y, Shin Y, Kloc M, Rajkovic A: Premature ovarian failure in nobox-deficient mice is caused by defects in somatic cell invasion and germ cell cyst breakdown. J Assist Reprod Genet 2011;28:583–589.
97 Qin Y, Choi Y, Zhao H, Simpson JL, Chen ZJ, Rajkovic A: NOBOX homeobox mutation causes premature ovarian failure. Am J Hum Genet 2007;81:576–581.
98 Qin Y, Shi Y, Zhao Y, Carson SA, Simpson JL, Chen ZJ: Mutation analysis of NOBOX homeodomain in Chinese women with premature ovarian failure. Fertil Steril 2009;91(4 suppl):1507–1509.
99 Bouilly J, Bachelot A, Broutin I, Touraine P, Binart N: Novel NOBOX loss-of-function mutations account for 6.2% of cases in a large primary ovarian insufficiency cohort. Hum Mutat 2011;32:1108–1113.
100 Bouilly J, Roucher-Boulez F, Gompel A, Bry-Gauillard H, Azibi K, Beldjord C, Dode C, Bouligand J, Guiochon Mantel A, Hecart AC, et al: New NOBOX mutations identified in a large cohort of women with primary ovarian insufficiency decrease KIT-L expression. J Clin Endocrinol Metab 2014;100:994–1001.
101 Pelusi C, Ikeda Y, Zubair M, Parker KL: Impaired follicle development and infertility in female mice lacking steroidogenic factor 1 in ovarian granulosa cells. Biol Reprod 2008;79:1074–1083.
102 Philibert P, Leprieur E, Zenaty D, Thibaud E, Polak M, Frances AM, Lespinasse J, Raingeard I, Servant N, Audran F, et al: Steroidogenic factor-1 (SF-1) gene mutation as a frequent cause of primary amenorrhea in 46,XY female adolescents with low testosterone concentration. Reprod Biol Endocrinol 2010;8:28.
103 Lourenco D, Brauner R, Lin L, De Perdigo A, Weryha G, Muresan M, Boudjenah R, Guerra-Junior G, Maciel-Guerra AT, Achermann JC, et al: Mutations in *NR5A1* associated with ovarian insufficiency. N Engl J Med 2009;360:1200–1210.
104 Janse F, de With LM, Duran KJ, Kloosterman WP, Goverde AJ, Lambalk CB, Laven JS, Fauser BC, Giltay JC; Dutch Primary Ovarian Insufficiency Consortium: Limited contribution of *NR5A1* (SF-1) mutations in women with primary ovarian insufficiency (POI). Fertil Steril 2012;97;141–146.e142.
105 Jiao X, Qin Y, Li G, Zhao S, You L, Ma J, Simpson JL, Chen ZJ: Novel *NR5A1* missense mutation in premature ovarian failure: detection in Han Chinese indicates causation in different ethnic groups. PLoS One 2013;8;e74759.
106 Qin Y, Jiao X, Dalgleish R, Vujovic S, Li J, Simpson JL, Al-Azzawi F, Chen ZJ: Novel variants in the *SOHLH2* gene are implicated in human premature ovarian failure. Fertil Steril 2014;101:1104–1109.e6.
107 Zhao S, Li G, Dalgleish R, Vujovic S, Jiao X, Li J, Simpson JL, Qin Y, Ivanisevic M, Ivovic M, et al: Transcription factor SOHLH1 potentially associated with primary ovarian insufficiency. Fertil Steril 2015;103:548–553.e5.
108 Bayram Y, Gulsuner S, Guran T, Abaci A, Yesil G, Gulsuner HU, Atay Z, Pierce SB, Gambin T, Lee M, et al: Homozygous loss-of-function mutations in SOHLH1 in patients with nonsyndromic hypergonadotropic hypogonadism. J Clin Endocrinol Metab 2015;100:E808–E814.
109 Feng R, Sang Q, Kuang Y, Sun X, Yan Z, Zhang S, Shi J, Tian G, Luchniak A, Fukuda Y, et al: Mutations in TUBB8 and human oocyte meiotic arrest. N Engl J Med 2016;374:223–232.
110 Qin Y, Guo T, Li G, Tang TS, Zhao S, Jiao X, Gong J, Gao F, Guo C, Simpson JL, et al: CSB-PGBD3 mutations cause premature ovarian failure. PLoS Genet 2015;11:e1005419.
111 Reddy P, Liu L, Adhikari D, Jagarlamudi K, Rajareddy S, Shen Y, Du C, Tang WL, Hamalainen T, Peng SL, et al: Oocyte-specific deletion of *Pten* causes premature activation of the primordial follicle pool. Science 2008;319:611–613.

112 Shimizu Y, Kimura F, Takebayashi K, Fujiwara M, Takakura K, Takahashi K: Mutational analysis of the PTEN gene in women with premature ovarian failure. Acta Obstet Gynecol Scand 2009;88:824–825.
113 Zhao Z, Qin Y, Ma J, Zhao H, Li J, Wang L, Ren C, Che L, Chen ZJ: *PTEN* gene analysis in premature ovarian failure patients. Acta Obstet Gynecol Scand 2011;90:678–679.
114 Tsuda M, Sasaoka Y, Kiso M, Abe K, Haraguchi S, Kobayashi S, Saga Y: Conserved role of nanos proteins in germ cell development. Science 2003; 301:1239–1241.
115 Qin Y, Zhao H, Kovanci E, Simpson JL, Chen ZJ, Rajkovic A: Mutation analysis of NANOS3 in 80 Chinese and 88 Caucasian women with premature ovarian failure. Fertil Steril 2007;88:1465–1467.
116 Wu X, Wang B, Dong Z, Zhou S, Liu Z, Shi G, Cao Y, Xu Y: A *NANOS3* mutation linked to protein degradation causes premature ovarian insufficiency. Cell Death Dis 2013;e825.
117 Kreidberg JA, Sariola H, Loring JM, Maeda M, Pelletier J, Housman D, Jaenisch R: WT-1 is required for early kidney development. Cell 1993;74: 679–691.
118 Gao F, Zhang J, Wang X, Yang J, Chen D, Huff V, Liu YX: Wt1 functions in ovarian follicle development by regulating granulosa cell differentiation. Hum Mol Genet 2014;23:333–341.
119 Wang H, Li G, Zhang J, Gao F, Li W, Qin Y, Chen ZJ: Novel WT1 Missense mutations in Han Chinese women with premature ovarian failure. Sci Rep 2015;5:13983.
120 Rajareddy S, Reddy P, Du C, Liu L, Jagarlamudi K, Tang W, Shen Y, Berthet C, Peng SL, Kaldis P, et al: p27kip1 (cyclin-dependent kinase inhibitor 1B) controls ovarian development by suppressing follicle endowment and activation and promoting follicle atresia in mice. Mol Endocrinol 2007;21;2189–2202.
121 Ojeda D, Lakhal B, Fonseca DJ, Braham R, Landolsi H, Mateus HE, Restrepo CM, Elghezal H, Saad A, Laissue P: Sequence analysis of the *CDKN1B* gene in patients with premature ovarian failure reveals a novel mutation potentially related to the phenotype. Fertil Steril 2011;95:2658–2660.e1.
122 Wang B, Ni F, Li L, Wei Z, Zhu X, Wang J, Cao Y, Ma X: Analysis of cyclin-dependent kinase inhibitor 1B mutation in Han Chinese women with premature ovarian failure. Reprod Biomed Online 2010;21:212–214.
123 Zhao Z, Wei D, Mu Y, Qin Y, Li G, Cui L, Chen ZJ: Mutational analysis of SKP2 and P27 in Chinese Han women with premature ovarian failure. Reprod Biomed Online 2013;27:104–106.
124 Kevenaar ME, Themmen AP, Laven JS, Sonntag B, Fong SL, Uitterlinden AG, de Jong FH, Pols HA, Simoni M, Visser JA: Anti-Müllerian hormone and anti-Mullerian hormone type II receptor polymorphisms are associated with follicular phase estradiol levels in normo-ovulatory women. Hum Reprod 2007;22:1547–1554.
125 Wang HQ, Takakura K, Takebayashi K, Noda Y: Mutational analysis of the mullerian-inhibiting substance gene and its receptor gene in Japanese women with polycystic ovary syndrome and premature ovarian failure. Fertil Steril 2002;78:1329–1330.
126 Hui ES, Udofa EA, Soto J, Vanderhoof VH, Zachman K, Tong ZB, Nelson LM: Investigation of the human stem cell factor KIT ligand gene, KITLG, in women with 46,XX spontaneous premature ovarian failure. Fertil Steril 2006;85:1502–1507.
127 Watkins WJ, Umbers AJ, Woad KJ, Harris SE, Winship IM, Gersak K, Shelling AN: Mutational screening of *FOXO3A* and *FOXO1A* in women with premature ovarian failure. Fertil Steril 2006;86:1518–1521.
128 Choi Y, Qin Y, Berger MF, Ballow DJ, Bulyk ML, Rajkovic A: Microarray analyses of newborn mouse ovaries lacking Nobox. Biol Reprod 2007;77: 312–319.
129 Zhang J, Tam WL, Tong GQ, Wu Q, Chan HY, Soh BS, Lou Y, Yang J, Ma Y, Chai L, et al: Sall4 modulates embryonic stem cell pluripotency and early embryonic development by the transcriptional regulation of *Pou5f1*. Nat Cell Biol 2006;8:1114–1123.
130 Wang B, Li L, Ni F, Song J, Wang J, Mu Y, Ma X and Cao Y: Mutational analysis of SAL-Like 4 (*SALL4*) in Han Chinese women with premature ovarian failure. Mol Hum Reprod 2009;15: 557–562.
131 Simpson JL: Disorders of the gonads, genital tract, and genitalia; in Rimoin D, Pyeritz R, Korf B (eds): Emery and Rimoin's. Principles and Practice of Medical Genetics. Cambridge, Academic Press, 2015, chapt 88, pp 1–45.
132 Allingham-Hawkins DJ, Babul-Hirji R, Chitayat D, Holden JJ, Yang KT, Lee C, Hudson R, Gorwill H, Nolin SL, Glicksman A, et al: Fragile X premutation is a significant risk factor for premature ovarian failure: the International Collaborative POF in Fragile X study – preliminary data. Am J Med Genet 1999;83:322–325.
133 Wittenberger MD, Hagerman RJ, Sherman SL, McConkie-Rosell A, Welt CK, Rebar RW, Corrigan EC, Simpson JL, Nelson LM: The FMR1 premutation and reproduction. Fertil Steril 2007;87: 456–465.
134 Bussani C, Papi L, Sestini R, Baldinotti F, Bucciantini S, Bruni V, Scarselli G: Premature ovarian failure and fragile X premutation: a study on 45 women. Eur J Obstet Gynecol Reprod Biol 2004; 112:189–191.
135 Conway GS, Payne NN, Webb J, Murray A, Jacobs PA: Fragile X premutation screening in women with premature ovarian failure. Hum Reprod 1998;13:1184–1187.
136 Guo T, Qin Y, Jiao X, Li G, Simpson JL, Chen ZJ: FMR1 premutation is an uncommon explanation for premature ovarian failure in Han Chinese. PLoS One 2014;9;e103316.
137 Ishizuka B, Okamoto N, Hamada N, Sugishita Y, Saito J, Takahashi N, Ogata T, Itoh MT: Number of CGG repeats in the *FMR1* gene of Japanese patients with primary ovarian insufficiency. Fertil Steril 2011;96:1170–1174.
138 Gersak K, Meden-Vrtovec H, Peterlin B: Fragile X premutation in women with sporadic premature ovarian failure in Slovenia. Hum Reprod 2003;18: 1637–1640.
139 Crisponi L, Deiana M, Loi A, Chiappe F, Uda M, Amati P, Bisceglia L, Zelante L, Nagaraja R, Porcu S, et al: The putative forkhead transcription factor FOXL2 is mutated in blepharophimosis/ptosis/epicanthus in blepharophimosis/ptosis/epicanthus inversus syndrome. Nat Genet 2001;27:159–166.
140 Beysen D, Vandesompele J, Messiaen L, De Paepe A, De Baere E: The human FOXL2 mutation database. Hum Mutat 2004;24:189–193.

141 Harris SE, Chand AL, Winship IM, Gersak K, Aittomäki K, Shelling AN: Identification of novel mutations in FOXL2 associated with premature ovarian failure. Mol Hum Reprod 2002;8:729–733.
142 Chatterjee S, Modi D, Maitra A, Kadam S, Patel Z, Gokrall J, Meherji P: Screening for *FOXL2* gene mutations in women with premature ovarian failure: an Indian experience. Reprod Biomed Online 2007;15:554–560.
143 Ni F, Wen Q, Wang B, Zhou S, Wang J, Mu Y, Ma X, Cao Y: Mutation analysis of *FOXL2* gene in Chinese patients with premature ovarian failure. Gynecol Endocrinol 2010;26:246–249.
144 De Baere E, Lemercier B, Christin-Maitre S, Durval D, Messiaen L, Fellous M, Veitia R: *FOXL2* mutation screening in a large panel of POF patients and XX males. J Med Genet 2002;39:e43.
145 Gong Y, Krakow D, Marcelino J, Wilkin D, Chitayat D, Babul-Hirji R, Hudgins L, Cremers CW, Cremers FP, Brunner HG, et al: Heterozygous mutations in the gene encoding noggin affect human joint morphogenesis. Nat Genet 1999;21;302–304.
146 Kosaki K, Sato S, Hasegawa T, Matsuo N, Suzuki T, Ogata T: Premature ovarian failure in a female with proximal symphalangism and Noggin mutation. Fertil Steril 2004;81:1137–1139.
147 Laissue P, Christin-Maitre S, Bouchard P, Fellous M, Veitia RA: Mutations in the *NOG* gene are not a common cause of nonsyndromic premature ovarian failure. Clin Endocrinol 2007;66:900.
148 Bonomi M, Somigliana E, Cacciatore C, Busnelli M, Rossetti R, Bonetti S, Paffoni A, Mari D, Ragni G, Persani L: Blood cell mitochondrial DNA content and premature ovarian aging. PLoS One 2012;7:e42423.
149 May-Panloup P, Chretien MF, Jacques C, Vasseur C, Malthiery Y, Reynier P: Low oocyte mitochondrial DNA content in ovarian insufficiency. Hum Reprod 2005;20:593–597.
150 Tong ZB, Sullivan SD, Lawless LM, Vanderhoof V, Zachman K, Nelson LM: Five mutations of mitochondrial DNA polymerase-gamma (POLG) are not a prevalent etiology for spontaneous 46,XX primary ovarian insufficiency. Fertil Steril 2010;94:2932–2934.
151 Pagnamenta AT, Taanman JW, Wilson CJ, Anderson NE, Marotta R, Duncan AJ, Bitner-Glindzicz M, Taylor RW, Laskowski A, Thorburn DR, et al: Dominant inheritance of premature ovarian failure associated with mutant mitochondrial DNA polymerase gamma. Hum Reprod 2006;21:2467–2473.
152 Jenkinson EM, Rehman AU, Walsh T, Clayton-Smith J, Lee K, Morell RJ, Drummond MC, Khan SN, Naeem MA, Rauf B, et al: Perrault syndrome is caused by recessive mutations in CLPP, encoding a mitochondrial ATP-dependent chambered protease. Am J Hum Genet 2013;92:605–613.
153 Pierce SB, Chisholm KM, Lynch ED, Lee MK, Walsh T, Opitz JM, Li W, Klevit RE, King MC: Mutations in mitochondrial histidyl tRNA synthetase HARS2 cause ovarian dysgenesis and sensorineural hearing loss of Perrault syndrome. Proc Natl Acad Sci USA 2011;108:6543–6548.
154 Pierce SB, Gersak K, Michaelson-Cohen R, Walsh T, Lee MK, Malach D, Klevit RE, King MC, Levy-Lahad E: Mutations in *LARS2*, encoding mitochondrial leucyl-tRNA synthetase, lead to premature ovarian failure and hearing loss in Perrault syndrome. Am J Hum Genet 2013;92:614–620.
155 Kang H, Lee SK, Kim MH, Song J, Bae SJ, Kim NK, Lee SH, Kwack K: Parathyroid hormone-responsive B1 gene is associated with premature ovarian failure. Hum Reprod 2008;23:1457–1465.
156 Knauff EA, Franke L, van Es MA, van den Berg LH, van der Schouw YT, Laven JS, Lambalk CB, Hoek A, Goverde AJ, Christin-Maitre S, et al: Genome-wide association study in premature ovarian failure patients suggests ADAMTS19 as a possible candidate gene. Hum Reprod 2009;24:2372–2378.
157 Pyun JA, Cha DH, Kwack K: *LAMC1* gene is associated with premature ovarian failure. Maturitas 2012;71:402–406.
158 Oldenburg RA, van Dooren MF, de Graaf B, Simons E, Govaerts L, Swagemakers S, Verkerk JM, Oostra BA, Bertoli-Avella AM: A genome-wide linkage scan in a Dutch family identifies a premature ovarian failure susceptibility locus. Hum Reprod 2008;23:2835–2841.
159 Caburet S, Zavadakova P, Ben-Neriah Z, Bouhali K, Dipietromaria A, Charon C, Besse C, Laissue P, Chalifa-Caspi V, Christin-Maitre S, et al: Genome-wide linkage in a highly consanguineous pedigree reveals two novel Loci on chromosome 7 for non-syndromic familial premature ovarian failure. PLoS One 2012;7:e33412.
160 Qin CR, Chen SL, Yao JL, Li T, Wu WQ: Haplotype and mutation analysis of the *TGFBR3* gene in Chinese women with idiopathic premature ovarian failure. Gynecol Endocrinol 2012;28:63–67.
161 Aboura A, Dupas C, Tachdjian G, Portnoi MF, Bourcigaux N, Dewailly D, Frydman R, Fauser B, Ronci-Chaix N, Donadille B, et al: Array comparative genomic hybridization profiling analysis reveals deoxyribonucleic acid copy number variations associated with premature ovarian failure. J Clin Endocrinol Metab 2009;94:4540–4546.
162 Quilter CR, Karcanias AC, Bagga MR, Duncan S, Murray A, Conway GS, Sargent CA, Affara NA: Analysis of X chromosome genomic DNA sequence copy number variation associated with premature ovarian failure (POF). Hum Reprod 2010;25:2139–2150.
163 Dudding TE, Lawrence O, Winship I, Froyen G, Vandewalle J, Scott R, Shelling AN: Array comparative genomic hybridization for the detection of submicroscopic copy number variations of the X chromosome in women with premature ovarian failure. Hum Reprod 2010;25:3159–3160, author reply 3160–3161.
164 Ledig S, Ropke A, Wieacker P: Copy number variants in premature ovarian failure and ovarian dysgenesis. Sex Dev 2010;4:225–232.
165 Knauff EA, Blauw HM, Pearson PL, Kok K, Wijmenga C, Veldink JH, van den Berg LH, Bouchard P, Fauser BC, Franke L: Copy number variants on the X chromosome in women with primary ovarian insufficiency. Fertil Steril 2011;95:1584–1588.e1.
166 McGuire MM, Bowden W, Engel NJ, Ahn HW, Kovanci E, Rajkovic A: Genomic analysis using high-resolution single-nucleotide polymorphism arrays reveals novel microdeletions associated with premature ovarian failure. Fertil Steril 2011;95:1595–1600.

167 Chen ZJ, Zhao H, He L, Shi Y, Qin Y, Li Z, You L, Zhao J, Liu J, Liang X, et al: Genome-wide association study identifies susceptibility loci for polycystic ovary syndrome on chromosome 2p16.3, 2p21 and 9q33.3. Nat Genet 2011;43:55–59.
168 Shi Y, Zhao H, Cao Y, Yang D, Li Z, Zhang B, Liang X, Li T, Chen J, Shen J, et al: Genome-wide association study identifies eight new risk loci for polycystic ovary syndrome. Nat Genet 2012;44:1020–1025.
169 Uno S, Zembutsu H, Hirasawa A, Takahashi A, Kubo M, Akahane T, Aoki D, Kamatani N, Hirata K, Nakamura Y: A genome-wide association study identifies genetic variants in the CDKN2BAS locus associated with endometriosis in Japanese. Nat Genet 2010;42:707–710.
170 Jiang M, Aittomäki K, Nilsson C, Pakarinen P, Iitia A, Torresani T, Simonsen H, Goh V, Pettersson K, de la Chapelle A, et al: The frequency of an inactivating point mutation (566C–>T) of the human follicle-stimulating hormone receptor gene in four populations using allele-specific hybridization and time-resolved fluorometry. J Clin Endocrinol Metab 1998;83:4338–4343.
171 Aittomäki K, Herva R, Stenman UH, Juntunen K, Ylostalo P, Hovatta O, de la Chapelle A: Clinical features of primary ovarian failure caused by a point mutation in the follicle-stimulating hormone receptor gene. J Clin Endocrinol Metab 1996;81:3722–3726.
172 Voican A, Bachelot A, Bouligand J, Francou B, Dulon J, Lombes M, Touraine P, Guiochon-Mantel A: *NR5A1* (SF-1) mutations are not a major cause of primary ovarian insufficiency. J Clin Endocrinol Metab 2013;98:E1017–E1021.
173 Philibert P, Paris F, Lakhal B, Audran F, Gaspari L, Saad A, Christin-Maitre S, Bouchard P, Sultan C: *NR5A1* (SF-1) gene variants in a group of 26 young women with XX primary ovarian insufficiency. Fertil Steril 2013;99:484–489.

Joe Leigh Simpson
March of Dimes Foundation
1275 Mamaroneck Avenue
White Plains, NY 10605 (USA)
E-Mail jsimpson@marchofdimes.com

Vogt PH (ed): Genetics of Human Infertility. Monogr Hum Genet.
Basel, Karger, 2017, vol 21, pp 40–56 (DOI: 10.1159/000477277)

Genetics of Klinefelter Syndrome: Experimental Exploration

Joachim Wistuba · Cristin Brand · Michael Zitzmann · Oliver S. Damm

Centre of Reproductive Medicine and Andrology, University of Muenster, Muenster, Germany

Abstract

Klinefelter syndrome (KS) is a frequent male sex-chromosomal trisomy (47,XXY) of heterogeneous phenotype (infertility, hypogonadism, gynecomastia, disturbed bone metabolism, diabetes, cognitive deficits and, vascular and cardiac problems) and variable severity. In all patients, germ cell loss and hypergonadotropic hypogonadism is observed. Morbidity and mortality are increased, but so far KS is strongly underdiagnosed. Clinical studies have suggested that changes such as DNA methylation and X-chromosomal and autosomal gene expression are affected. Mouse models resembling the human KS are of great advantage as only few genes escape from X-inactivation, likely causative and sufficient to induce a phenotype closely resembling the human disorder. Here, we report the expression of X-chromosomal escapee genes in 41,XX^{Y*} mice which are shared with men (*Utx, Kdm5c, Eif2s3x, Ddx3x*). A tissue-, gene-, and development-specific expression profile was observed. We discuss the need for improved diagnostics as many patients go undetected. Novel diagnostics and the development of cryobanking with the aim of preserving fertility have recently initiated a debate on prenatal diagnosis and the counselling of patients for tissue storage as a reserve. Diagnosis tools are needed, as evidence indicates that KS should be encountered early has increased.

Klinefelter syndrome (KS) is a frequent (1–2: 1,000) male sex-chromosomal trisomy caused by a supernumerary X chromosome due to meiotic nondisjunctions (Fig. 1). Approximately 80% of affected men show a karyotype of 47,XXY; the remaining exhibit higher grade X-chromosomal aneuploidies [1]. The condition results in a heterogeneous phenotype of variable severity. Prominent features of KS are infertility, hypogonadism, gynecomastia, disturbed bone metabolism, diabetes, and cognitive deficits [2–4]. Recently, reduced diameters of arteries, cardiovascular problems (pulmonary embolism, vascular diseases), and shortened QTc intervals have also been associated with the condition in a proportion of KS men, contributing to the increased morbidity and mortality [5–7]. In all patients, a progressive germ cell loss leading to infertility and hypergonadotropic hypogonadism is observed.

The disorder-related symptoms only progress slowly to the full phenotype. In fetuses, there is evidence for androgen insufficiency, but only for a minority of cases and the incidence for underdeveloped genitalia and cryptorchidism appears increased in KS boys at birth. In common, there is a normal activation of the hypothalamic-pituitary-

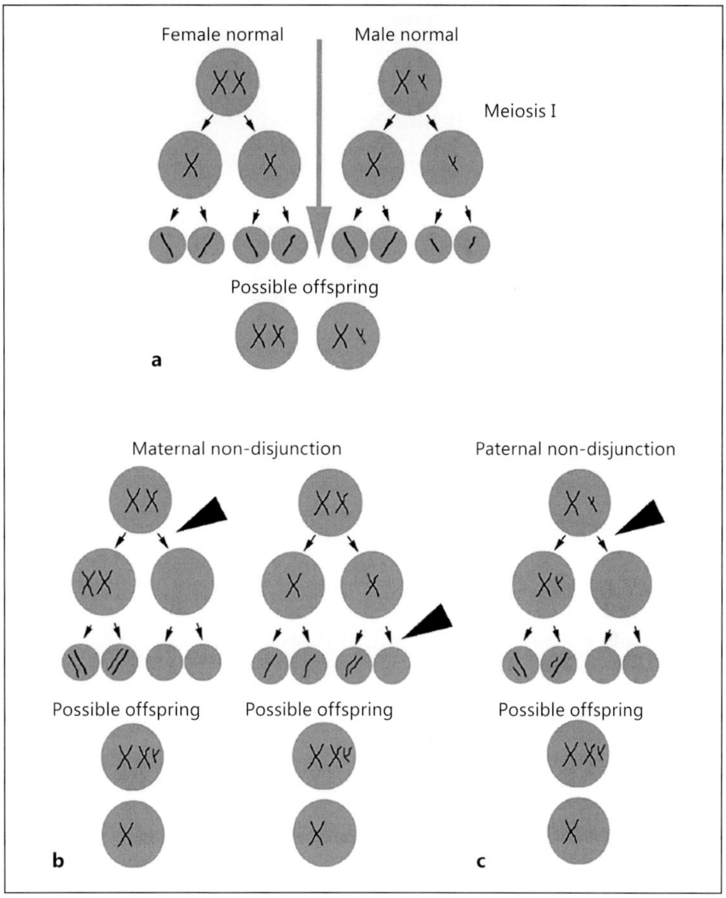

Fig. 1. Overview of possible parental origins of the supernumerary X chromosome by nondisjunction events (arrowheads). **a** Healthy state: haploid gametes lead to offspring with a normal karyotype. **b** Maternal nondisjunction in first (left) or second (right) meiotic division can lead to offspring with the XXY (KS) or XO (Turner syndrome) karyotype. **c** Paternal nondisjunction events in first meiotic division can result in offspring with an XXY and XO karyotype.

gonadal axis during infancy indicating functional somatic testicular Sertoli cells (SCs) and Leydig cells (LCs). However, slower penile growth, the lack of testis growth and less spermatogonia (consistent with findings in the mouse model [8]) point to early androgen deficiency [9]. Pre- and peripubertal hormone levels (anti-Müllerian hormone and inhibin) become irregular and point to the commencement of SC dysfunction. At this time testicular malfunction and hypergonadotropic hypogonadism become overt as the testes remain small and gonadotropins exceed normal ranges. This phenotype becomes pronounced in adulthood [9].

Novel assisted reproductive techniques, such as micro testicular sperm extraction, revealed a substantial percentage of KS men to exhibit small foci of intact spermatogenesis from which – in approximately 50% of patients – testicular sperm could be used to father children by intracytoplasmic sperm injection [10]. Thus, KS men are no longer infertile per se, but might become fathers if supported by assisted reproductive techniques. However, no marker for successful sperm retrieval has been defined yet and the beneficial effects of certain medications to enhance sperm retrieval are not proven.

Currently, it is debated whether focal spermatogenesis reflects a germ line micromosaicism, i.e., that differentiating germ cells have a corrected karyotype [11]. However, this has not been unequivocally solved and is lacking systematic analysis.

Diagnosis of Klinefelter Syndrome

No routine neonatal screening exists for KS and, thus, the disorder is highly underdiagnosed. Postnatally, only 25% of KS patients and – more rarely – 3% of prepubertal boys are diagnosed [12, 13]. This is partly due to the fact that the identification of affected individuals is limited with regard to clinical signs. However, anthropometric measures and the body composition of KS patients can be altered. Associations of those signs with the CAG repeat length of the androgen receptor and a decreased intrauterine testosterone have been suggested [14, 15].

Noninvasive prenatal testing might increase the rate of successful diagnosis substantially, by up to 10-fold [9]. Early diagnosis could lead to a better medical as well as psychological care for KS boys. However, possible stigmatization (e.g., parents or peers) must be taken into account and balanced against the putative benefits of an early diagnosis. For example, the prenatal KS diagnosis often results in elective termination of the pregnancy in approximately half of cases [16–18].

The discrepancy between the expected incidence and diagnosed cases was debated during the 2nd International Workshop on KS. Extrapolating older data, the consensus was that three-quarters of patients must be undetected. This remains unexplained, as due to increased mortality and morbidity the likelihood of being diagnosed by treating clinicians should be higher than it currently is. Whether this is due to milder phenotypes could be resolved by pre- or perinatal screening and subsequent follow-up [4].

Since infertility is common in KS and germ cell loss occurs before puberty, early detection of the syndrome could improve fertility preservation by storing sperm and/or less differentiated germ cell stages collected from semen samples or testicular sperm extraction. As the testicular phenotype develops early, attempts to preserve fertility should be undertaken as early as possible [8, 9, 19]. In prepubertal boys, taking biopsies and cryopreservation followed by in vitro differentiation of present immature germ cell stages has been suggested [20]. In terms of fertility preservation in KS beyond the use of ejaculates or testicular samples, first approaches have been developed with the future aim of rescuing the germ line of KS boys without gametes but still a number of undifferentiated germ cells. Methods for the isolation of spermatogonia from testicular biopsies have been investigated [21]. These are promising considering that harvesting, culture, and differentiation in novel 3-dimensional culture systems of such cells might become possible [22]. This progress has recently initiated a debate on whether clinical counselling of patients should include the offer of optional tissue cryobanking in order to provide a reserve for when KS boys have grown up and might wish to become fathers [20].

Morbidity and Mortality in Klinefelter Syndrome

Morbidity and mortality are increased in KS but the question remains as to whether this is due to the disorder as such or to a poorer socioeconomic status as a consequence of poorer cognitive performance, or whether a combination of both provokes higher mortality. Bojesen et al. [23] analyzed over 1,000 KS men and more than 100,000 controls from Danish registries, and found that KS men had fewer partnerships and entered them later, had a lower educational level, lower income, and were retired younger. Furthermore, KS patients had worse outcomes for all socioeconomic trajectories and increased mortality [23].

Although the neuropsychological phenotype is variable, neurocognitive deficits and increased psychiatric morbidity influence the socioeconomic status of many KS men, who are known to perform poorer in cognitive tests. This has led to the suggestion that they should be offered both special education and psychological treatment [24]. When brain morphology and neuropsychology were analyzed in KS patients, those with skewed X chromosome inactivation presented a smaller global brain matter volume [24].

In summary, the condition seems to affect cognitive abilities, as has also been experimentally confirmed in mouse models. However, the concomitant poorer socioeconomic conditions also seem to enhance mortality. On reviewing clinical studies it becomes evident that further research is needed, in particular experimental manipulation aiming at mechanistic insights, which can be achieved using a mouse model.

Mouse Models for the Experimental Exploration of Klinefelter Syndrome

Mouse models derived from of the strain B6Ei. LT-Y* with a supernumerary X chromosome (karyotypes 41,XXY or 41,XX^{Y*}; Fig. 2) resembling human KS [25, 26] have been successfully established (a comparison between mouse models as well as between models and patients can be found in Wistuba [27]; features of 41,XX^{Y*} mice that resemble the human phenotype are summarized in Table 1). For 41,XX^{Y*} male mice ("KS mice"), it was demonstrated that body proportions are altered, and that cognitive problems and hypergonadotropic hypogonadism occur in adulthood [27, 28]. The endocrine phenotype was suggested to be related to a disturbed function and/or maturation of LCs, resulting in an insufficient response to stimulation. However, contradictory findings were revealed in the 41,XX^{Y*} mice by demonstrating mature and (hyper)reactive LCs. Furthermore, intratesticular testosterone values were similar to controls in mice and patients [29, 30].

The 41,XX^{Y*} mouse model also resembles progressive germ cell loss and infertility [8, 28]. Germ cell loss is believed to manifest postnatally and to be complete around puberty. This was challenged by findings in mice and men. Firstly, in a study analyzing the time course of germ cell loss in 41,XX^{Y*} mice, the number of undifferentiated germ cells was already reduced at birth and linked to an altered protein expression of spermatogonial stem cell (SSC) markers. Lin28 and Pgp9.5 expression were no longer detected after 3 days postpartum (3 dpp) and 5 dpp, respectively. At this time point undifferentiated spermatogonia can still be observed in the seminiferous epithelium, however these were immunonegative [8]. Lin28 regulation implements a network of several miRNAs, such as miR-125b and miR-let7g, which are normally expressed in a complementary pattern. However, this pattern was found to be completely disturbed in 41,XX^{Y*} mice [8].

Focal spermatogenesis was also observed in 41,XX^{Y*} mice exhibiting few tubules with differentiating germ cells [8] (Fig. 3). In tubules with germ cells, the expression of Lin28 and Pgp9.5 was corrected. Based on these findings, a revised model for prenatal germ cell loss was developed in the KS mouse model and preliminary evidence suggests that germ cell loss also starts earlier than previously thought in humans [9]. The model hypothesized that a first wave of germ cell death occurs already in the embryonic phase during colonization of the gonad. A second phase includes gonocyte propagation followed by a third phase, when surviving germ cells enter but fail to complete meiosis due to chromosomal imbalance, except for a few germ cells which can eventually undergo full spermatogenesis [8]. It has to be stated that this model still requires confirmation, for example by proving the cell ploidy using fluorescence in situ hybridization (FISH). Unfortunately, in contrast to human subjects, FISH is technically more challenging and focal spermatogenesis far less frequent in KS mice.

As the supernumerary X chromosome is the underlying disorder, gene dosage effects provoking the phenotypical features are likely. In the following discussion we will therefore focus on X-inactivation and X-chromosomal genes that are plausible candidates for being causative of related changes.

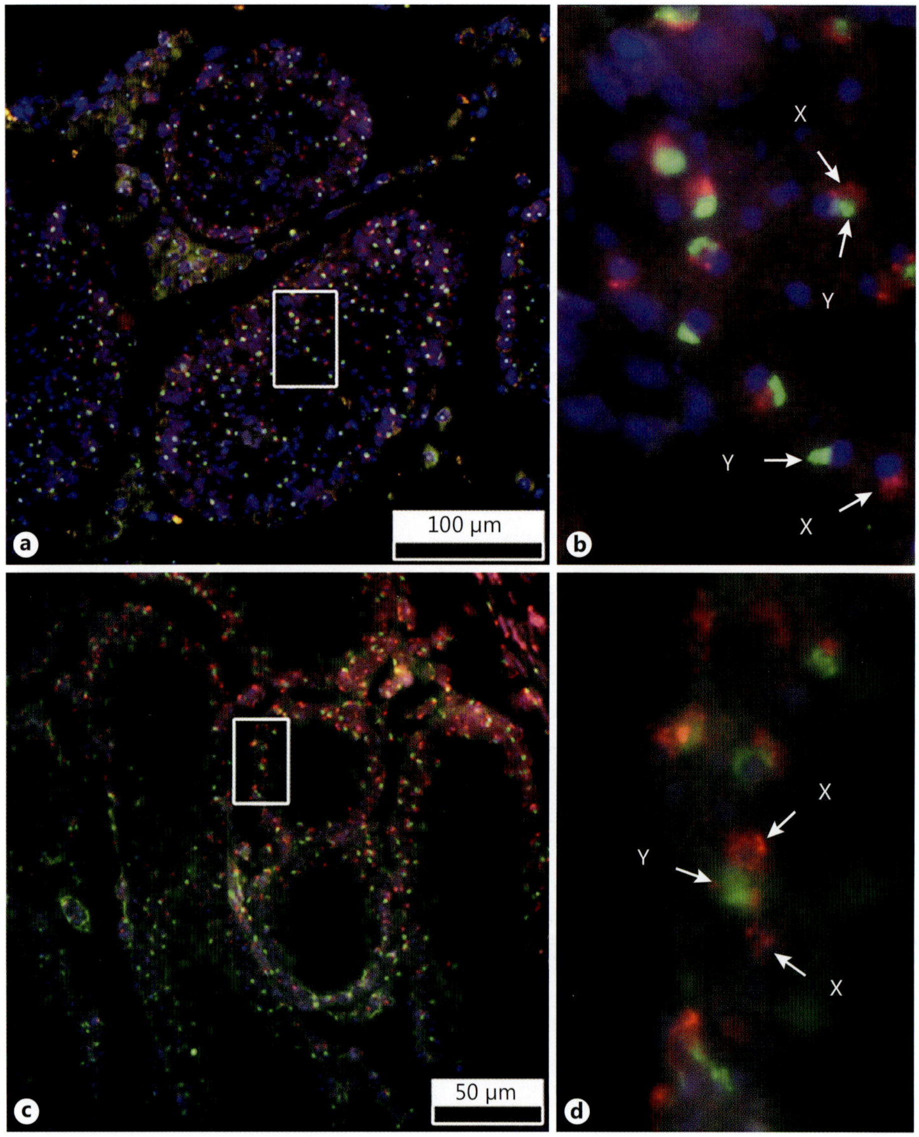

Fig. 2. FISH on testicular tissue. X (red) and Y chromosomes (green; probes by Cambio, Cambridge, UK) in cell nuclei (blue, DAPI). Overview (**a**) and detail (**b**) of sex chromosomes in an adult 40,XY* mouse. Overview (**c**) and detail (**d**) of a pubertal 41,XX^{Y}* mouse (21 dpp), presenting 1 Y and 2 X chromosomes in the cell nuclei.

Table 1. Comparative survey of KS features resembled in the 41,XX^{Y*} mouse model (updated from Kitamura et al. [13])

Feature	41,XX^{Y*} mice	KS 47,XXY patient
Body proportions	heavier, bigger	bigger, changed proportions
Androgenization	impaired	impaired
Serum testosterone	reduced (lower limit)	reduced (lower limit)
Intratesticular testosterone	normal	normal
Serum LH	elevated	elevated
Serum FSH	elevated	elevated
Cognition/behavior	affected	affected
Germ cell loss	starting in utero	pre- and peripubertal(?)
LC number	hyperplasia	hyperplasia
LC steroidogenesis in vitro	elevated	elevated
LC marker gene expression	elevated	not addressed
Bone metabolism	impaired	impairment frequently observed
X-inactivation	~50% (normal)	~50% (normal)
Life expectancy	normal	reduced by ~2 years
Incidence of mosaicism	not observed (linked to the model)	10–20%
Germ cell maturation?/spermatogenesis	single cases observed	focally in up to ~50% of patients
Phenotype	homogenous	heterogenous (except natural infertility and hypogonadism)
X-linked escapee genes	3%	15%
Parental origin of supernumerary X	only paternally	equally distributed
Vascularization	altered	altered
Cardiovascular risk	not observed (linked to the model)	increased

KS, Klinefelter syndrome; LH, luteinizing hormone; FSH, follicle-stimulating hormone; LC, Leydig cell.

Genetic Aspects of Klinefelter Syndrome: Evidence from Clinical Studies

It had been suggested from a small cohort of 10 men that autosomal expression is influenced by the supernumerary X chromosome [9] (480 autosomal genes were found to be upregulated and 200 to be downregulated), and transcriptome analyses indicated that the SCs and LCs of patients are deregulated. Furthermore, DNA methylation was also found to be affected. These findings drove the hypothesis that the aneuploidy itself may provoke specific changes of autosomal genes in various tissues [9]. The pathophysiological link between a supernumerary X chromosome and clinical phenotypes was addressed in the Epigenetics, X-Chromosomal Features and Clinical Applications in KS Trial (EXAKT), a prospective project involving over 130 KS patients at the Department of Clinical Andrology of the University of Münster, Germany. Following the hypothesis that differentially expressed genes (DEGs) are related to the phenotype, 36 X-chromosomal and autosomal DEGs were identified, putting KS patients into a unique genetic setting (Fig. 4). A higher number of DEGs were seen in a much smaller cohort consisting of boys and adolescents compared to the large cohort with adult KS men. This provides an interesting aspect for research: DEG expression of KS men in comparison to

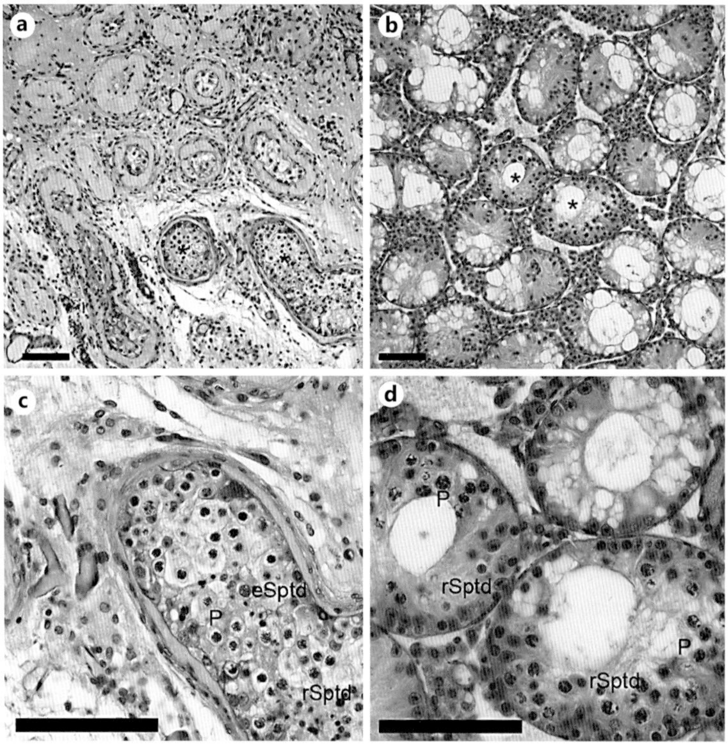

Fig. 3. Corresponding testicular cross-sections (periodic acid-Schiff reagent and hemalaun staining) from KS patients and a 41,XX^{Y*} mouse. Overview (**a**) and detail (**b**) of tissue from a KS patient. Tubules are predominantely of SCO type and have thickened lamina propria; LCs exhibit hyperplasia. A few tubules show focal spermatogenesis (asterisks). Overview (**c**) and detail (**d**) of testicular tissue of a 41,XX^{Y*} mouse. Some tubules exhibit focal spermatogenesis (asterisks). P, pachytene spermatocytes; rSptd, eSptd, round and elongated spermatids, respectively. Scale bars, 100 µm.

normal men may be less pronounced with advancing age. Thus, a time-dependent correction mechanism for gene expression may be active in KS. The genetic state was associated with clinical differences such as elevated insulin resistance, enhanced inflammatory and procoagulatory status, higher waist circumference, and dyslipidemia. Analyzing electrocardiograms, shorter (in some patients pathologically shortened) QTc intervals were observed [6, 7]. The authors concluded that the aberrant expression of X-chromosomal genes is associated with and likely causative for the clinical phenotype [7, 31].

X Inactivation and Escapee Genes

Sex determination in mammals is genetically dependent by the combination of sex chromosomes: XY in males and XX in females. The main difference between the sex chromosomes is the amount of genetic content, i.e., the genetic information of an X chromosome is comparable to that of autosomes, while the Y chromosome contains only 1% of the total DNA of a nucleus and bears less information [32]. The differences in sex chromosome-linked expression need to be equalized. For gene dosage compensation, only 1 X chromosome is supposed active in somatic cells, making them functionally monosomic for X. While males carry only 1 active X chromosome (X_a), a silencing process of the second X chromosome, called X inactivation, is needed in females due to the high dosage of X-linked genes and, thus, only 1 X chromosome can escape from silencing [33, 34]. Silencing, an epigenetic process in the blastocyst, occurs in the 10- to 20-cell epiblast lineage immediately before gastrulation [35]. Once an X chromosome is selected for silencing, its status is thought to remain in all descendants of this cell during life.

The X-inactivation center is the main regulatory region for X-inactivation [36], controlling the process of silencing by X chromosome counting, random X chromosome choice, and the initiation of silencing along approximately 1,000 X-linked genes [37]. Furthermore, despite encoding 4 nontranslated RNAs (*Xist, Tsix, Jpx, Ftx*) [36], it offers a binding site for blocking factors and regulatory proteins.

The X inactive specific transcript (*Xist*) is of crucial importance for X-inactivation and gene dosing [31, 38]. In every cell with more than 1 X chromosome, this noncoding RNA is transcribed from the *XIST* gene of the inactivated chromosome (X_i). The X-inactivation occurs by the transcription of the *Xist* RNA from X_i, which spreads over the whole X_i chromosome [39]. On the contrary, *Xist* transcription is repressed on the activated X chromosome by action of the noncoding antisense RNA *Tsix* [40]. Once the X chromosome inactivation is established, this noncoding RNA is solely expressed from X_a.

Impaired X-inactivation was suspected to underlie KS in both patients and 41,XX^{Y*} mice, until it was demonstrated that the inactivation of the supernumerary X chromosome in KS is correct and comparable to healthy females [31, 38]. A diagnostic method based on these findings was recently introduced for patients [41]. As the supernumerary X chromosome is correctly silenced in KS men, genes escaping from inactivation are most likely related to the phenotype. These are the only candidates differently expressed, i.e., only these escapee genes are expressed in a female pattern but in a male physiological environment [31]. Thus, all putative molecular cascades originate in the active presence of these relatively few genes that finally provoke (either by regulatory mechanisms or directly) the phenotype. Using 41,XX^{Y*} mice for expression analysis of those "escapee" genes, a tissue- and gene-specific expression profile was revealed, oscillating over development [31]. Approximately 15% of X-linked genes (mainly clustered in the pseudoautosomal region 1, PAR 1, of the short arm of the X chromosome [42]) in humans remain active and cause the transcriptome differences between 46,XY males and 46,XX females, but also between 46,XY males and 47,XXY KS men. In contrast, only about 3% of murine X-linked genes escape from inactivation. Additionally, the presence of a Y chromosome puts KS men into a special setting, as epigenetic features and clinical characteristics of 46,XX men, who present a very rare condition, are fundamentally different to KS [43].

Escapee Gene Expression: Lessons from the Mouse Model

More than 150 genes escape from silencing of the human X chromosome, rendering the exploration of genotype-phenotype correlations difficult. In contrast, only 13 genes were found to escape from X-inactivation in mice, and of those only 10 are encoding proteins [31, 26, 42]. Recently, X-inactivation in mice was shown to vary amongst mouse tissues and hints for both tissue and cell line-specific escapes from X-inactivation were reported [44]. However, this small number in 41,XX^{Y*} mice is sufficient to induce a phenotype resembling the human disorder [13, 15]. This enables genotype-phenotype correlations to be drawn much easier than in the human, e.g., X-chromosomal gene dosage was previously reported to directly influence social behavior and vasopressin expression in mice [45]. Both species have only 4 escapees in common, namely *Utx* (also known as *Kdm6a,* histone demethylase, di- and trimethylation of histone 3), *Kdm5c* (ubiquitous demethylase, linked to mental retardation), *Eif2s3x* (eukaryotic translation initiation factor 2, involved in cell cycle regulation), and *Ddx3x* (putatively involved in spermatogenesis and also in brain function) [31]. These genes are the most

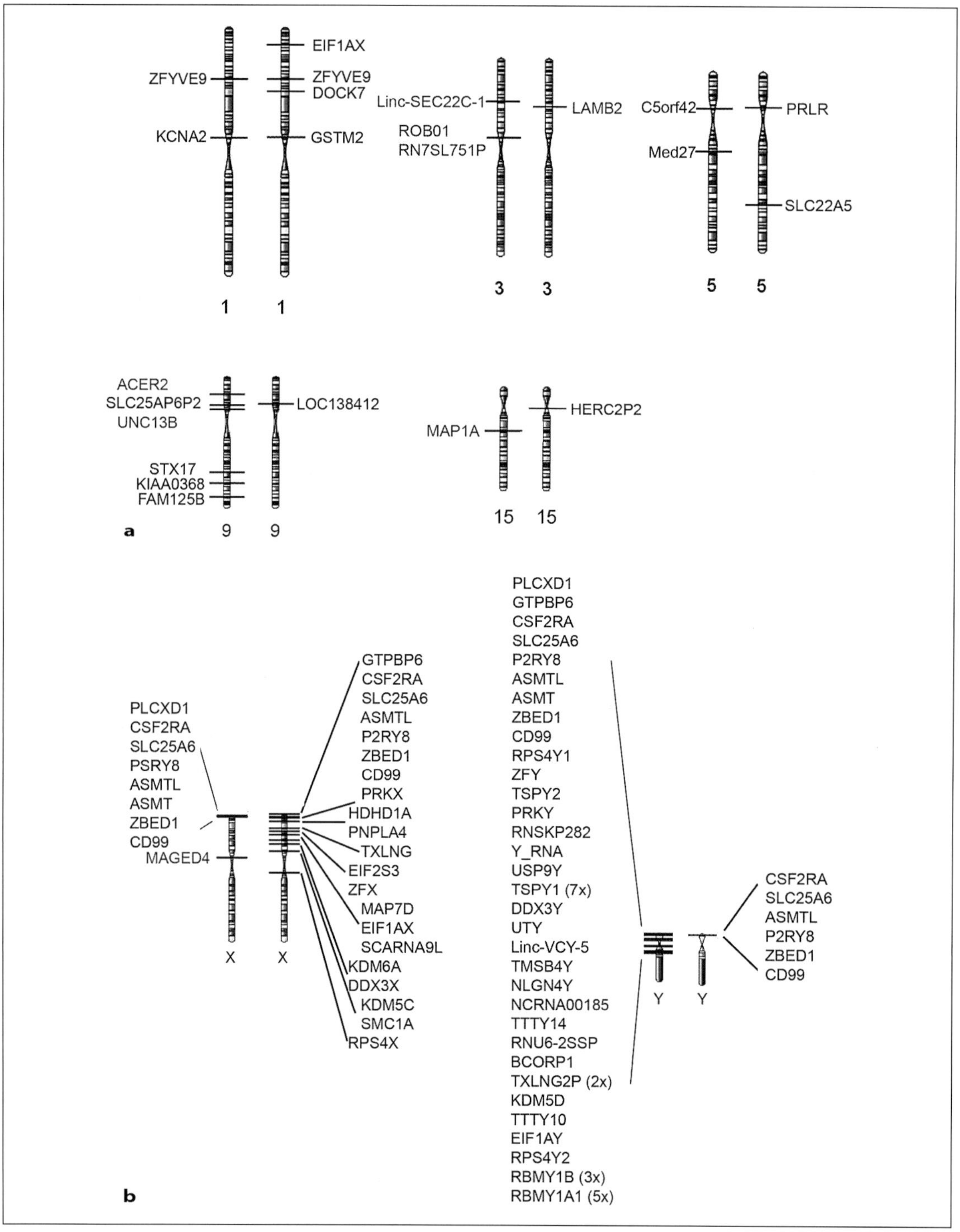

Fig. 4. Gene expression of KS patients differs from healthy males (M) and females (F) regarding autosomes (1, 3, 5, 9, 15; **a**) and heterosomes (**b**). Genes given in black indicate a higher expression and those in gray a lower expression in KS patients. The 4 X-linked escapees (*UTX [KDM6A]*, *KDM5C*, *EIF2S3X*, *DDX3X*) are overexpressed in KS compared to healthy males.

interesting for analysis in the mouse to gain insights into genotype-phenotype relations [31]. Using 41,XX^{Y*} mice for expression analysis of these "escapee" genes, a tissue- and gene-specific expression profile was revealed and suggested to be the genetic basis of the phenotypical changes [26, 31].

We addressed the quantitative expression of the "escapees" *Kdm6a*, *Kdm5c*, *Eif2s3x*, *Ddx3x*, and the silenced X-linked control gene *Pgk1* between birth and adulthood (1, 3, 5, 10, 14, 21 dpp and >30 weeks) in various tissues in 41,XX^{Y*} and female and male control mice (Fig. 5). For the heart (Fig. 5a), all escapee genes were generally expressed more highly in 41,XX^{Y*} mice compared to male controls, mimicking the female pattern with variable expression profiles during development. These differences were sometimes already significant from birth onwards (*Eif2s3x*, *Kdm6a*) but appeared at the latest by day 7 (*Kdm5c*). Due to high variations between the individuals, significant differences should be interpreted carefully due to the known heterogeneous X chromosomal gene expression in female mammals [42]. During postnatal development, the differences were relatively variable in the first week but generally tended to decrease slightly from 7 dpp onwards in all karyotypes, which is particularly interesting for *Kdm6a* (*Utx*), a key player in heart and vessel formation [46], both of which are thought to be affected by the disorder. Interestingly, its expression was comparable at 1 dpp in 41,XX^{Y*} and 40,XY* mice. Liver expression profiles of the escapee genes revealed the weakest differences becoming only sporadically significant after a few days, although in general expression in 41,XX^{Y*} mice appeared intermediate when compared to the male and female controls (Fig. 5b). Expression patterns for all genes increased during 1–21 dpp and dropped strongly (*Kdm6a*, *Eif2s3x*) or moderately (*Kdm5c*, *Ddx3x*) afterwards. Compared to 40,XY* males, the expression in 41,XX^{Y*} males was elevated for *Kdm6a* at 10 and 21 dpp, for *Kdm5c* at 3 dpp, and for *Eif2s3x* at 21 dpp. A difference in *Ddx3x* expression was detected between females and 40,XY* males only at 1 dpp. Expression in the brain (Fig. 5c) during development contrasted with previous reports [31] in which all escapees were found to be overexpressed in KS mice only. Here, *Kdm6a*, *Kdm5c*, *Eif2s3x* were higher in females and 41,XX^{Y*} males, resembling the mimicking pattern also observed in the heart for both significant expression differences between the karyotypes as well as the general pattern of expression, including the slight drop towards adulthood. Although these data would support the supposed "femalization" of 41,XX^{Y*} males, repeated experiments and larger groups are needed, especially because of the putative role of *Kdm5c* for cognitive deficits [47]. The expression of *Kdm6a* and *Kdm5c* remained constant between 21 dpp and adulthood, while *Eif2s3x* and *Ddx3x* increased in 41,XX^{Y*} and 40,XX mice. Increased levels of the 4 genes similar to 40,XX mice were detected in 41,XX^{Y*} mice for *Eifs3x* until 10 dpp, for *Kdm6a* until 7 dpp, and for *Kdm5c* until 5 dpp. In adults, expression of *Kdm6a*, *Kdm5c*, and *Eif2s3x* was comparable to females. Not surprisingly, marked differences for expression in testis samples from 10 dpp onwards were found as by that time in XY* mice germ cell differentiation has started, while in 41,XX^{Y*} the germ line is continuously attenuated (Fig. 5d). *Ddx3x*, *Eif2s3x*, and *Kdm6a* expression decreased in 41,XX^{Y*} and 40,XY* mice, and was the lowest at adult age. For *Kdm5c*, expression levels oscillated, reaching the lowest level in adulthood. Expression levels in 41,XX^{Y*} males were always higher than those of 40,XY* mice. For *Kdm6a*, a significant difference was already detected at 1 dpp. Values for mRNA differ significantly between the karyotypes from 7 dpp onwards, when germ cell differentiation starts and testicular cell composition changes. Thus, any postnatal comparison is thought to be invalid and interpretation impossible as the altered testicular composition of 41,XX^{Y*} animals at birth requires in utero analyses [8].

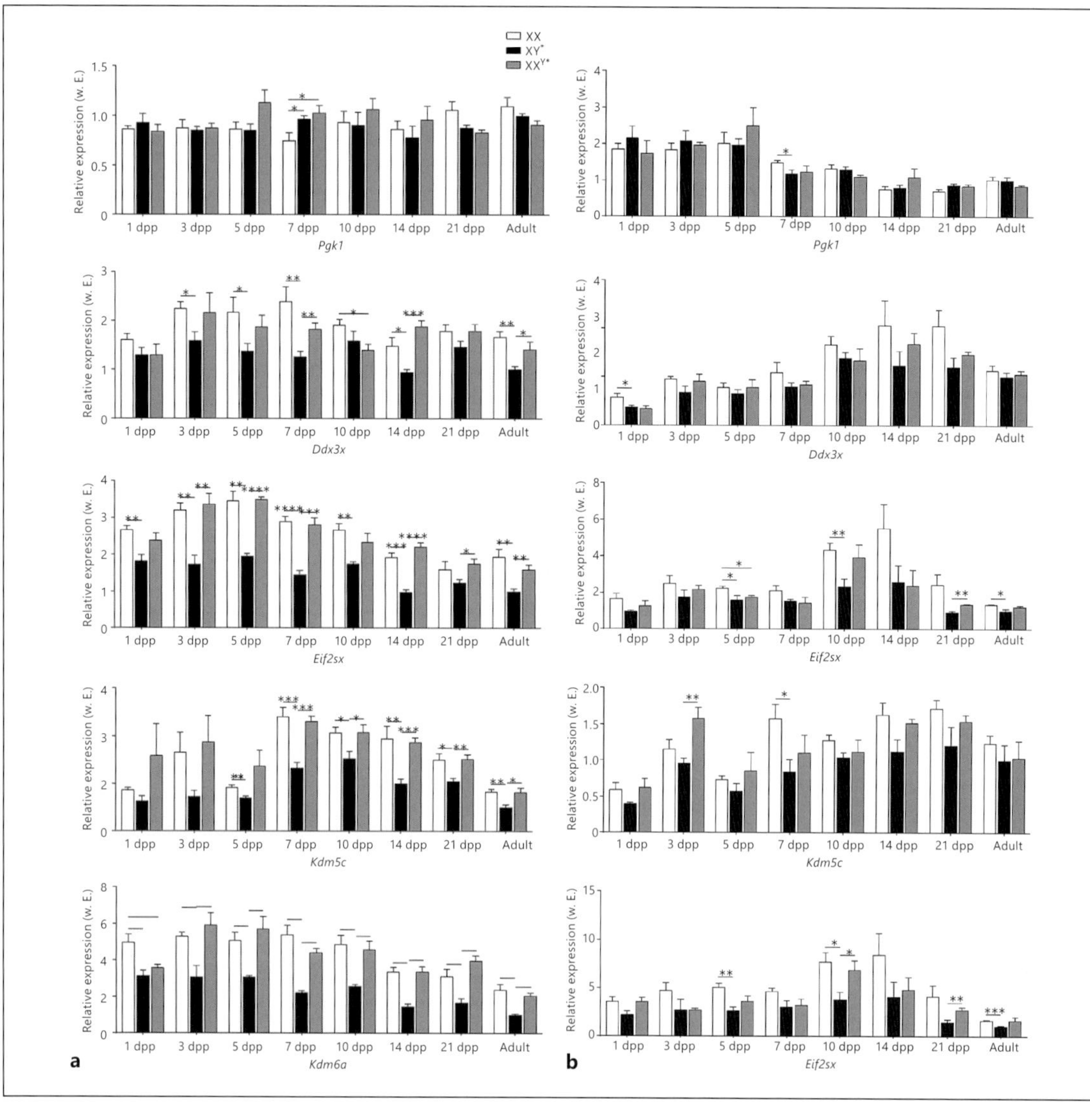

Fig. 5. a Quantitative mRNA expression of escapee genes in the heart of 41,XX^{Y*}, 40,XY*, and 40,XX mice: expression of *Pgk1, Ddx3x, Eif2s3x, Kdm5c, Kdm6a (Utx)*. The silenced X-linked *Pgk1* served as the control; the latter are escapees. Data were normalized by defining the expression of the adult 40,XY* littermate as 1. Values are shown as the mean + SEM in females and 41,XX^{Y*} males between 1 and 7 dpp. Variable *Kdm5c* expression was found whilst expression of the other genes analyzed was constant before dropping from 7 dpp to adulthood. Escapee expressions in male mice were similar at 1 dpp but diverged from 3 dpp onwards, when 41,XX^{Y*} profiles became similar to those of females. Expression of *Kdm5c* and *Ddx3x* (from 3 dpp onwards) in KS mice was comparable to female patterns during development. Due to high interanimal variations, significant differences occurred from 7 dpp. **b** Escapee gene expression in liver tissue of 41,XX^{Y*}, 40,XY*, and 40,XX mice. Expression patterns for all genes increased between 1 and 21 dpp and dropped strongly (*Kdm6a [Utx]*, *Eif2s3x*) or moderately (*Kdm5c, Ddx3x*) until adulthood. Expression levels of *Kdm6a* and *Eif2s3x* were greater on 5 and 10 dpp in female and in 40,XY* male controls in adulthood. For *Kdm5c*, this holds only true on 7 dpp. In comparison to 40,XY*, the expression levels in 41,XX^{Y*} males were elevated for *Kdm6a* at 10 and 21 dpp, for *Kdm5c* at 3 and for *Eif2s3x* at 21 dpp. Only at 1 dpp, a significant difference in *Ddx3x* expression was detected between females and 40,XY* males. * $p < 0.05$; ** $p < 0.01$; *** $p < 0.001$; **** $p < 0.0001$. w. E., arbitrary unit.

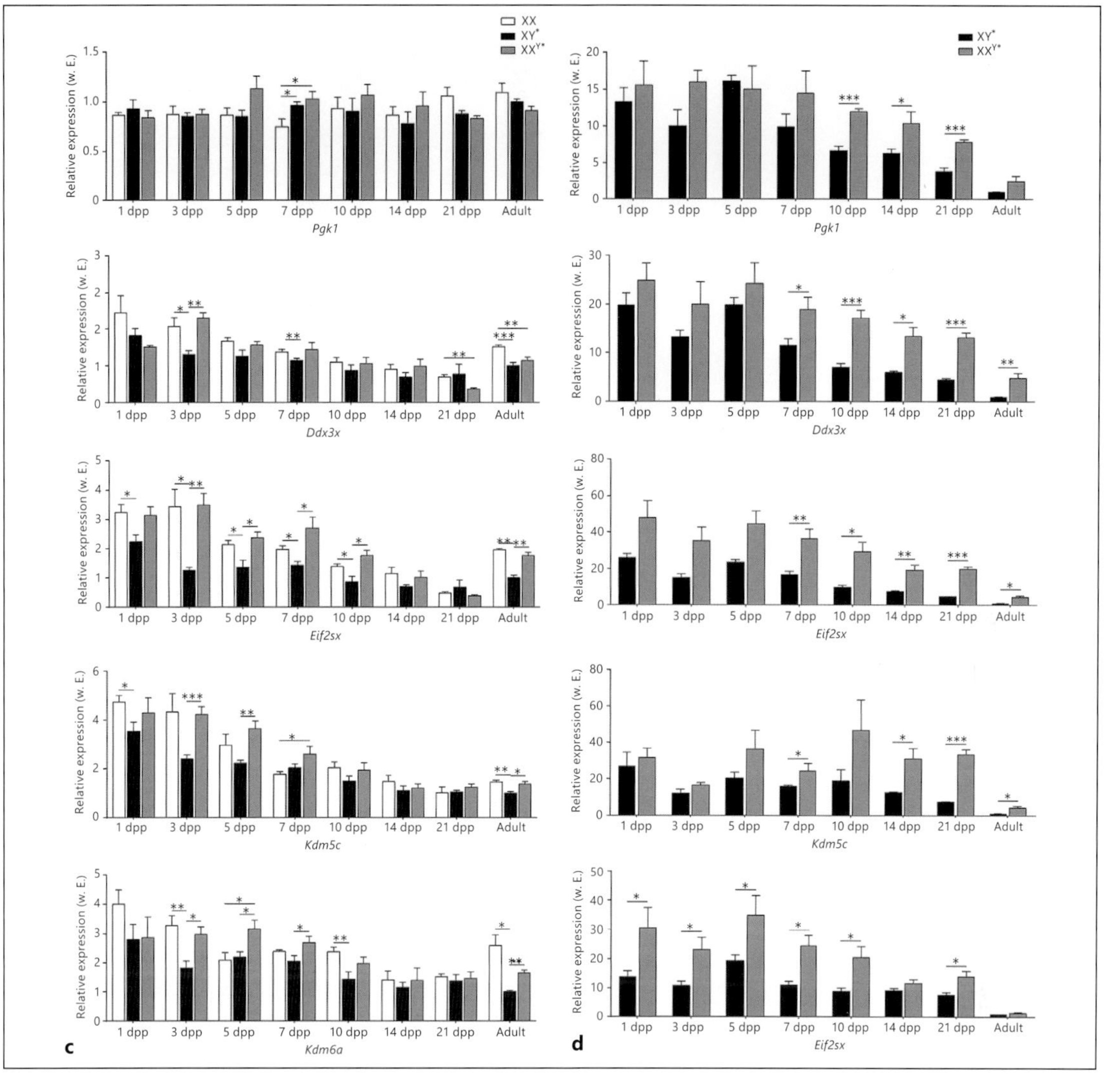

Fig. 5. c Escapee gene expression in the brain tissue of 41,XX^{Y}*, 40,XY*, and 40,XX mice. *Pgk1* expression pattern for KS and healthy controls pointed to a correct X-inactivation. The expression levels of *Kdm6a* (*Utx*) and *Kdm5c* remained constant between 21 dpp and adulthood, while the RNAs levels of *Eif2s3x* and *Ddx3x* in 41,XX^{Y}* and 40,XX mice increased. Striking changes in expressions were detected in 41,XX^{Y}* mice on 1 and 3 dpp. Compared with healthy littermates, increased levels of the 4 genes similar to those of female mice were detected. This observation is true for *Eifs3x* until 10 dpp, for *Kdm6a* until 7 dpp, and for *Kdm5c* until 5 dpp. In later developmental stages, the level of expression was between 40,XY* and 40,XX mice or even higher than female levels. Expression levels of 41,XX^{Y}* mice were never lower than levels of 40,XY* mice. In the adult KS animals, expression levels of *Kdm6a*, *Kdm5c*, and *Eif2s3x* were similar to females. **d** Escapee gene expression in the testis of 41,XX^{Y}* and 40,XY* mice. *Ddx3x*, *Eif2s3x*, and *Kdm6a* expression decreased in 41,XX^{Y}* and 40,XY* mice and was lowest in adult age. For *Kdm5c*, expression levels showed an oscillating profile and values reached the lowest level in adulthood. Expression levels of 41,XX^{Y}*males were always higher than those of 40,XY* mice. For *Kdm6a* (*Utx*), a significant difference between these 2 groups was detected from 1 dpp onwards. mRNA expression levels for all genes differed between the karyotypes from 7 dpp onwards, i.e., the starting point of germ cell differentiation and due to the discrepancy of testicular cell composition between the groups. * $p < 0.05$; ** $p < 0.01$; *** $p < 0.001$; **** $p < 0.0001$. w. E., arbitrary unit.

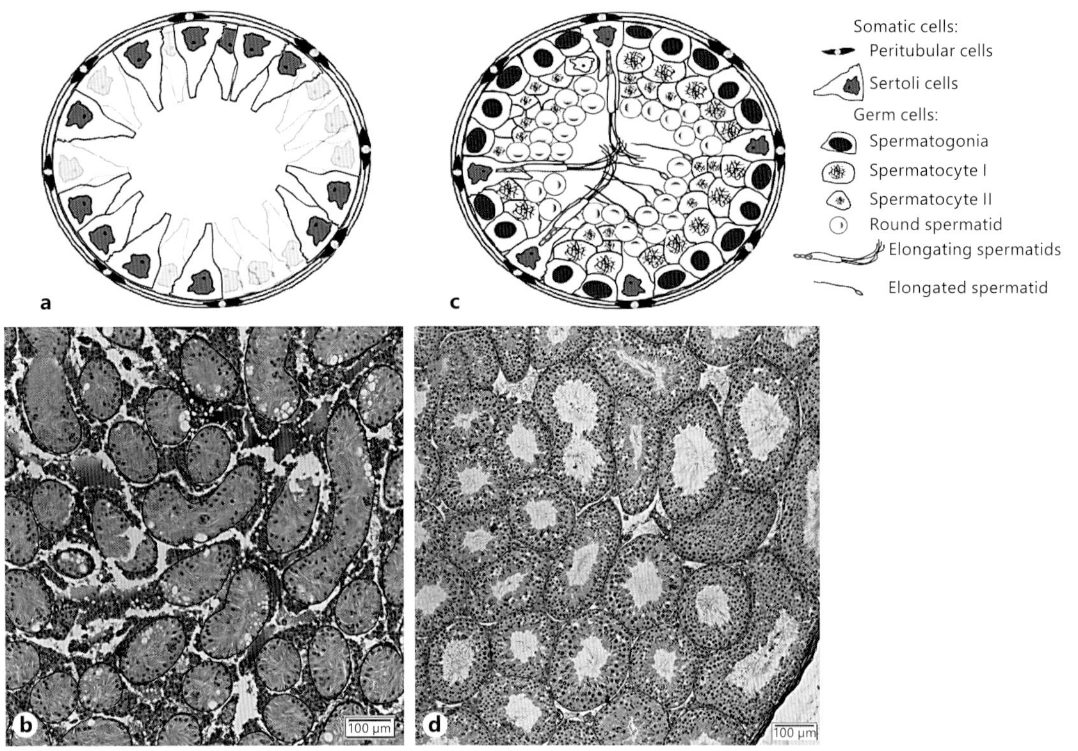

Fig. 6. Cellular composition of tubules of $41,XX^{Y*}$ and 40,XY* mice. **a**, **b** Scheme and corresponding histology of testicular tissue in a KS mouse: tubules predominantly consist of peritubular and SCs showing an SC-only status. **c**, **d** Scheme and corresponding histology of testicular tissue of a healthy 40,XY* mouse with complete spermatogenesis.

Consequences of the Supernumerary X Chromosome for the Male Phenotype

Similar to observations in patients, the influence of sex chromosomal (aneuploidy) effects on various metabolic processes has been demonstrated. As changes were shown concerning learning and memory recognition in mouse models [27], behavioral disturbances were confirmed also for male sexual behavior and a feminization was observed, associated with certain gene expression patterns in the brain [48]. Moreover, (partly sex-specific) differences in locomotion, adiposity, and the lipoprotein/cholesterol metabolism were proven to depend on the heterosomes and are therefore prone to be affected in sex chromosomally trisomic mice [49–51]. Thus, the imbalance between the sex chromosomes appears to be metabolically difficult in general and is reflected by the clinical features.

Consequently, the testis has to be seen as the most severely affected organ since it reflects the genotype-phenotype relation of this condition the strongest (Fig. 6). Both testicular functions, the maintenance of the male endocrine milieu, and the production of gametes are consistently affected. Therefore, the logical target for the exploration of gene dosage effects is the analysis of gene expression and the functional response of testicular cell types. The availability of mouse models, the option to analyze gene expression patterns and somatic cell responses, and a close cooperation between clinics and basic science should result in the direct translation of findings into a clinical context [7, 30, 52].

Germ cell function is dependent on direct contact to SCs and, vice versa, SC function depends on the presence of germ cells. Little is known about SC-germ cell interactions on the molecular level under KS conditions. SCs, LCs, and peritubular cells provide factors essential for migration, stem cell retention, and for the regulation of SSC functions [53]. Amongst such factors, recent studies have revealed that the chemokine (C-X-C motif) ligand 12 (*Cxcl12*) – an SC product – is involved in the migratory processes by which the primordial germ cells (PGCs) detect the niche.

SC function in KS mice is at least sufficient to support the germ cells of a normal karyotype, independent of the presence of an additional X chromosome in SCs [54, 55]. However, it was found that during the testicular degeneration observed in KS, SCs also degenerate over time [3]. This observation is in line with our mouse data demonstrating that SC numbers are altered during postnatal development [8]. Taken together, the altered SC physiology needs detailed analyses already during prenatal development.

Germ line propagation and differentiation is in particular affected by the consequences of the chromosomal aberration. Thus, processes occurring specifically in the germ line might be altered by the chromosomal imbalance, i.e., the PGC and the SSC system development. In vitro studies have shown that aneuploid undifferentiated germ cells died when isolated from embryonic gonads and only those with a randomly corrected karyotype survived in culture [8, 27]. Thus, SSCs with an aberrant karyotype must have entered a default pathway during the intrauterine phase, and at the latest in the perinatal period. When only germ cells with a corrected karyotype survive in vitro after they were isolated from the embryonic gonad, while aberrant germ cells die over time, the question arises as to why, in vivo, the germ cell loss progresses postnatally [8]. Even if a few aberrant germ cells are still present perinatally in the testis, a certain proportion of those present at birth should be of the correct karyotype and the population of spermatogonial cells should at least remain stable even if they are not propagating. Hence, correction by random propulsion explains the survival of a reduced population of PGCs [27, 54]. Subsequently, gonocytes can survive into the postnatal period, with some expressing all relevant markers correctly and driving the foci of spermatogenesis. Systematic evaluation of these phenotypic changes during development in utero is only possible in a mouse model per se.

Testicular angiogenesis, the establishment of the male germ line, and the differentiation of the LC population are closely linked during early development. Blood vessels situated proximately are a prerequisite for SSC niche formation and for a correct localization of LC clusters [55]. Thus, impaired angiogenesis and vascularization may contribute to germ cell reduction.

By recruiting endothelial progenitor cells, new vessels form through a process called vasculogenesis. The initial vascular network is later modified by growth, i.e., by angiogenesis building the majority of embryonic blood vessels, a process that remains crucially important also in the adult. The formation and modulation of the blood vessel system are regulated by numerous signaling molecules. Among these, the vascular endothelial growth factor signaling pathway is involved in vasculogenesis and angiogenesis [56]. During embryonic development, vascularization of the testis also starts when cords are separated in parallel from the surrounding tissue, the later interstitial compartment. When the coelomic vessel has been built between embryonic day 10.5 and 11.5, it serves as the origin for the extension of other vessels that finally generate the testicular vascular system [57].

The altered blood vessel situation described by Foresta et al. [5] and our own finding of a significantly reduced and altered vascularization of testicular tissue in 41,XX^{Y*} mice [30], prompted us to hypothesize that hampered testicular blood flow could provoke a disturbed blood supply. Consequently, impaired vascularization would contribute to the endocrine phenotype, as transport of hormones from the peripheral circulation into (Luteinizing hormone) as well as out of the testicular tissue (testosterone) might be affected.

In fact, adult KS men are regularly diagnosed in fertility clinics due to infertility. The standard for detection is karyotyping. However, other testing procedures have been described in recent years, including the Xist RNA assay that has been used for diagnosis since 1994. Subsequently, a novel qPCR assay which allows the detection of a supernumerary X chromosome by using primer for unmethylated Xist is even more sensitive [41]. Furthermore, MLPA (multiplex ligation-dependent probe amplification) [58] and the detection of the copy numbers of X-linked AR-receptors by qPCR [59] are expedient approaches. However, these methods require special expertise and devices. Recently, a method for population-based screening using dried blood samples already collected for the national newborn screening program was postulated [60]. In addition, noninvasive prenatal diagnosis of fetal chromosomal aneuploidy was proposed to be promising for KS diagnosis already during pregnancy [61]. Nevertheless, improved and in particular early diagnosis tools are needed, as the consequences of the disorder – increased morbidity and mortality – should be encountered as early as possible.

Conclusion

KS has been addressed clinically and experimentally for more than 70 years. Astonishingly, most relevant and novel insights have been provided only recently during the last 2 decades, for example that KS men cannot be considered infertile per se, and should also be counselled for potential cardiovascular risk. This is due to new methods regarding gene expression, but also to the availability of experimental models. Thus, apart from improved diagnosis and patient care, it is of enormous importance to extend the experimental exploration of the syndrome in order to further increase the life quality of affected men.

Acknowledgements

Parts of the data presented were obtained during a project funded by the DFG (WI2723/4-1) and from the Medical Faculty (IZKF CRA03/09). The data on gene expression during development in mice were obtained by Katharina Körner, whom we gratefully acknowledge.

References

1 Tüttelmann F, Gromoll J: Novel genetic aspects of Klinefelter's syndrome. Mol Hum Reprod 2010;16:386–395.

2 Lanfranco F, Kamischke A, Zitzmann M, Nieschlag E: Klinefelter's syndrome. Lancet 2004;364:273–283.

3 Aksglaede L, Juul A: Testicular function and fertility in men with Klinefelter syndrome: a review. Eur J Endocrinol 2013; 168:R67–R76.

4 Nieschlag E, Ferlin A, Gravholt CH, Gromoll J, Köhler B, Lejeune H, Rogol AD, Wistuba J: The Klinefelter syndrome: current management and research challenges. Andrology 2016;4:545–549.

5 Foresta C, Caretta N, Palego P, Ferlin A, Zuccarello D, Lenzi A, Selice R: Reduced artery diameters in Klinefelter syndrome. Int J Androl 2012;35:720–725.

6 Jørgensen IN, Skakkebaek A, Andersen NH, Pedersen LN, Hougaard DM, Bojesen A, Trolle C, Gravholt CH: Short QTc interval in males with klinefelter syndrome-influence of CAG repeat length, body composition, and testosterone replacement therapy. Pacing Clin Electrophysiol 2015;38:472–482.

7 Zitzmann M, Bongers R, Werler S, Bogdanova N, Wistuba J, Kliesch S, Gromoll J, Tüttelmann F: Gene expression patterns in relation to the clinical phenotype in Klinefelter syndrome. J Clin Endocrinol Metab 2015;100:E518–E523.

8 Werler S, Demond H, Ehmcke J, Damm OS, Middendorff R, Gromoll J, Wistuba J: Early loss of germ cells is associated with fading expression of Lin28, a spermatogonial stem cell marker in the 41,XXY* mouse model for Klinefelter Syndrome. Reproduction 2014;147:253–264.

9 Davis SM, Rogol AD, Ross JL: Testis development and fertility in boys with Klinefelter syndrome. Endocrinol Metab Clin North Am 2015;44:843–865.

10 Fullerton G, Hamilton M, Maheshwari A: Should non-mosaic Klinefelter syndrome men be labelled as infertile in 2009? Hum Reprod 2010;25:588–597.

11 Sciurano RB, Luna Hisano CV, Rahn MI, Brugo Olmedo S, Rey Valzacchi G, Coco R, Solari AJ: Focal spermatogenesis originates in euploid germ cells in classical Klinefelter patients. Hum Reprod 2009;24:2353–2360.

12 Bojesen A, Juul S, Gravholt CH: Prenatal and postnatal prevalence of Klinefelter syndrome: a national registry study. J Clin Endocrinol Metab 2003;88:622–626.

13 Kitamura M, Matsumiya K, Koga M, Nishimura K, Miura H, Tsuji T, Matsumoto M, Okamoto Y, Okuyama A: Ejaculated spermatozoa in patients with non-mosaic Klinefelter's syndrome. Int J Urol 2000;7:88–92, discussion 93–94.

14 Zitzmann M, Depenbusch M, Gromoll J, Nieschlag E: X-chromosome inactivation patterns and androgen receptor functionality influence phenotype and social characteristics as well as pharmacogenetics of testosterone therapy in Klinefelter patients. J Clin Endocrinol Metab 2004;89:6208–6217.

15 Chang S, Skakkebæk A, Trolle C, Bojesen A, Hertz JM, Cohen A, Hougaard DM, Wallentin M, Pedersen AD, Østergaard JR, Gravholt CH: Anthropometry in Klinefelter syndrome – multifactorial influences due to CAG length, testosterone treatment and possibly intrauterine hypogonadism. J Clin Endocrinol Metab 2015;100:E508–E517.

16 Ataman E, Cogulu O, Durmaz A, Karaca E, Durmaz B, Akin H, Ozkinay F: The rate of sex chromosome aneuploidies in prenatal diagnosis and subsequent decisions in Western Turkey. Genet Test Mol Biomarkers 2012;16:150–153.

17 Forrester MB, Merz RD: Pregnancy outcome and prenatal diagnosis of sex chromosome abnormalities in Hawaii, 1986–1999. Am J Med Genet A 2003;15; 119A:305–310.

18 Mansfield C, Hopfer S, Marteau TM: Termination rates after prenatal diagnosis of Down syndrome, spina bifida, anencephaly, and Turner and Klinefelter syndromes: a systematic literature review. Prenat Diagn 1999;19:808–812.

19 Rohayem J, Fricke R, Czeloth K, Mallidis C, Wistuba J, Krallmann C, Zitzmann M, Kliesch S: Age and markers of Leydig cell function, but not of Sertoli cell function predict the success of sperm retrieval in adolescents and adults with Klinefelter's syndrome. Andrology 2015; 3:868–875.

20 van Saen D, Gies I, de Schepper J, Tournaye H, Goossens E: Can pubertal boys with Klinefelter syndrome benefit from spermatogonial stem cell banking? Hum Reprod 2012;27:323–330.

21 Kossack N, Terwort N, Wistuba J, Ehmcke J, Schlatt S, Schöler H, Kliesch S, Gromoll J: A combined approach facilitates the reliable detection of human spermatogonia in vitro. Hum Reprod 2013;28:3012–3025.

22 Stukenborg JB, Schlatt S, Simoni M, Yeung CH, Elhija MA, Luetjens CM, Huleihel M, Wistuba J: New horizons for in vitro spermatogenesis? An update on novel three-dimensional culture systems as tools for meiotic and postmeiotic differentiation of testicular germ cells. Mol Hum Reprod, 2009;15:521–529.

23 Bojesen A, Stochholm K, Juul S, Gravholt CH: Socioeconomic trajectories affect mortality in Klinefelter syndrome. J Clin Endocrinol Metab 2011; 96:2098–2104.

24 Skakkebæk A, Wallentin M, Gravholt CH: Neuropsychology and socioeconomic aspects of Klinefelter syndrome: new developments. Curr Opin Endocrinol Diabetes Obes 2015;22:209–216.

25 Eicher EM, Hale DW, Hunt PA, Lee BK, Tucker PK, King TR, Eppig JT, Washburn LL: The mouse Y* chromosome involves a complex rearrangement, including interstitial positioning of the pseudoautosomal region. Cytogenet Cell Genet 1991;57:221–230.

26 Wistuba J, Werler S, Lewejohann L: Mouse models for the exploration of Klinefelter's syndrome; in Conn PM (ed): Animal Models for the Study of Human Diseases. Amsterdam, Elsevier, 2013, vol 1, pp 759–784.

27 Wistuba J: Animal models for Klinefelter's syndrome and their relevance for the clinic. Mol Hum Reprod 2010;16: 375–385.

28 Lewejohann L, Damm O, Luetjens CM, Hämäläinen T, Simoni M, Nieschlag E, Gromoll J, Wistuba J: Impaired recognition memory in male mice with a supernumerary X chromosome. Physiol Behav 2009;96:23–29.

29 Wistuba J, Luetjens CM Dittmann M, Werler S, Poplinski A, Damm O, Stukenborg JB Hämäläinen T, Simoni M, Gromoll J: Male 41, XXY* mice as a model for Klinefelter syndrome: hyperactivation of Leydig cells. Endocrinology 2010; 151:2898–2910.

30 Tüttelmann F, Damm OS, Luetjens CM, Baldi M, Zitzmann M, Kliesch S, Nieschlag E, Gromoll J, Wistuba J, Simoni M: Intratesticular testosterone is increased in men with Klinefelter syndrome and may not be released into the bloodstream owing to altered testicular vascularization – a preliminary report. Andrology 2014;2:275–281.

31 Werler S, Poplinski A, Gromoll J, Wistuba J: Expression of genes escaping from X-inactivation in the 41, XX^{Y*} mouse model for Klinefelter's syndrome. Acta Paed 2011;100:885–891.

32 Liu Z, Venkatesh SS, Maley CC: Sequence space coverage, entropy of genomes and the potential to detect non-human DNA in human samples. BMC Genomics 2008;9:509.

33 Rastan S, Robertson EJ: X-chromosome deletions in embryo-derived (EK) cell lines associated with lack of X-chromosome inactivation. J Embryol Exp Morphol 1985;90:379–388.

34 Barakat TS, Jonkers I, Monkhorst K, Gribnau J: X-changing information on X inactivation. Exp Cell Res 2010;10;316: 679–687.

35 Okamoto I, Otte AP, Allis CD, Reinberg D, Heard E: Epigenetic dynamics of imprinted X inactivation during early mouse development. Science 2004;303:644–649.
36 Chureau C, Prissette M, Bourdet A, Barbe V, Cattolico L, Jones L, Eggen A, Avner P, Duret L: Comparative sequence analysis of the X-inactivation center region in mouse, human, and bovine. Genome Res 2002;12:894–908.
37 Brown CJ, Lafreniere RG, Powers VE, Sebastio G, Ballabio A, Pettigrew AL, Ledbetter DH, Levy E, Craig IW, Willard HF: Localization of the X inactivation centre on the human X chromosome in Xq13. Nature 1991;349:82–84.
38 Poplinski A, Wieacker P, Kliesch S, Gromoll J: Severe XIST hypomethylation clearly distinguishes (SRY+) 46,XX-maleness from Klinefelter syndrome. Eur J Endocrinol 2010;162:169–175.
39 Csankovszki G, Panning B, Bates B, Pehrson J R Jaenisch R: Conditional deletion of Xist disrupts histone macroH2A localization but not maintenance of X inactivation. Nat Genet 1999;22:323–324.
40 Lee JT, Davidow LS, Warshawsky D: *Tsix*, a gene antisense to Xist at the X-inactivation centre. Nat Gen 1999;21: 400–404.
41 Mehta A, Mielnik A, Schlegel PN, Paduch DA: Novel methylation specific real-time PCR test for the diagnosis of Klinefelter syndrome. Asian J Androl 2014;16:684–688.
42 Carrel L, Willard HF: X-inactivation profile reveals extensive variability in X-linked gene expression in females. Nature 2005;434:400–404.
43 Vorona E, Zitzmann M, Gromoll J, Schüring AN, Nieschlag E: Clinical, endocrinological, and epigenetic features of the 46,XX male syndrome, compared with 47,XXY Klinefelter patients. J Clin Endocrinol Metab 2007;92:3458–3465.
44 Berletch JB, Ma W, Yang F, Shendure J, Noble WS, Disteche CM, Deng X: Escape from X inactivation varies in mouse tissues. PLoS Genet 2015;18;11:e1005079.
45 Cox KH, Quinnies KM, Eschendroeder A, Didrick PM, Eugster EA, Rissman EF: Number of X-chromosome genes influences social behavior and vasopressin gene expression in mice. Psychoneuroendocrinology 2015;51:271–281.
46 Lee S, Lee JW, Lee SK: UTX, a histone H3-lysine 27 demethylase, acts as a critical switch to activate the cardiac developmental program. Dev Cell 2012; 22: 25–37.
47 Kramer JM, van Bokhoven H: Genetic and epigenetic defects in mental retardation. Int J Biochem Cell Biol 2009;41: 96–107.
48 Ngun TC, Ghahramani NM, Creek MM, Williams-Burris SM, Barseghyan H, Itoh Y, Sánchez FJ, McClusky R, Sinsheimer JS, Arnold AP, Vilain E: Feminized behavior and brain gene expression in a novel mouse model of Klinefelter syndrome. Arch Sex Behav 2014;43:1043–1057.
49 Link JC, Chen X, Prien C, Borja MS, Hammerson B, Oda MN, Arnold AP, Reue K: Increased high-density lipoprotein cholesterol levels in mice with XX versus XY sex chromosomes. Arterioscler Thromb Vasc Biol 2015;35:1778–1786.
50 Chen X, McClusky R, Itoh Y, Reue K, Arnold AP: X and Y chromosome complement influence adiposity and metabolism in mice. Endocrinology 2013;154: 1092–1104.
51 Chen X, Williams-Burris SM, McClusky R, Ngun TC, Ghahramani N, Barseghyan H, Reue K, Vilain E, Arnold AP: The Sex Chromosome Trisomy mouse model of XXY and XYY: metabolism and motor performance. Biol Sex Differ 2013;4:15.
52 Westernströer B, Terwort N, Ehmcke J, Wistuba J, Schlatt S, Neuhaus N: Profiling of Cxcl12 receptors, Cxcr4 and Cxcr7 in murine testis development and a spermatogenic depletion model indicates a role for Cxcr7 in controlling Cxcl12 activity. PLoS One 2014; 9:e112598.
53 Vialard F, Bailly M, Bouazzi H, Albert M, Pont JC, Mendes V, Bergere M, Gomes DM, de Mazancourt P, Selva J: The high frequency of sperm aneuploidy in Klinefelter patients and in nonobstructive azoospermia is due to meiotic errors in euploid spermatocytes. J Androl 2012;33:1352–1359.
54 Yoshida S, Sukeno M, Nabeshima Y: A vasculature-associated niche for undifferentiated spermatogonia in the mouse testis. Science 2007;317:1722–1726.
55 Patel-Hett S, D'Amore PA: Signal transduction in vasculogenesis and developmental angiogenesis. Int J Dev Biol 2011;55:353–363.
56 Brennan J, Capel B: One tissue, two fates: molecular genetic events that underlie testis versus ovary development. Nat Rev Genet 2004;5:509–521.
57 Yan JB, Xu M, Xiong C, Zhou DW, Ren ZR, Huang Y, Mommersteeg M, van Beuningen R, Wang YT, Liao SX, Zeng F, Wu Y, Zeng YT: Rapid screening for chromosomal aneuploidies using array-MLPA. BMC Med Genet 2011;12:68.
58 Ottesen AM, Garn ID, Aksglaede L, Juul A, Rajpert-De Meyts E: A simple screening method for detection of Klinefelter syndrome and other X-chromosome aneuploidies based on copy number of the androgen receptor gene. Mol Hum Reprod 2007;13:745–750.
59 Aksglaede L, Garn ID, Hollegaard MV, Hougaard DM, Rajpert-De Meyts E, Juul A: Detection of increased gene copy number in DNA from dried blood spot samples allows efficient screening for Klinefelter syndrome. Acta Paediatr 2012;101:e561–e563.
60 Lo YM: Noninvasive prenatal detection of fetal chromosomal aneuploidies by maternal plasma nucleic acid analysis: a review of the current state of the art. BJOG 2009;116:152–157.
61 Samango-Sprouse C, Keen C, Sadeghin T, Gropman A: The benefits and limitations of cell-free DNA screening for 47, XXY (Klinefelter syndrome). Prenat Diagn 2017;37:497–501.

Dr. Joachim Wistuba
Centre of Reproductive Medicine and Andrology, University of Muenster, Albert-Schweitzer Campus 1, Building D11
DE–48149 Muenster (Germany)
E-Mail joachim.wistuba@ukmuenster.de

Vogt PH (ed): Genetics of Human Infertility. Monogr Hum Genet.
Basel, Karger, 2017, vol 21, pp 57–73 (DOI: 10.1159/000477278)

Human Y Chromosome and Male Infertility: Forward and Back from Azoospermia Factor Chromatin Structure to Azoospermia Factor Gene Function

Peter H. Vogt • U. Bender • J. Zimmer • T. Strowitzki

Reproduction Genetics Unit, Department of Gynecological Endocrinology and Reproductive Medicine, University of Heidelberg, Heidelberg, Germany

Abstract

In the euchromatic part of the long arm of the human Y chromosome (Yq11) at least 13 Y genes encoding proteins and expressed in male germ cells were found in 3 distinct genomic Y regions frequently deleted in infertile men with idiopathic azoospermia, i.e., for unknown reasons no mature sperm were found in their semen fluid. Accordingly, they were designated as azoospermia factor (AZF) regions: AZFa, AZFb, and AZFc. Additionally, 10 Y genes called "testis-specific transcript Y" (*TTTY*) genes were mapped in the same AZF intervals. They belong to the long non-coding RNA gene pool in human germ cells because they seem to lack any protein-coding potential. Distinct chromatin regions in Yq11 overlapping with AZFb and AZFc are supposed to be involved in the premeiotic X and Y chromosome pairing and inactivation process controlling male germ cell meiosis. It can thus be assumed that the germ line function of the AZF loci in Yq11 may be not only based on the expression of some germ cell proteins, but also on the expression of some germ cell-specific *TTTY* transcripts and a locally dynamic and specific chromatin folding structure probably controlled by some germ cell-specific nuclear proteins.

The azoospermia factor (AZF) locus in Yq11 was first recognised by observation of microscopically visible terminal deletions of the long arm of the Y chromosome in 6 patients with azoospermia, i.e., with no mature sperm in their ejaculate [1]. They included the complete polymorphic heterochromatin block in distal Yq (Yq12) and were assumed to also affect the neighbouring distal euchromatic Y long arm region (Yq11.23). It has been suggested that some function of the distal Yq heterochromatin blocks human male fertility despite the commonly observed polymorphism length in Yq12 [2]. Careful molecular analyses then revealed more individual breakpoints extending along the complete euchromatic long Y arm region (Yq11) in infertile men with AZF-Yq11 aberrations, and histological analyses of their individual testicular pathology displayed a severe disruption of spermatogenesis at different development phases [3]. This suggested an essential function of AZF during premeiotic and postmeiotic human male germ cell development, and consequently that this genetic locus should encode more than 1 Y gene functionally involved in the complex human male germ cell differentiation process.

Their location in Yq11 could first be distinguished after having established detailed molecular deletion maps of genomic Y DNA in a number of infertile patients with distinct aberrant Yq11 regions and collected in different research groups. These maps were based on the distinct location of Y-specific DNA probes selected from different Y chromosome clone libraries and the analyses of their presence or absence on DNA blots of a series of genomic DNA samples extracted from infertile men with microscopically visible Yq11 deletions and rearrangements [4–6]. On this molecular level, for the first time, we observed some interstitial microdeletions in Yq11 when screening azoospermic men with a normal-looking Y chromosome and a normal 46,XY karyotype [7, 8]. At that time, interstitial microdeletions were already found in comparable dynamic chromosome regions of different autosomes [9]. This therefore raised the question of whether the genomic region(s) of this AZF locus could be better focussed when mapping the location of more interstitial microdeletions in Yq11 on the Y chromosome of azoospermic men with a normal karyotype (46,XY).

This became possible after more detailed molecular interval maps of the human Y chromosome could be generated using the novel PCR technology with specific primer pairs which generate numerous sequence tagged sites (STSs) along the complete human Y chromosome [10–12].

In the first large STS deletion screening study using the genomic DNA samples of 370 infertile men with idiopathic azoospermia – all with a normal 46,XY karyotype – numerous interstitial Yq11 microdeletions were revealed, especially in distal Yq11. Of greatest interest was the identification of 3 microdeletions which cluster with similar breakpoints in 3 distinct molecular intervals in Yq11 [13]. They were "de novo" mutation events, i.e., occurring only in the patients' Y chromosomes. Inspection of the testicular histology of these patients revealed disruption of their spermatogenesis at 3 distinct developmental phases. The 3 Yq11 microdeletions overlapped with the location of AZF in Yq11; they were tentatively coined "AZFa," "AZFb," and "AZFc," respectively. A complete Sertoli cell-only (SCO) syndrome was observed in all patients with deletion of the complete AZFa interval mapped in proximal Yq11 (Yq11.21). Only Sertoli cells, but no germ cells, were visible in the tubules of their testis tissue sections. Arrest at meiosis was observed in the testis tissue of all patients with deletion of the complete AZFb interval mapped distal to AZFa in Yq11.22. The populations of spermatogonia and primary spermatocytes in all testis tubules analysed were in the normal range; however, no postmeiotic germ cells were identified. A gradual inhibition of the postmeiotic spermatid maturation process with individually variable testicular pathologies was found in patients with the most frequently occurring AZFc deletions mapped in distal Yq11 (Yq11.23). In most tubules, only Sertoli cells were identified, but in some tubules germ cells of different developmental stages were clearly visible and the occurrence of mature sperm cells, albeit in a low number, was observed repeatedly. This testicular pathology has also been described as SCO type II, or mixed atrophy [14].

Some patients with a "de novo" AZFc deletion were still able to produce small numbers of mature sperm in their ejaculate (i.e., "severe oligozoospermia"), while some patients were found to have inherited their AZFc deletions from their fathers [15–18]. It could therefore be concluded that the primary pathology of an AZFc deletion is most likely not an SCO syndrome but hypospermatogenesis [13]. Some more interstitial Y deletions were found in and outside of AZFa, b, and c in Yq11, but most of them were also present on the father's Y chromosome [19]. This confirmed the presence of some polymorphic sequence regions in Yq11 as expected [2]. Polymorphic genomic mutations are, however, most likely not associated with the occurrence of azoospermia in these infertile patients.

The molecular complexity of the genomic structure in Yq11 and the functional gene content of each AZF microdeletion became established after knowledge of the complete genomic Y sequence in Yq11 [20]. Twenty-three Y genes expressed in human testis and located in 1 of the AZF deletion intervals were registered. These include 13 protein-coding genes specifically expressed in testicular tissue (5 single copy, 8 multicopy) and 10 so-called testis-specific transcript Y (*TTTY*) genes (5 single copy, 5 multicopy; Fig. 1). At that time (2003), the *TTTY* genes were considered to be non-functional, although these RNAs contained distinct exon structures and significant lengths of "open reading frames" for potential protein coding were reported [20].

The human Y chromosome that was first sequenced is now called the "reference sequence" (http://www.ncbi.nlm.nih.gov/nuccore/NC_000024.10). Today we know that it is only 1 of more than 1,200 distinct Y sequences now analysed. They are spread with different rates worldwide in all human populations [21]. The Y reference sequence originates from the donation of a genomic DNA sample by an anonymous man in California with an unknown fertility status and belongs to Y lineage R1* [22]. All Y lineages could be schematically ordered in 1 large pedigree due to distinct patterns of single nucleotide variations combined with distinct lengths of STR (small tandem repeat) blocks found along the genomic sequence of the short and long Y arm. This indicates that they have evolved from an ancient common ancestor and form stable "haplogroups" due to the lack of meiotic crossing over events between the X and Y chromosome during their continuous evolution in the different human population pedigrees [23–25].

Here we aim to update the reader on the functional complexity of the AZF locus in Yq11. We begin with a comprehensive description of its putatively germ line-specific dynamic chromosome structure probably supported by expression of at least some *TTTY* genes, followed by a critical description of putative function(s) of the single AZFa, AZFb, and AZFc genes proposed to be required for the human spermatogenesis process. For the latter purpose, some PCR multiplex assays were developed which allow the detection of any single AZF gene deletion and to distinguish distinct AZF breakpoint border regions found on the Y chromosome of infertile men with respectively complete and partial AZFa, AZFb, and AZFc deletions [26]. They have been composed according to the guidelines provided by the European Academy of Andrology (EAA) and the European Molecular Quality Network (EMQN; www.emqn.org), respectively.

Impairment of Dynamic Azoospermia Factor Chromosome Structure in Men with Infertility

It has been shown in mice that pairing of the sex chromosomes in premeiotic male germ cells is required for their further differentiation during meiosis and postmeiotic spermatid development [27]. It starts during the DNA replication phase with B spermatogonia increasing their nuclei and becomes visible by long chromosome threads in the leptotene phase of spermatocytes. During this process, the Y chromosome decondenses and starts to pair with the X chromosome at their DNA homologous sequence domains called pseudoautosomal regions (PARs). They are located at the tip of the short and long chromosome arms (XpYp: PAR1; XqYq: PAR2) and display a high recombination frequency [28]. In humans, pairing of both sex chromosomes proceeds in a gradient beyond the PARs, including eventually the complete short Y arm and at least the proximal part of Yq11 (Fig. 2a) [29, 30]. These extensive premeiotic X-Y paring structures, which were confirmed by different research groups, can explain why induction of a high frequency of double strand breaks required for subsequent XY chromosome pairing and recombination in PAR1 and PAR2 also extends into the neighbouring

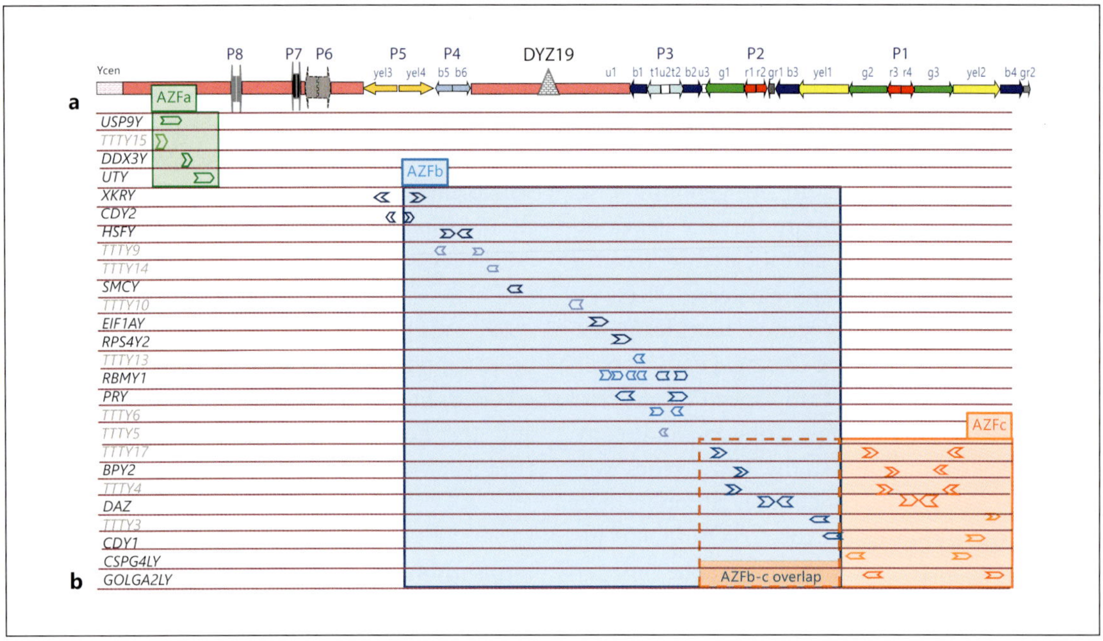

Fig. 1. a Schematic view of the euchromatic part of the long arm of the human Y chromosome (Yq11) using the colour code of Kuroda-Kawaguchi et al. [126]. Pink marks the Y sequence region still with visible homology to the X sequence. In AZFb it is split by DYZ19, a heterochromatic tandem repetitive sequence block of 400 kb. Yq11 is composed mainly by 8 palindromes (P1–P8) composed by large repetitive sequence blocks with high sequence homology (>99.7%), which are also called "amplicons" [126]. **b** The extension of the AZFa, AZFb, and overlapping AZFc deletion intervals are marked by distinct colours. The extension of the AZFb-c overlap is marked by a stippled box. Their gene content including the no protein-encoding *TTTY* gene copies are listed on the left and mapped in the AZF intervals according to their relative position, including their distinct polarities.

proximal non-homologous short Y arm [31]. It also explains the putative molecular origin of a number of distinct Xp-Yp translocations in mice and men, all causing male infertility.

In the late pachytene stage, the pairing structure of X and Y chromosomes then forms a compact chromatin structure also called the X-Y body [30], which is visible with a light microscope (Fig. 2b). The X-Y body displays no transcriptional activity and this meiotic sex chromosome inactivation (MSCI) is required for the subsequent meiotic division events [32]. Consequently, any disruption of this X-Y pairing gradient in male germ cells results in male infertility. Causative disrupting agents are mainly XY aneuploidies and structural rearrangements [33].

Recently, it has been proposed that distinct chromatin regions in Yq11 overlapping with the genomic AZFb and AZFc intervals might also be functional for this premeiotic X and Y chromosome pairing process. In premeiotic germ cells of azoospermic men with distinct AZF microdeletions, distortion of the X-Y pairing structure was observed with Y chromosomes containing AZFb [34] and AZFc microdeletions [35], and earlier with overlapping AZFb-c deletions [36]. AZFb deletions seem to interfere with the initiation of meiotic recombination [34, 36], whereas Y chromosomes with AZFc deletions displayed an extended zygotene stage and reduced condensation at pachytene [35]. These data suggest that meiotic arrest, the major testicular pathology of infertile

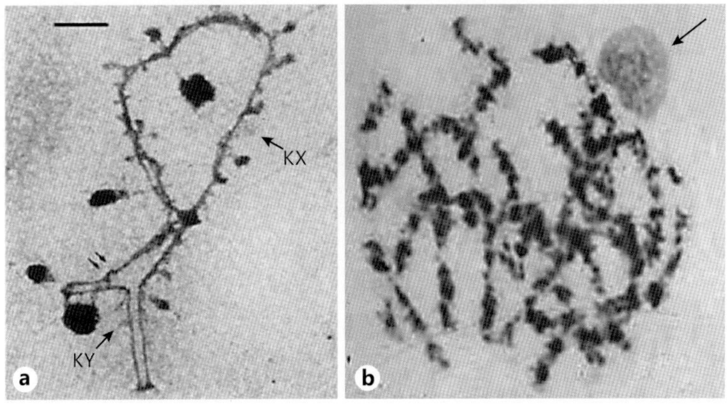

Fig. 2. Human X-Y pairing structures before (**a**) and at meiosis (**b**) according to the microscopic analysis of Solari [29] on meiotic chromosome spreads with the electron microscope (**a**) and light microscope (**b**). In the early pachytene phase (**a**), the X and Y chromosome axes can pair beyond their homologous sequence region called PAR1 and the Y centromere including at least part of the Y long arm. Scale bar, 1 μm. During the late pachytene phase (**b**), X and Y forms a compact chromatin structure, also called the X-Y body or, more commonly, "sex vesicle." However, note that this last term is wrong because no membranous vesicle is formed around the X-Y body in the spermatocyte nucleus.

men with complete AZFb deletion, might not be mainly caused by any AZFb gene deletion, but rather by deletion of a locus-specific and dynamic chromatin structure located in the genomic AZFb and AZFc region.

This would revitalise an old hypothesis on the germ line function of AZF proposed to include not only functional AZF proteins, but also a specific AZF chromatin folding code controlling the condensation cycle of the Y chromosome in the male germ line [37, 38]. Assemblies of tandem repetitive sequence blocks organised in large locus-specific repetitive sequence structures like those found in AZFb and AZFc (Fig. 1) should indeed be able to fold the underlying chromatin in locus-specific domains [39, 40].

Three large heterochromatic sequence blocks, DYZ17, DYZ18, and DYZ19, were mapped in Yq11 by sequence analyses [20]. Two border the euchromatic Yq11 long arm region distal to the centromere (DYZ17) and proximal to the large and polymorphic Yq12 heterochromatin block (DYZ18), respectively. DYZ19 is located in AZFb (Fig. 1) and occasionally visible under the microscope as the small G(iemsa) dense band – Yq11.22 – of human metaphase spreads. Whereas DYZ17 and DYZ18 are composed by multiple tandem repetitive GGAAT sequence units, DYZ19 contains 3,200 tandem repetitive copies of a basic 125-nt long sequence unit in a 400-kb long heterochromatic sequence block [20]. These heterochromatic sequence blocks can be considered as putative candidate regions for a specific chromatin folding code involved in the general decondensation process of the Y long arm during premeiotic male germ cell development [41].

However, nothing is yet known about a putative dynamic decondensation-condensation cycle of the DYZ17/DYZ18 chromatin structures, nor that of DYZ19 in AZFb during the X-Y pairing process. Neither has it been determined whether the compact DYZ19 chromatin structure in AZFb has some control function for the expression of the most neighboured AZFb protein-coding genes, *SMCY* and *EIF1AY*, respectively (Fig. 1). This has recently been shown for some polymorphic heterochromatic sequence blocks located on the Y chromosome of *Drosophila* controlling expression of the neighbouring Y-encoded protein genes expressed in male germ cells [42].

In proximal AZFb, we probably found another putative locus-specific chromatin structure in the b(lue)5 and b(lue)6 amplicons forming the P4 palindrome. Both amplicons contain significant homology regions to a germ cell-specific transcript (*dhMiF1*) expressed on the lampbrush loops of the Y chromosome of *D. hydei* and designated earlier as the pYH6 sequence family [43]. Their major sequence cluster (pY6H14, pYH34, pYH54, pYH64, pYH65) was found on both arms of the P4 palindrome [Keil et al., unpubl. data], which also include the protein-coding *HSFY* genes overlapping in their 3′UTR in antisense with the *TTTY9* gene copies (Fig. 1) also expressed only in male germ cells [44]. Most interestingly, the multicopy pY6H65 sequence in P4 was also found in the other b amplicons (b1-b4) in AZFb and AZFc, respectively, suggesting a common evolutionary origin [Emig and Vogt, in preparation]. Future experiments will now have to analyse the chromatin structure dynamic in these b amplicons especially in the P4 palindrome. Lange et al. [45] reported that the P4 palindrome might be a hotspot for breakage and structural rearrangements to form dicentric chromosome structures.

AZFa Locus and Gene Deletions and Male Infertility

The genomic extension of the AZFa locus in proximal Yq11 can be estimated by its conserved chromatin domain with the same gene order in mouse, cat, porcine, and non-human primates [46]. It extends about 1,150 kb and is bordered by STS sY85 and sY89 (12.526.311 nts: start of sY85 and 13.675.643 nts: end of sY89), respectively, according to the recent human Y chromosome sequence edition: NC000024.10. It includes 3 protein encoding genes, *DDX3Y*, *USP9Y*, *UTY*, and 1 of the testis-specific transcription units, *TTTY15* (Fig. 1).

An intrachromosomal recombination event between 2 homologous retroviral sequence blocks (HERV15yq1 and HERV15yq2) deletes 792 kb of this AZFa region [47–49]. No somatic pathology was observed in men with this large Y deletion; however, they had a severe testicular pathology. Men with AZFa deletion suffer from a complete germ cell aplasia, also called SCO syndrome. Consequently, it was proposed that at least 1 of the Y genes deleted in this genomic Y interval, *USP9Y*, *DDX3Y*, *TTTY15*, might already be involved in male germ cell development during early human embryogenesis. AZFa deletions are frequently observed in men with complete SCO syndrome (9–55%) [50–52].

To analyse which of the AZFa Y gene deletions is indeed associated with the observed severe testicular pathology, SCO patients with single gene "de novo" deletion events in AZFa would be most informative. The first "de novo" AZFa gene deletion was found with *USP9Y*. Its deletion was found to be associated with a postmeiotic disruption phase of spermatogenesis [53]. This was confirmed later by expression analysis of the USP9Y protein being predominantly in spermatids [46]. Natural transmission of some *USP9Y* mutations, including complete deletion in an Italian pedigree [54, 55], then revealed that disruption of the putative function of the *USP9Y* gene during the postmeiotic male germ cell development might not be essential for male fertility. Consequently, *USP9Y* could be excluded as a major *AZFa* gene, which is required to be functional during foetal germ cell development.

Single *DDX3Y* gene deletions were reported in some infertile men from northern Italy, and their testicular pathologies included the SCO syndrome [56]. Later observation of DDX3Y protein expression in foetal male germ cells revealed its initiation during the 17th gestation week [57]. After birth its expression was concentrated in the so-called Ap(ale) spermatogonia, and after puberty in the cytoplasm of Ap and Ad(ark) spermatogonia located at the basal membrane [57, 58].

In xenograft experiments within the mouse germ line transfected with human transgenes, including an active *DDX3Y* gene, it was recently shown that the DDX3Y protein in this germ line supports the maintenance and differentiation of the germ line spermatogonia stem cell fraction after puberty [59]. These experiments significantly support a function of *DDX3Y* in human male germ cells also after puberty. The molecular targets of DDX3Y in human spermatogonia are not yet known. It might be involved as translational control factor for other still unknown germ cell transcripts with extended and structural complex 5′UTRs. This conclusion could be drawn because it was found for all other RNA helicases of the DDX3 protein subfamily conserved from yeast to men [60].

One might thus predict that any AZFa deletion including the *DDX3Y* gene on the human Y chromosome will indeed cause an early disruption of human spermatogenesis, which finally results in the complete absence of germ cells in the testis tubules after puberty.

It remains an open question whether expression of the third AZFa gene, *UTY*, can interfere with the testicular phenotype of an AZFa deletion including only *USP9Y* and *DDX3Y*. UTY belongs to the large family of H3K27me2/3 histone demethylases with a JmjC domain, which are known to be involved in male germ cell development of the mouse (JMJD1A, also known as JHDM2A) [61, 62] and JMJD1C [63]. JMJD3, the third member of the UTX/UTY subfamily of JmjC domain-containing proteins (also called KDM6B), was found to be expressed in mouse spermatogonia stem cells [64]. We recently found a pattern of UTY expression in foetal male germ cells and after puberty in spermatogonia at the basal membrane, comparable with that of the DDX3Y protein [Vogt, in preparation]. It would therefore be interesting to analyse a putative functional interaction of both these AZFa proteins in the premeiotic human male germ cells.

AZFb Gene Deletions and Male Infertility

The molecular extension of complete AZFb deletions causing meiotic arrest were originally defined by absence of a set of genomic STS markers mapped schematically in linear order of a molecular deletion interval map [13]. Later sequence analysis revealed that the proximal border of this microdeletion was mainly located in a palindrome of 2 large repetitive sequence blocks with nearly identical sequence structures, coined P5 palindrome [65]. The distal border line was also found in a palindrome with 2 highly homologous 92-kb-long sequence blocks. This was embedded within a large repetitive sequence block called "yellow amplicon" located in the AZFc deletion interval (see the section relating to AZFc, below). It was designated P1.2 because the yellow amplicon was part of the large P1 palindrome in AZFc (Fig. 1); AZFb deletions thus overlap with AZFc deletions. In proximal AZFb, the break fusion events were proximally mapped 30 kb proximal to the centre of the P5 palindrome and distally 25 kb proximal to the centre of the P1.2 palindrome [65]. Small homologous sequence domains within these sequence regions suggest that AZFb deletions are caused by homologous recombination events like AZFa deletions. Classical AZFb deletions are therefore sometimes also designated as "P5/proximal-P1" or P5/P1.2 deletions [65]. However, non-homologous recombinations that also cause complete AZFb deletions and even larger microdeletions, additionally encompassing nearly the complete AZFc interval, have been identified [65]. The molecular extensions of these so-called AZFb+c deletions are not the sum of an AZFb and AZFc deletion, but are shorter because the distal breakpoints in AZFc are located in the short P1.1 palindrome embedded in the distal yellow amplicon in AZFc. Classical AZFc deletions end in the more distally located repetitive sequence block called "b(lue) 4" amplicon (Fig. 1).

Classical AZFb deletions caused by P5/P1.2 recombination encompass a 6.2-Mb-long genomic Y sequence including 6 protein-encoding Y genes, *EIFA1Y*, *HSFY* (2 functional copies), *PRY* (2 functional copies), *RBMY* (6 functional copies), *RPS4Y*, and *SMCY* (also known as *JARID1D* or *KDM5D*), which are deleted completely in patients with this Y chromosome aberration. Additionally, 1 copy of *CDY2* and *XKRY* is located in the proximal AZFb P5 palindrome, and copies of the AZFc gene families, *BPY1* (1 copy), *DAZ* (2 copies), and *CDY1* (1 copy), are in the distal overlapping AZFb/c interval. Complete AZFb deletions also include 9 Y genes of the *TTTY* class (Fig. 1).

It has not yet been clarified whether any of these AZFb genes are causative agents for the testicular pathology because disruption of the chromatin folding structure in AZFb might be already sufficient to cause meiotic arrest of the patients' germ cells (see the section on the AZF chromosome structure, above). To obtain a final answer to this basic question, PCR multiplex assays for diagnosing deletions of each single AZFb gene separately are obviously required [26, 66, 67].

This focus is feasible, especially in AZFb, because multiple genomic deletions were found in this genomic Y interval on the Y chromosome of infertile men which were significantly smaller than those of the "classical" AZFb and AZFc microdeletions that were described first [13]. Some of them were not associated with the infertility phenotype because they were also found as polymorphic length variants on the Y chromosome of fertile men from different populations [68]. Therefore, AZFb genes in these polymorphic AZFb subdomains could be excluded as causative agents for the meiotic arrest pathology. A short summary of single AZFb gene deletion results analysed so far is given here in alphabetical order.

EIF1AY protein expression was mainly found in the testis and ovary (http://www.genecards.org/). Like DDX3Y it is functional in the efficiency control of the ribosomal translation initiation process. However, single *EIF1AY* gene deletions associated with male infertility have not yet been found.

HSFY protein is expressed in many germ cells (spermatogonia, zygotic spermatocytes, elongated spermatids) and also in Sertoli cells [69]. Complete *HSFY* deletion (2 gene copies) were found to be inherited over many generations in some families with hypospermatogenesis in southern France [66]. They are therefore most likely not candidates for causing the major AZFb pathology (meiotic arrest).

PRY protein expression was found in spermatids and spermatozoa, and the PRY fraction positively staining spermatozoa increased from 1.5 to 51.2% in sperm samples with increased apoptotic DNA degradation [70]. This protein phosphatase is therefore assumed to be involved in the apoptotic degradation of non-functional spermatozoa. Since PRY protein was not detected in premeiotic germ cells, its contribution to the testicular pathology of men with AZFb deletion (meiotic arrest) is questionable. Single *PRY* gene deletions are difficult to identify [71]. The 2 functional gene copies have a high sequence homology because they are located in the P3 palindrome of AZFb (Fig. 1).

RBMY protein is expressed only in the male germ line and predominantly in premeiotic germ cells [72]. It probably provides spermatogonia and early spermatocytes with a germ cell-specific splicing cofactor interacting in a multiprotein complex with other splicing factors, such as 9G8, SRp20, SRp30c, and TRA-2β [72, 73]. It is interesting that its X homolog, RBMX, cannot functionally replace RBMY because only the RBMY RNA binding domain recognises stem-loop structures in RNAs with a $C^A/_UCAA$ consensus sequence [74]. It can therefore be assumed that the RBMY protein structure evolved from that of

RBMX by evolutionarily selection for a male germ line-specific splicing factor functional in human germ cells before meiosis [72]. Single *RBMY* gene deletions are difficult to assess because at least 6 functional gene copies are located in the P3 palindrome of AZFb near the *PRY* genes (Fig. 1).

RPS4Y2 is mainly expressed in testis tissue containing germ cells and in the prostate [75]. The gene evolved by duplication from *RPS4Y1* located on the short Y arm during primate evolution [76]. Single *RPS4Y2* gene deletions have not been found in infertile men. Whether and where the protein is required for human male germ cell development is therefore not yet known.

SMCY protein can form a complex with MSH5, a critical meiosis-regulatory protein, and immunohistochemical analyses with murine testicular tissue sections revealed co-localisation of both proteins at a specific meiotic stage of spermatogenesis [77]. Like RBMY, it can therefore be considered as a major candidate for causing the AZFb testicular pathology. However, *SMCY* (now designated *KDM5Y* because it is recognised as a functional histone demethylase) gene deletions have not yet been found in infertile men.

More informative in revealing the AZFb genes that cause meiotic arrest if disrupted has been the description of a "de novo" partial AZFb deletion on the Y chromosome of an infertile man in China who suffers from a severe oligoasthenoterato (OAT) syndrome [78]. It encompassed the complete deletion of *HSFY*, *SMCY*, *EIF1AY*, and *RPS4Y2*, but did not remove the *PRY* and *RBMY* gene copies, suggesting that only these 2 AZFb genes, but not *HSFY*, *SMCY*, *EIF1AY*, and *RPS4Y2* are required for meiotic human germ cell development.

The description of another partial AZFb deletion also found in an infertile patient with OAT syndrome excluded the *PRY* genes as major AZFb genes because this deletion was found to be inherited from father to son and included the complete P2 and P3 amplicon in the distal AZFb region with 2 *DAZ* gene copies, both functional *PRY* copies, and 4 *RBMY* gene copies [79]. This leaves the possibility of a major AZFb gene now only open for *RBMY*, since on the Y chromosome of this OAT patient 2 *RBMY* gene copies were still present [79].

The exclusion of *EIFA1Y*, *HSFY*, *RPS4Y*, and *SMCY* as major AZFb genes was confirmed by our own diagnostic experience in applying PCR multiplex AZF gene deletion assays. We found a partial AZFb deletion on the Y chromosome of a man with severe OAT syndrome, again encompassing *EIFA1Y*, *RPS4Y*, and *SMCY*, but no *RBMY* genes and only 1 copy of *PRY* [Vogt et al., in preparation]. Nevertheless, we cannot yet exclude that the Y genes deleted may contribute to the observed aberrant OAT sperm phenotype of these patients.

More partial AZFb deletions associated with variable testicular histologies but not meiotic arrest and with distal breakpoints concentrated in the overlapping genomic AZFb-AZFc interval have been described in the literature [80–82]. Unfortunately, most of them did not address the basic question of whether the observed partial AZFb microdeletion was "de novo," and thus only found on the patients' Y chromosomes, or polymorphic because it was also found on the Y chromosomes of their fertile fathers. Nevertheless, no partial AZFb deletion was identified with complete deletion of all *RBMY* gene copies and a testicular pathology less severe than meiotic arrest.

We can thus surmise that only the *RBMY* gene family might have an essential function during meiosis for the human male germ cell. It probably controls some germ cell-specific splicing processes of transcripts occurring in germ cells predominantly before meiosis and required for the meiotic cell divisions. Moreover, partial *RBMY* gene deletion might be associated with the OAT syndrome (see above) because expression of the RBMY protein was also found in postmeiotic round and elongating spermatids and in the midpiece region of sperm [83].

In this context, it is worthwhile reporting the exceptional case of an infertile man with complete

AZFb+c deletion but with a testicular histology usually only found in patients with partial AZFb or AZFc deletions, since the postmeiotic marker genes, *PRM1* and *TNP1*, were found to be expressed and the patient produced a low number of mature sperm [84]. The haplogroup of this Y chromosome derived from the Y-L* lineage, which is rare in Western Europe and North American male populations, but predominant in Asia, Pakistan, and India. The authors therefore assume that some genetic modifier(s) must be present on the Y chromosome of this man or on other chromosomes supporting the meiotic pairing process in the patient's spermatocytes, and thereby probably replacing any functional requirement for an intact genomic AZFb region with some *RBMY* genes.

Based on this overview, we can assume that the genomic Y region encompassed by the AZFb microdeletion in the Y reference sequence with haplogroup R1* might be highly variable on the Y chromosomes derived from other Y lineages located predominantly only in Africa, Asia, or Australia, as already suggested earlier by Jobling et al. [68]. Indeed, some hot-spot regions for polymorphic Y chromosomal breaks and rearrangements were found especially in distal AZFb near the *PRY* and *RBMY* gene copies in or near the P3 palindrome. They result in a number of complete *PRY* deletions and partial *RBMY* gene copy deletions, which looks to be compatible with normal male fertility [85].

In summary, it might therefore be possible that the major testicular pathology, complete meiotic arrest, found in infertile patients with complete AZFb microdeletion is based primarily on the disruption of some specific chromatin structure in AZFb extending at this phase of male germ cell development to arrange a proper start of the premeiotic X-Y pairing structure. Expression of the germ cell-specific splicing factors encoded by the *RBMY* gene family during the same germ line phase might not be required for the subsequent meiotic cell divisions, but probably are functional by supporting the efficiency of this process.

AZFc Gene Deletions and Male Infertility

Similar considerations might help to reveal the functional contribution of the polymorphic gene content of the genomic AZFc region, sometimes inherited from fathers to sons [15, 16]. Complete AZFc microdeletions were found with high frequency (5–15%), however, only in genomic DNA samples of infertile men with a severe reduction in sperm number (<10 million per mL ejaculate) and including the OAT syndrome [22, 86–88]. These studies clearly show that complete AZFc deletions interfere with the spermatogenic maturation process, reducing its efficiency and causing hypospermatogenesis as the primary mutation effect. Age-dependent secondary mutation effects might – but must not – eventually cause a complete absence of mature spermatozoa (i.e., azoospermia) in the man's semen fluid [13, 88].

This raised similar questions to those concerning the AZFb genes – which AZFc gene, if any, is functionally required for human male germ cell development, and do AZFc genes only improve the efficiency of this complex cellular differentiation process?

All AZFc gene families are composed by more than 1 gene copy, and partial AZFc deletions reducing the copy number were also found in fertile men. It has been shown that the impact of any partial AZFc deletion on the efficiency of the spermatogenic process mainly depends on the patient's Y chromosomal haplogroup [86, 89–91]. The frequency of the different Y haplogroups found in a given human population might therefore be the result of a balancing selection aimed to optimise the male fertility function of the Y chromosomal AZF locus in each population, thus driving male reproductive fitness [92, 93]. The observed genomic deletion and amplification mechanisms in the locus-specific repetitive sequence blocks on the short and long arm of the Y chromosome in men, which create large palindromes, might be considered as efficient driving tools [94, 95].

The most prominent partial AZFc deletions became the so-called gr-gr deletions, meaning any partial AZFc deletion caused by recombination within the 3 green, g1, g2, g3, and 4 red, r1, r2, r3, r4, amplicons in AZFc [22, 98]. At least 14 independent recombination events in these amplicons have already been found in distinct Y lineages. Some seem to cause male infertility, while some do not [22, 96, 97]. It is therefore surprising that clinical protocols aimed to reveal a gr-gr recombination events interfering with patient fertility only use 1 STS marker (sY1291). This sY marker is located at the red2-grey1 border site [22, 98] and always deleted in men with a gr-gr partial AZFc deletion independent from his fertility status.

Another popular approach to distinguishing the heterogeneity of gr-gr recombinations in AZFc is the numbering of FISH signals specifically marking the number of green and red amplicons on the Y chromosome in the lymphocyte nuclei with green and red fluorescent spots visible under the microscope [98]. However, the large heterogeneity of recombination sites in the red and green amplicons now found on the Y chromosome of fertile men and infertile men in different human populations cannot be resolved with this diagnostic tool, but only by sequence analyses [99–101].

It has been shown that complete AZFc microdeletions do not interfere with the premeiotic male germ cell development; numbers of spermatogonia and spermatocytes in the testis tubules are comparable to those of fertile men [102]. It can therefore be concluded that expression of any AZFc gene is only required during the postmeiotic spermatid maturation process. In a population-based survey of 20,000 Y chromosomes derived from fertile and infertile men with different Y haplogroups it has been recently shown that the risk for male infertility increased 145-fold in men with complete AZFc microdeletion, whereas partial AZFc deletions designated gr-gr, b1-b3, and b2-b3, respectively, would only double the infertility risk depending on the Y haplogroup [101]. Similar results were previously found in a study of partial AZFc deletions in fertile and infertile men in Portugal [103], China [104], and France [105]. However, there might be some exceptions since another study in China claimed that b2-b3 partial AZFc deletions show a higher risk for spermatogenic failure than complete AZFc microdeletions [106], and a study in Italy claimed that gr-gr deletions in AZFc are significantly increased in men with a lower sperm count [107].

Most AZF deletion studies do not answer the question of whether the partial AZFc microdeletion identified has occurred "de novo," i.e., is present only on the patient's Y chromosome or is also present on the Y chromosome of the father or other fertile male family members. Therefore, it is difficult to assess which of these partial AZFc microdeletions diagnosed by the presence or absence of a couple of STS and single nucleotide variation markers has an impact on the clinical observed phenotype of the patient's infertility. Since no study has described the exact break-fusion sequence of the proposed ampliconic recombination site, the question remains open regarding which of the AZFc genes, when expressed in the testis tubules, is really functionally required for the development of the human postmeiotic male germ cells. It would be most interesting in this context to reveal some spermatogenic impairment associated with failure of expression of the *BPY2, CDY1*, and *DAZ* gene copies in the postmeiotic germ cells of these patients, since these genes are known to be expressed during spermatid maturation and in mature sperm.

The *BPY2* gene family contains 3 gene copies (*BPY2.1–3*) with an identical exon structure and were mapped to the green amplicons (g1–g3) in distal Yq11 (Fig. 1). They have evolved only recently during primate evolution and encode a basic protein of 13.9 kDa, found after meiosis in the nuclei of round spermatids and sperm [108]. It was therefore suggested that these basic proteins are functionally important for maintaining the sperm fertilisation capacity. This view gains support through a specific interaction of BPY2 protein with UBE3A, a ubiquitin protein ligase [109], and with VCY2IP-1 associated with the sperm tail microtubules [110].

The *CDY* genes (2 copies in AZFc in the yellow amplicons) were also shown to be expressed only in testis tissue and expression of the protein was mainly observed in spermatids [111]. CDY proteins are functionally histone acetyltransferases with a strong preference for histone H4 localised in the nuclei of maturing spermatids. This suggests that they functionally contribute to the specific histone hyperacetylation process in late spermatids, resulting in a more open chromatin structure, which is required to facilitate the spermatogenic histone replacement by transition proteins and protamines.

The number of *DAZ* gene copies in the red amplicons in AZFc can change between 2 and 8 copies on the Y chromosome of fertile men depending on the Y lineage [98, 112, 113]. Their exon structures are variable, especially in the number of their exon 7 variants, which are also called "DAZ repeats" [99, 114, 115]. DAZ repeats are known to be important RNA binding partners [116]. All *DAZ* gene copies present in the AZFc region were shown to become translated, forming a pattern of polymorphic protein variants expressed in the postmeiotic human male germ cells [117]. Alternative splicing of distinct *DAZ* transcripts can additionally increase the number of polymorphic DAZ proteins.

The most prominent DAZ protein interacting partner with a putative function in the postmeiotic male germ cells might be the DAZAP1 protein first expressed in midpachytene spermatocytes then in round and elongated spermatids shuttling between the nucleus and cytoplasm during postmeiotic germ cell maturation [118]. Since this protein specifically recognises the DAZ repeat (i.e., variable number of exon 7 sequence variants) encoded peptide region [116], its binding potential can be efficiently modulated by the number of DAZ repeat copies in each DAZ protein variant expressed after meiosis. In mice, DAZAP1 controls the postmeiotic splicing efficiency of CREM, CRISP2, and POT1a transcripts in germ cells [119]. However, DAZ proteins are absent in mice because the AZFc locus evolved on the Y chromosome first during primate evolution.

It is therefore most likely that the genomic Y region containing AZFc and its *DAZ* gene family in humans evolved and became established on the Y chromosome during a consecutive duplication-diversification process from their autosomal ancestors, *DAZL* on chromosome 3 and *BOLL* (also known as *BOULE*) on chromosome 2 [120], thereby extending and/or improving their functional profile in the male germ cells. Expression of BOLL and DAZL proteins was mainly found in germ cells before meiosis [121], whereas DAZ proteins were mainly expressed during the postmeiotic germ cell phase in late spermatids and spermatozoa [122].

Considering the great heterogeneity of *DAZ* gene deletions in fertile and infertile men (see above), we assume that DAZ proteins are not essential for the terminal differentiation process of male germ cells, but may be required for their optimal function. In immunostaining experiments using antibodies probably specific for DAZ2, we found DAZ immunoreactivity in the innermost layer of the mature sperm cell epithelium, preferentially in their so-called residual bodies immediately prior to spermiation and in the tails of ejaculated spermatozoa [122]. From these findings, we can deduce a function for DAZ proteins in the RNA metabolism of late spermatids, presumably in the storage or transport of testis-specific mRNAs, the translation of which is repressed until the formation of mature spermatozoa.

Functional Aspects of the Testis-Specific *LNC* Transcripts (*TTTY*) in AZFa, AZFb, and AZFc

Sequence analysis of the human Y reference sequence also revealed a number of Y genes in the 3 AZF regions which are expressed only in testis tissue but supposed to have no protein-encoding potential, despite containing longer open reading frames [20]. They were designated as testis transcript unit Y (*TTTY*) genes and can be classified as belonging to the long non-coding (*LNC*) transcript genes. Thirteen *TTTY* genes were single copy, 12

TTTY genes were probably duplicated due to their location in palindromes; 2 *TTTY* genes, *TTTY4* and *TTTY17*, had 3 copies. The map of those located in AZFa, AZFb, and AZFc is shown in Figure 1. In AZFc, we discovered by sequence comparison that *TTTY4* and *TTTY17* were both derived from ancient tandem repetitive sequence units related to the β-satellite sequence family. Interestingly, their exon structures could be compared to that of the embedded *BPY2* genes, suggesting an evolutionary pathway for development of the protein-encoding *BPY2* genes from an ancient β-satellite sequence unit on the Y chromosome of primates with development of the flanking *TTTY4* and *TTTY17* structures as stable intermediates.

One way to reveal a potential protein-coding potential in *LNC* genes would be inspection for the presence of some known functional protein domains in the open reading frames identified using the Prosite database (http://prosite.expasy.org/). Until now, we were not able to mark any functional protein domain in the exon structures of *TTTY* transcripts located in AZFb and/or AZFc.

The function of *TTTY* gene expression during human spermatogenesis might therefore be on the transcript level, like many other *LNC* genes with tissue-specific transcripts now mapped to the X chromosome and the autosomes [123]. Accordingly, *TTTY* transcription might be involved in opening and extending the AZFb chromatin structure during the premeiotic X-Y pairing process (see the above section relating to AZF chromosomes). An enhancer function of a testis-specific long non-coding RNA expressed only in mouse spermatocytes was recently found 3.4 kb upstream of the mouse testicular cell adhesion molecule1 (*Tcam1*) gene [124]. Major candidates in AZFb would be the *TTTY9* copies in the P4 palindrome overlapping the distal part of the *HSFY* genes in opposite polarity, *TTTY5*, *TTTY6*, *and TTTY13*, in the P3 palindrome embedded in the *RBMY* and *PRY* gene copies, and *TTTY4* and *TTTY17* flanking the *BPY2* gene copies (Fig. 1). *TTTY13* transcription might also contribute to the observed instability of the human Y chromosome only in the P3 palindrome [45] because its transcription seems to be controlled by HERV (human endogenous retroviral)-related sequence domains belonging to the HERV-K14C sequence family [125].

References

1 Tiepolo L, Zuffardi O: Localization of factors controlling spermatogenesis in the nonfluorescent portion of the human Y chromosome long arm. Hum Genet 1976;34:119–124.

2 Unnérus V, Fellmann J, de la Chapelle A: The length of the human Y chromosome. Cytogenet 1967;6:213–227.

3 Vogt P, Keil R, Kirsch S: The AZF-function of the human Y chromosome during spermatogenesis; in Chandley AC, Summer A (eds): Chromosomes Today. London, Chapman & Hall, 1993, vol 11, pp 227–239.

4 Vergnaud G, Page DC, Simmler MC, Brown L, Rouyer F, Noel B, Botstein D, de la Chapelle A, Weissenbach J: A deletion map of the human Y chromosome based on DNA hybridization. Am J Hum Genet 1986;38:109–124.

5 Bardoni B, Zuffardi O, Guioli S, Ballabio A, Simi P, Cavalli P, Grimoldi MG, Fraccaro M, Camerino G: A deletion map of the human Yq11 region: implications for the evolution of the Y chromosome and tentative mapping of a locus involved in spermatogenesis. Genomics 1991;11:443–451.

6 O'Reilly AJ, Affara NA, Simpson E, Chandler P, Goulmy E, Ferguson-Smith MA: A molecular deletion map of the Y chromosome long arm defining X and autosomal homologous regions and the localisation of the HYA locus to the proximal region of the Yq euchromatin. Hum Mol Genet 1992;1:379–385.

7 Ma K, Sharkey A, Kirsch S, et al: Towards the molecular localisation of the AZF locus: mapping of microdeletions in azoospermic men within 14 subintervals of interval 6 of the human Y chromosome. Hum Mol Genet 1992;1:29–33.

8 Vogt P, Chandley AC, Hargreave TB, et al: Microdeletions in interval 6 of the Y chromosome of males with idiopathic sterility point to disruption of AZF, a human spermatogenesis gene. Hum Genet 1992;89:491–496.

9 Schinzel A: Microdeletion syndromes, balanced translocations, and gene mapping. J Med Genet 1988;25:454–462.

10 Vollrath D, Foote S, Hilton A, et al: The human Y chromosome: a 43-interval map based on naturally occurring deletions. Science 1992;258:52–59.

11 Kirsch S, Keil R, Edelmann A, et al: Molecular analysis of the genomic structure of the human Y chromosome in the euchromatic part of its long arm (Yq11). Cytogen Cell Genet 1996;75:197–206.
12 Najmabadi H, Huang V, Yen P, Subbarao MN, Bhasin D, Banaag L, Naseeruddin S, de Kretser DM, Baker HW, McLachlan RI, et al: Substantial prevalence of microdeletions of the Y-chromosome in infertile men with idiopathic azoospermia and oligozoospermia detected using a sequence-tagged site-based mapping strategy. J Clin Endocrinol Metab 1996;81:1347–1352.
13 Vogt PH, Edelmann A, Kirsch S, et al: Human Y chromosome azoospermia factors (AZF) mapped to different subregions in Yq11. Hum Mol Gent 1996;5: 933–943.
14 Luetjens CM, Gromoll J, Engelhardt M, von Eckardstein S, Bergmann M, Nieschlag E, Simoni M: Manifestation of Y-chromosomal deletions in the human testis: a morphometrical and immunohistochemical evaluation. Hum Reprod 2002;17:2258–2266.
15 Calogero AE, Garofalo MR, Barone N, Longo GA, De Palma A, Fichera M, Rappazzo G, D'Agata R, Vicari E: Spontaneous transmission from a father to his son of a Y chromosome microdeletion involving the deleted in azoospermia (DAZ) gene. J Endocrinol Invest 2002; 25:631–634.
16 Kühnert B, Gromoll J, Kostova E, Tschanter P, Luetjens CM, Simoni M, Nieschlag E: Case report: natural transmission of an AZFc Y-chromosomal microdeletion from father to his sons, Hum Reprod 2004;19:886–888.
17 Zhu XB, Liu YL, Zhang W, Ping P, Cao XR, Liu Y, Huang YR, Li Z: Vertical transmission of the Yq AZFc microdeletion from father to son over two or three generations in infertile Han Chinese families. Asian J Androl 2010;12:240–246.
18 Li LL, Zhu YZ, Yu XW, Wang RX, Hu ZM, Liu RZ: Pedigrees of infertile Chinese men with Y chromosome microdeletions derived from natural transmission and de novo mutation. Genet Mol Res 2015;4:1932–1941.
19 Pryor JL, Kent-First M, Muallem A, Van Bergen AH, Nolten WE, Meisner L, Roberts KP: Microdeletions in the Y chromosome of infertile men. N Engl J Med 1997;20:534–539.
20 Skaletsky H, Kuroda-Kawaguchi T, Minx PJ, et al: The male-specific region of the human Y chromosome is a mosaic of discrete sequence classes. Nature 2003;423:825–837.
21 Poznik GD, Xue Y, Mendez FL, et al: Punctuated bursts in human male demography inferred from 1,244 worldwide Y-chromosome sequences. Nat Genet 2016;48:593–599.
22 Vogt PH: AZF deletions and Y chromosomal haplogroups: history and update based on sequence. Hum Reprod Update 2005;11:319–336.
23 The Y Chromosome Consortium: A nomenclature system for the tree of human Y-chromosomal binary haplogroups. Genome Res 2002;12:339–348.
24 Hallast P, Batini C, Zadik D, et al: The Y-chromosome tree bursts into leaf: 13,000 high-confidence SNPs covering the majority of known clades. Mol Biol Evol 2015;32:661–673.
25 Jobling MA, Tyler-Smith C: Human Y chromosome variation in the genome-sequencimg era. Nat Rev Genet 2017;18: 485–497.
26 Vogt PH, Bender U: Human Y chromosome microdeletion analysis by PCR multiplex protocols identifying only clinically relevant AZF microdeletions; in Carrell DT, Aston KI (eds): Spermatogenesis: Methods and Protocols. New York, Humana Press, 2013, pp 187–204.
27 Burgoyne PS, Mahadevaiah SK, Sutcliffe MJ, Palmer SJ: Fertility in mice requires X-Y pairing and a Y-chromosomal "spermiogenesis" gene mapping to the long arm. Cell 1992;11:391–398.
28 Kauppi L, Barchi M, Baudat F, Romanienko PJ, Keeney S, Jasin M: Distinct properties of the XY pseudoautosomal region crucial for male meiosis. Science 2011;331:916–920.
29 Solari AJ: The behavior of the XY pair in mammals. Int Rev Cytol 1974;38:273–317.
30 Solari AJ: Synaptic behaviour and recombination nodules in the human XY pair. Genetica 1988;77:149–158.
31 Decarpentrie F, Ojarikre OA, Mitchell MJ, Burgoyne PS: Recombination between the mouse Y chromosome short arm and an additional Y short arm-derived chromosomal segment attached distal to the X chromosome PAR. Chromosoma 2016;125:177–188.
32 Royo H, Polikiewicz G, Mahadevaiah SK, Prosser H, Mitchell M, Bradley A, de Rooij DG, Burgoyne PS, Turner JM: Evidence that meiotic sex chromosome inactivation is essential for male fertility. Curr Biol 2010;20:2117–2123.
33 Mohandas TK, Speed RM, Passage MB, Yen PH, Chandley AC, Shapiro LJ: Role of the pseudoautosomal region in sex-chromosome pairing during male meiosis: meiotic studies in a man with a deletion of distal Xp. Am J Hum Genet 1992; 51:526–533.
34 Perrin J, Metzler-Guillemain C, Karsenty G, Grillo JM, Mitchell MJ, Guichaoua MR: Meiotic arrest at the midpachytene stage in a patient with complete azoospermia factor b deletion of the Y chromosome. Fertil Steril 2006;85:494.e5–e8.
35 Geoffroy-Siraudin C, Aknin-Seiffer I, Metzler-Guillemain C, Ghalamoun-Slaimi R, Bonzi MF, Levy R, Guichaoua MR: Meiotic abnormalities in patients bearing complete AZFc deletion of Y chromosome. Hum Reprod 2007;22: 1567–1572.
36 Yogev L, Segal S, Zeharia E, Gamzu R, Maymon BB, Paz G, Botchan A, Hauser R, Yavetz H, Kleiman SE: Sex chromosome alignment at meiosis of azoospermic men with azoospermia factor microdeletion. J Androl 2004;25:110–116.
37 Armstrong SJ, Kirkham AJ, Hulten MA: XY chromosome behaviour in the germ-line of the human male: a FISH analysis of spatial orientation, chromatin condensation and pairing. Chromosome Res 1994;2:445–452.
38 Vogt PH, Edelmann A, Hirschmann P, et al: The azoospermia factor (AZF) of the human Y chromosome in Yq11: function and analysis in spermatogenesis. Reprod Fertil Dev 1995;7:685–693.
39 Vogt P: Potential genetic functions of tandem repeated DNA sequence blocks in the human genome are based on a highly conserved "chromatin folding code." Hum Genet 1990;84:301–336.
40 Vogt P: Code domains in tandem repetitive DNA sequence structures. Chromosoma 1992;101:585–589.
41 Speed RM, Vogt P, Kohler MR, et al: Chromatin condensation behaviour of the Y chromosome in the human testis. I. Evidence for decondensation of distal Yq in germ cells prior to puberty with a switch to Sertoli cells in adults. Chromosoma 1993;102:421–427.

42 Branco AT, Tao Y, Hartl DL, Lemos B: Natural variation of the Y chromosome suppresses sex ratio distortion and modulates testis-specific gene expression in *Drosophila simulans*. Heredity 2013; 111:8–15.

43 Vogt P, Keil R, Köhler M, Lengauer C, Lewe D, Lewe G: Selection of DNA sequences from interval 6 of the human Y chromosome with homology to a Y chromosomal fertility gene sequence of *Drosophila hydei*. Hum Genet 1991;86: 341–349.

44 Vogt PH, Falcao CL, Hanstein R, Zimmer J: The AZF proteins. Int J Androl 2008;31:383–394.

45 Lange J, Skaletsky H, van Daalen SK, Embry SL, Korver CM, Brown LG, Oates RD, Silber S, Repping S, Page DC: Isodicentric Y chromosomes and sex disorders as byproducts of homologous recombination that maintains palindromes. Cell 2009;138:855–869.

46 Vogt PH, Ditton HJ, Kamp C, Zimmer J: Structure and function of AZFa locus in human spermatogenesis; in Lau YFC, Chan WY (eds): The Y Chromosome and Male Germ Cell Biology in Health and Diseases. Hackensack, World Scientific, 2007, pp 91–125.

47 Blanco P, Shlumukova M, Sargent CA, et al: Divergent outcomes of intrachromosomal recombination on the human Y chromosome: male infertility and recurrent polymorphism. J Med Genet 2000; 37:752–758.

48 Kamp C, Hirschmann P, Voss H, et al: Two long homologous retroviral sequence blocks in proximal Yq11 cause AZFa microdeletions as a result of intrachromosomal recombination events. Hum Mol Genet 2000;9:2563–2572.

49 Sun C, Skaletsky H, Rozen S, et al: Deletion of azoospermia factor a (AZFa) region of human Y chromosome caused by recombination between HERV15 proviruses. Hum Mol Genet 2000;9: 2291–2296.

50 Foresta C, Ferlin A, Garolla A, Moro E, Pistorello M, Barbaux S, Rossato M: High frequency of well-defined Y-chromosome deletions in idiopathic Sertoli cell-only syndrome. Hum Reprod 1998; 13:302–307.

51 Blagosklonova O, Fellmann F, Clavequin MC, Roux C, Bresson JL: AZFa deletion in Sertoli cell-only syndrome: a retrospective study. Mol Hum Reprod 2000; 6:795–799.

52 Kamp C, Huellen K, Fernandes S, Sousa M, Schlegel PN, Mielnik A, Kleiman S, Yavetz H, Krause W, Kupker W, Johannisson R, Schulze W, Weidner W, Barros A, Vogt PH: High deletion frequency of the complete AZFa sequence in men with Sertoli-cell-only syndrome. Mol Hum Reprod 2001;7:987–994.

53 Qureshi SJ, Ross AR, Ma K, Cooke HJ, Intyre MA, Chandley AC, Hargreave TB: Polymerase chain reaction screening for Y chromosome microdeletions: a first step towards the diagnosis of genetically-determined spermatogenic failure in men. Mol Hum Reprod 1996;2:775–779.

54 Krausz C, Degl'Innocenti S, Nuti F, et al: Natural transmission of USP9Y gene mutations: a new perspective on the role of AZFa genes in male fertility. Hum Mol Genet 2006;15:2673–2681.

55 Luddi A, Margollicci M, Gambera L, et al: Spermatogenesis in a man with complete deletion of *USP9Y*. N Engl J Med 2009;360:881–885.

56 Foresta C, Ferlin A, Moro E: Deletion and expression analysis of AZFa genes on the human Y chromosome revealed a major role for DBY in male infertility. Hum Mol Genet 2000;9:1161–1169.

57 Gueler B, Sonne SB, Zimmer J, Hilscher B, Hilscher W, Graem N, Rajpert-De Meyts E, Vogt PH: AZFa protein DDX3Y is differentially expressed in male germ cells during development and in testicular tumours: new evidence for phenotypic plasticity of germ cells. Hum Reprod 2012;27:1547–1555.

58 Ditton HJ, Zimmer J, Kamp C, Rajpert-De Meyts E, Vogt PH: The *AZFa* gene DBY (*DDX3Y*) is widely transcribed but the protein is limited to the male germ cells by translation control. Hum Mol Genet 2004;13:2333–2341.

59 Ramathal C, Angulo B, Sukhwani M, Cui J, Durruthy-Durruthy J, Fang F, Schanes P, Turek PJ, Orwig KE, Reijo Pera R: *DDX3Y* gene rescue of a Y chromosome *AZFa* deletion restores germ cell formation and transcriptional programs. Sci Rep 2015;5:15041.

60 Sharma D, Jankowsky E: The Ded1/DDX3 subfamily of DEAD-box RNA helicases. Crit Rev Biochem Mol Biol 2014;49:343–360.

61 Okada Y, Scott G, Ray MK, Mishina Y, Zhang Y: Histone demethylase JHDM2A is critical for *Tnp1* and *Prm1* transcription and spermatogenesis. Nature 2007; 450:119–123.

62 Liu Z, Zhou S, Liao L, Chen X, Meistrich M, Xu J: Jmjd1a demethylase-regulated histone modification is essential for cAMP-response element modulator-regulated gene expression and spermatogenesis. J Biol Chem 2010;285:2758–2770.

63 Kuroki S, Akiyoshi M, Tokura M, Miyachi H, Nakai Y, Kimura H, Shinkai Y, Tachibana M: JMJD1C, a JmjC domain-containing protein, is required for long-term maintenance of male germ cells in mice. Biol Reprod 2013;93:1–9.

64 Iwamori N, Iwamori T, Matzuk MM: H3K27 demethylase, JMJD3, regulates fragmentation of spermatogonial cysts. PLoS One 2013;8:e72689.

65 Repping S, Skaletsky H, Lange J, Silber S, Van der Veen F, Oates RD, Page DC, Rozen S: Recombination between palindromes P5 and P1 on the human Y chromosome causes massive deletions and spermatogenic failure. Am J Hum Genet 2002;71:906–922.

66 Kichine E, Rozé V, Di Cristofaro J, Taulier D, Navarro A, Streichemberger E, Decarpentrie F, Metzler-Guillemain C, Lévy N, Chiaroni J, Paquis-Flucklinger V, Fellmann F, Mitchell MJ: *HSFY* genes and the *P4* palindrome in the *AZFb* interval of the human Y chromosome are not required for spermatocyte maturation. Hum Reprod 2012;27:615–624.

67 Alechine E, Corach D: High-throughput screening for spermatogenesis candidate genes in the AZFc region of the Y chromosome by multiplex real time PCR followed by high resolution melting analysis. PLoS One 2014;9:e97227.

68 Jobling MA, Samara V, Pandya A, Fretwell N, Bernasconi B, Mitchell RJ, Gerelsaikhan T, Dashnyam B, Sajantila A, Salo PJ, et al: Recurrent duplication and deletion polymorphisms on the long arm of the Y chromosome in normal males. Hum Mol Genet 1996;5:1767–1775.

69 Shinka T, Sato Y, Chen G, Naroda T, Kioshita K, Unemi Y, Tsujy K, Toida K, Iwamoto T, Nakahori Y: Molecular characterization of heat shock-like factor encoded on the human Y chromosome, and implications for male infertility. Biol Reprod 2003;71:297–306.

70 Stouffs K, Lissens W, Verheyen G, Van Landuyt L, Goossens A, Tournaye H, van Steirteghem A, Liebaers I: Expression pattern of the Y-linked PRY gene suggests a function in apoptosis but not in spermatogenesis. Mol Hum Reprod 2004;10:15–21.

71 Stouffs K, Lissens W, Van Landuyt L, Tournaye H, van Steirteghem A, Liebaers I: Characterization of the genomic organization, localization and expression of four PRY genes (PRY1, PRY2 and PRY4). Mol Hum Reprod 2001;7:603–610.
72 Elliott DJ: The role of potential splicing factors including RBMY, RBMX, hnRNPG-T and SSTAR proteins in spermatogenesis. Int J Androl 2004;27:328–334.
73 Dreumont N, Bourgeois CF, Lejeune F, Liu Y, Ehrmann IE, Elliott DJ, Stévenin J: Human RBMY regulates germline-specific splicing events by modulating the function of the serine/arginine-rich proteins 9G8 and Tra2-β. J Cell Sci 2010;123:40–50.
74 Skrisovska L, Bourgeois CF, Stefl R, Grellscheid SN, Kister L, Wenter P, Elliott DJ, Stevenin J, Allain FH: The testis-specific human protein RBMY recognizes RNA through a novel mode of interaction. EMBO Rep 2007;8:372–379.
75 Lopes AM, Miguel RN, Sargent CA, Ellis PJ, Amorim A, Affara NA: The human RPS4 paralogue on Yq11.223 encodes a structurally conserved ribosomal protein and is preferentially expressed during spermatogenesis. BMC Mol Biol 2010;11:33.
76 Andrés O, Kellermann T, López-Giráldez F, Rozas J, Domingo-Roura X, Bosch M: *RPS4Y* gene family evolution in primates. BMC Evol Biol 2008;142:1–12.
77 Akimoto C, Kitagawa H, Matsumoto T, Kato S: Spermatogenesis-specific association of SMCY and MSH5. Genes Cells 2008;13:623–633.
78 Shi YC, Cui YX, Zhou YC, Wei L, Jiang HT, Xia XY, Lu HY, Wang HY, Shang XJ, Zhu WM, Li XJ, Huang YF: A rare Y chromosome constitutional rearrangement: a partial AZFb deletion and duplication within chromosome Yp in an infertile man with severe oligoasthenoteratozoospermia. Int J Androl 2011;34:461–469.
79 Plotton I, Ducros C, Pugeat M, Morel Y, Lejeune H: Transmissible microdeletion of the Y-chromosome encompassing two DAZ copies, four RBMY1 copies, and both PRY copies. Fertil Steril 2010;94:2770.e11–e16.
80 Ferlin A, Moro E, Rossi A, Dallapiccola B, Foresta C: The human Y chromosome's azoospermia factor b (AZFb) region: sequence, structure, and deletion analysis in infertile men. J Med Genet 2003;40:18–24.
81 Costa P, Gonçalves R, Ferrás C, Fernandes S, Fernandes AT, Sousa M, Barros A: Identification of new breakpoints in AZFb and AZFc. Mol Hum Reprod 2008;14:251–258.
82 Soares AR, Costa P, Silva J, Sousa M, Barros A, Fernandes S: AZFb microdeletions and oligozoospermia – which mechanisms? Fertil Steril 2012;97:858–863.
83 Abid S, Sagare-Patil V, Gokral J, Modi D: Cellular ontogeny of RBMY during human spermatogenesis and its role in sperm motility. J Biosci 2013;38:85–92.
84 Longepied G, Saut N, Aknin-Seifer I, Levy R, Frances AM, Metzler-Guillemain C, Guichaoua MR, Mitchell MJ: Complete deletion of the AZFb interval from the Y chromosome in an oligozoospermic man. Hum Reprod 2010;25:265526–265563.
85 Balaresque P, Bowden GR, Parkin EJ, Omran GA, Heyer E, Quintana-Murci L, Roewer L, Stoneking M, Nasidze I, Carvalho-Silva DR, Tyler-Smith C, de Knijff P, Jobling MA: Dynamic nature of the proximal AZFc region of the human Y chromosome: multiple independent deletion and duplication events revealed by microsatellite analysis. Hum Mutat 2008;29:1171–1180.
86 Krausz C, Forti G, McElreavey K: The Y chromosome and male fertility and infertility. Int J Androl 2003;26:70–75.
87 Stahl PJ, Masson P, Mielnik A, Marean MB, Schlegel PN, Paduch DA: A decade of experience emphasizes that testing for Y microdeletions is essential in American men with azoospermia and severe oligozoospermia. Fertil Steril 2010;94:1753–1756.
88 Krausz C, Casamonti E: Spermatogenic failure and the Y chromosome. Hum Genet 2017;136:637–655.
89 Kuroki Y, Iwamoto T, Lee J, Yoshiike M, Nozawa S, Nishida T, Ewis AA, Nakamura H, Toda T, Tokunaga K, et al: Spermatogenic ability is different among males in different Y chromosome lineage. J Hum Genet 1999;44:289–292.
90 Krausz C, Quintana-Murci L, Rajpert-De Meyts E, Jorgensen N, Jobling MA, Rosser ZH, Skakkebaek NE, McElreavey K: Identification of a Y chromosome haplogroup associated with reduced sperm counts. Hum Mol Genet 2001;10:1873–1877.
91 McElreavey K, Quintana-Murci L: Male reproductive function and the human Y chromosome: is selection acting on the Y? Reprod Biomed Online 2003;7:17–23.
92 Gill TJ: Evolutionary genetics and infertility. Am J Reprod Immunol 2002;48:43–49.
93 Charlesworth B: The organization and evolution of the human Y chromosome. Genome Biol 2003;4:226.
94 Bhowmick BK, Satta Y, Takahata N: The origin and evolution of human ampliconic gene families and ampliconic structure. Genome Res 2007;17:441–450.
95 Bachtrog D: Y-chromosome evolution: emerging insights into processes of Y-chromosome degeneration. Nat Rev Genet 2013;14:113–124.
96 Krausz C, Escamilla AR, Chianese C: Genetics of male infertility: from research to clinic. Reproduction 2015;150:R159–R174.
97 Stouffs K, Lissens W, Tournaye H, Haentjens P: What about gr/gr deletions and male infertility? Systematic review and meta-analysis. Hum Reprod Update 2011;17:197–209.
98 Repping S, Skaletsky H, Brown L, van Daalen SK, Korver CM, Pyntikova T, Kuroda-Kawaguchi T, de Vries JW, Oates RD, Silber S, et al: Polymorphism for a 1.6-Mb deletion of the human Y chromosome persists through balance between recurrent mutation and haploid selection. Nat Genet 2003;35:247–251.
99 Vogt PH, Fernandes S: Polymorphic DAZ gene family in polymorphic structure of AZFc locus: artwork or functional for human spermatogenesis? APMIS 2003;111:115–126.
100 Repping S, Korver CM, Oates RD, Silber S, van der Veen F, Page DC, Rozen S: Are sequence family variants useful for identifying deletions in the human Y chromosome? Am J Hum Genet 2004;75:514–517, reply 517–519.
101 Rozen SG, Marszalek JD, Irenze K, Skaletsky H, Brown LG, Oates RD, Silber SJ, Ardlie K, Page DC: *AZFc* deletions and spermatogenic failure: a population-based survey of 20,000 Y chromosomes. Am J Hum Genet 2012;91:890–896.
102 Nickkholgh B, Korver CM, van Daalen SK, van Pelt AM, Repping S: AZFc deletions do not affect the function of human spermatogonia in vitro. Mol Hum Reprod 2015;21:553–562.

103 Navarro-Costa P, Pereira L, Alves C, Gusmão L, Proença C, Marques-Vidal P, Rocha T, Correia SC, Jorge S, Neves A, Soares AP, Nunes J, Calhaz-Jorge C, Amorim A, Plancha CE, Gonçalves J: Characterizing partial AZFc deletions of the Y chromosome with amplicon-specific sequence markers. BMC Genomics 2007;28:342.
104 Yang Y, Ma M, Li L, Zhang W, Chen P, Ma Y, Liu Y, Tao D, Lin L, Zhang S: Y chromosome haplogroups may confer susceptibility to partial AZFc deletions and deletion effect on spermatogenesis impairment. Hum Reprod 2008;23: 2167–2172.
105 Ravel C, Chantot-Bastaraud S, El Houate B, Rouba H, Legendre M, Lorenço D, Mandelbaum J, Siffroi JP, McElreavey K: Y-chromosome AZFc structural architecture and relationship to male fertility. Fertil Steril 2009; 92:1924–1933.
106 Lu C, Zhang J, Li Y, Xia Y, Zhang F, Wu B, Wu W, Ji G, Gu A, Wang S, Jin L, Wang X: The b2/b3 subdeletion shows higher risk of spermatogenic failure and higher frequency of complete AZFc deletion than the gr/gr subdeletion in a Chinese population. Hum Mol Genet 2009;18:1122–1130.
107 Giachini C, Laface I, Guarducci E, Balercia G, Forti G, Krausz C: Partial AZFc deletions and duplications: clinical correlates in the Italian population. Hum Genet 2008;124:399–410.
108 Tse JYM, Wong EYM, Cheung ANY, O WS, Tam PC, Yeung WSB: Specific expression of VCY2 in human male germ cells and its involvement in the pathogenesis of male infertility. Biol Reprod 2003;69:746–751.
109 Wong EYM, Tse JYM, Yao K-M, Lui VDH, Tam P-C, Yeung WSB: Identification and characterization of human VCY2-interacting protein: VCY2IP-1, a microtubule-associated protein-like protein. Biol Reprod 2004;70:775–784.
110 Wong EYM, Tse JYM, Yao K-M, Tam PC, Yeung WS: VCY2 protein interacts with the HECT domain of ubiqutitin-protein ligase. Biochem Biophys Res Commun 2002;296:1104–1111.
111 Lahn BT, Lan Tang Z, Zhou J, Barndt RJ, Parvinen M, Allis CD, Page DC: Previously uncharacterized histone acetyltransferases implicated in mammalian spermatogenesis. Proc Natl Acad Sci USA 2002;99:8707–8712.
112 Gläser B, Yen PH, Schempp W: Fibre-fluorescence in situ hybridization unravels apparently seven DAZ genes or pseudogenes clustered within a Y-chromosome region frequently deleted in azoospermic males. Chromosome Res 1998;6:481–486.
113 Fernandes S, Paracchini S, Meyer LH, Floridia G, Tyler-Smith C, Vogt PH: A large AZFc deletion removes *DAZ3/DAZ4* and nearby genes from men in Y haplogroup N. Am J Hum Genet 2004;74:180–187.
114 Saxena R, de Vries JW, Repping S, Alagappan RK, Skaletsky H, Brown LG, Ma P, Chen E, Hoovers JM, Page DC: Four *DAZ* genes in two clusters found in the *AZFc* region of the human Y chromosome. Genomics 2000;67:256–267.
115 Fernandes S, Huellen K, Goncalves J, Dukal H, Zeisler J, Rajpert De Meyts E, Skakkebaek NE, Habermann B, Krause W, Sousa M, et al: High frequency of DAZ1/DAZ2 gene deletions in patients with severe oligozoospermia. Mol Hum Reprod 2002;8:286–298.
116 Tsui S, Dai T, Roettger S, Schempp W, Salido EC, Yen PH: Identification of two novel proteins that interact with germ-cell-specific RNA-binding proteins DAZ and DAZL1. Genomics 2000;65:266–273.
117 Kim B, Lee Y, Kim Y, Lee KH, Chun S, Rhee K, Seo JT, Kim SW, Paick JS: Polymorphic expression of DAZ proteins in the human testis. Hum Reprod 2009;24:1507–1515.
118 Vera Y, Dai T, Hikim AP, Lue Y, Salido EC, Swerdloff RS, Yen PH: Deleted in azoospermia associated protein 1 shuttles between nucleus and cytoplasm during normal germ cell maturation. J Androl 2002;23:622–628.
119 Chen HY, Yu YH, Yen PH: DAZAP1 regulates the splicing of Crem, Crisp2 and Pot1a transcripts. Nucleic Acids Res 2013;41:9858–9869.
120 Xu EY, More FL, Pera RA: A gene family required for human germ cell development evolved from an ancient meiotic gene conserved in metazoans. Proc Natl Acad Sci USA 2001;98:7414–7419.
121 Fu XF, Cheng SF, Wang LQ, Yin S, De Felici M, Shen W: DAZ family proteins, key players for germ cell development. Int J Biol Sci 2015;11:1226–1235.
122 Habermann B, Mi HF, Edelmann A, Bohring C, Bäckert IT, Kiesewetter F, Aumüller G, Vogt PH: DAZ (deleted in azoospermia) genes encode proteins located in human late spermatids and in sperm tails. Hum Reprod 1998;13: 363–336.
123 Gaiti F, Calcino AD, Tanurdžić M, Degnan BM: Origin and evolution of the metazoan non-coding regulatory genome. Dev Biol 2016, Epub ahead of print.
124 Kurihara M, Shiraishi A, Satake H, Kimura AP: A conserved noncoding sequence can function as a spermatocyte-specific enhancer and a bidirectional promoter for a ubiquitously expressed gene and a testis-specific long noncoding RNA. J Mol Biol 2014;426: 3069–3093.
125 Sin HS, Koh E, Taya M, Iijima M, Sugimoto K, Maeda Y, Yoshida A, Iwamoto T, Namiki M: A novel Y chromosome microdeletion with the loss of an endogenous retrovirus related, testis specific transcript in AZFb region. J Urol 2011;186:1545–1552.
126 Kuroda-Kawaguchi T, Skaletsky H, Brown LG, Minx PJ, Cordum HS, Waterston RH, Wilson RK, Silber S, Oates R, Rozen S, Page DC: The AZFc region of the Y chromosome features massive palindromes and uniform recurrent deletions in infertile men. Nat Genet 2001;29:279–286.

Peter H. Vogt
Reproduction Genetics Unit, Department of Gynecological Endocrinology and Reproductive Medicine, University of Heidelberg
Im Neuenheimer Feld 440, DE–69120 Heidelberg (Germany)
E-Mail peter.vogt@med.uni-heidelberg.de

Vogt PH (ed): Genetics of Human Infertility. Monogr Hum Genet.
Basel, Karger, 2017, vol 21, pp 74–85 (DOI: 10.1159/000477279)

Genetics and Pathophysiology of the Cystic Fibrosis Transmembrane Conductance Regulator in Male Reproduction: New Evidence of a Direct Effect on the Male Germline

Aminata Touré

Institut Cochin, INSERM U1016, CNRS UMR8104, and Université Paris Descartes, Sorbonne Paris Cité, Paris, France

Abstract

The cystic fibrosis transmembrane conductance regulator (CFTR) gene encodes a cAMP-activated Cl^- and HCO_3^- channel, which is widely expressed in epithelial cells of the airways, as well as the digestive and reproductive tracts. Nearly 2,000 mutations in *CFTR* that affect CFTR function and/or expression have been identified. All these mutations are associated with cystic fibrosis (CF), which causes chronic lung infections and inflammation resulting in respiratory failure and digestive disorders. Some of these mutations have been identified in non-CF patients presenting male infertility due to congenital bilateral absence of the vas deferens (CBAVD), a phenotype considered to be a mild form of CF. Conflicting studies have also reported CFTR mutations in healthy non-CF patients with impaired sperm motility and numeration. In this review, the current knowledge of the molecular basis of CBAVD is briefly presented with a focus on CFTR function in epithelial cells of the genital tract. An emphasis is placed on recent findings from in vitro and in vivo mouse studies that reveal an unexpected expression and direct function of the CFTR channel in sperm cells.

The cystic fibrosis transmembrane conductance regulator (CFTR; MIM 602421) gene encodes a cAMP (cyclic adenosine monophosphate)-activated Cl^- and HCO_3^- channel which is widely expressed in epithelial cells of the airways, as well as the digestive and reproductive tracts [1]. Mutations that impair the function of CFTR are responsible for cystic fibrosis (CF; MIM 219700), an autosomal recessive disease, which affects 1 in 2,500 newborns in the Caucasian population. CF is the most common lethal genetic disease in this population [2–4]. Defective electrolyte transport due to CFTR mutations leads to the thickening and accumulation of mucus in the organs. This mainly causes chronic lung infections and inflammation, resulting in respiratory failure and digestive disorders in the patients [1]. The congenital bilateral absence of the vas deferens (CBAVD; MIM 277180) is another clinical symptom of CF and results in obstructive azoospermia and male infertility for 97% of CF patients [5].

Genetic analysis has allowed the identification of nearly 2,000 mutations in CFTR that affect CFTR

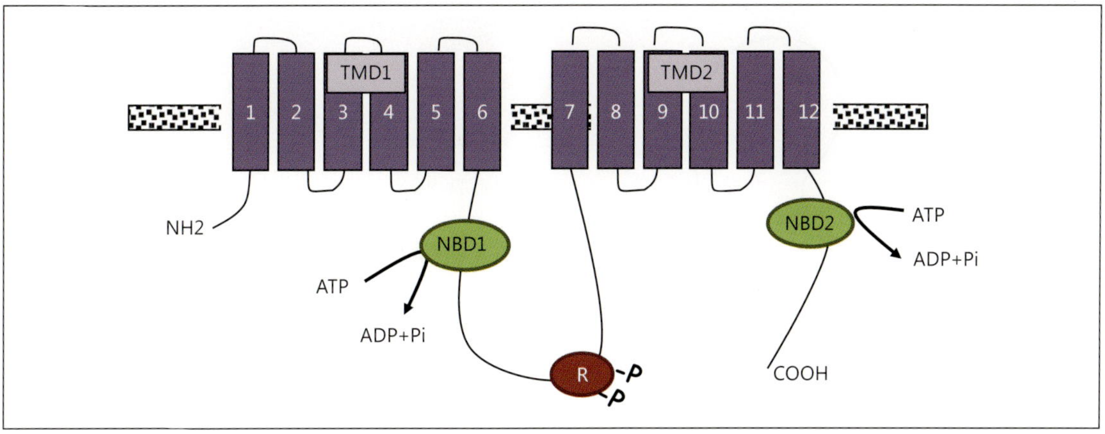

Fig. 1. Structure of the CFTR channel. The CFTR protein consists of 2 transmembrane domains, namely TMD1 and TMD2 (each containing 6 spans of alpha helices), 2 NBDs (NBD1 and NBD2), and a central regulatory domain (R-domain). CFTR functions as a cAMP-activated Cl^- and HCO_3^- channel, regulated by PKA-phosphorylation of the R-domain and ATP binding and hydrolysis at the 2 NBDs. TMD, transmembrane domain; NBD, nucleotide-binding domain; R, regulatory domain.

function and/or expression. Several mutations have been identified in patients that display CBAVD without any other clinical symptoms of CF. CFTR mutations have also been identified in nonobstructive azoospermia, oligozoospermia, and oligoasthenoteratozoospermia. This suggests that in addition to its function in epithelial cells of the genital tract, CFTR could also be required for proper sperm production and fertilization capacity. This review focuses on the genetics of CFTR in male reproduction. The current knowledge of the molecular basis of CBAVD is briefly presented, with a focus on the function of CFTR in epithelial cells of the genital tract. We will emphasize recent findings from in vitro and in vivo mouse studies that reveal unexpected expressions and a direct function for the CFTR channel in sperm.

CFTR: Structure, Function, and Pathophysiology

The CFTR gene is located on chromosome 7 (7q31.2). It comprises 27 exons spanning more than 190 kb and encodes a large transmembrane glycoprotein of 1,480 amino acids [6]. The CFTR protein consists of 2 transmembrane domains (each containing 6 spans of alpha helices), 2 nucleotide-binding domains (NBD1 and NBD2), and a central regulatory domain (R-domain; Fig. 1). CFTR is present at the surface of epithelial cells of many organs, including the lung, liver, pancreas, digestive tract, reproductive tract, and skin (Fig. 2). In these cells, CFTR functions as a cAMP activated Cl^- and HCO_3^- channel, regulated by PKA-phosphorylation of the R-domain, and ATP binding and hydrolysis at the 2 NBDs [1, 7].

Disruption of CFTR function results in the abnormal transport of chloride, which also affects sodium and water homeostasis across the epithelia resulting in thickened, viscous secretions [1, 8]. Mucus accumulation in the airways decreases mucociliary clearance and leads to chronic lung infections and inflammation. Indeed, the most common causes of death of CF patients are long-term breathing difficulties and cardiorespiratory complications. Abnormal secretion in the pancreas results in multiple digestive problems and nutrient malabsorption (Fig. 2). In addition, fertility impairment has been reported for both

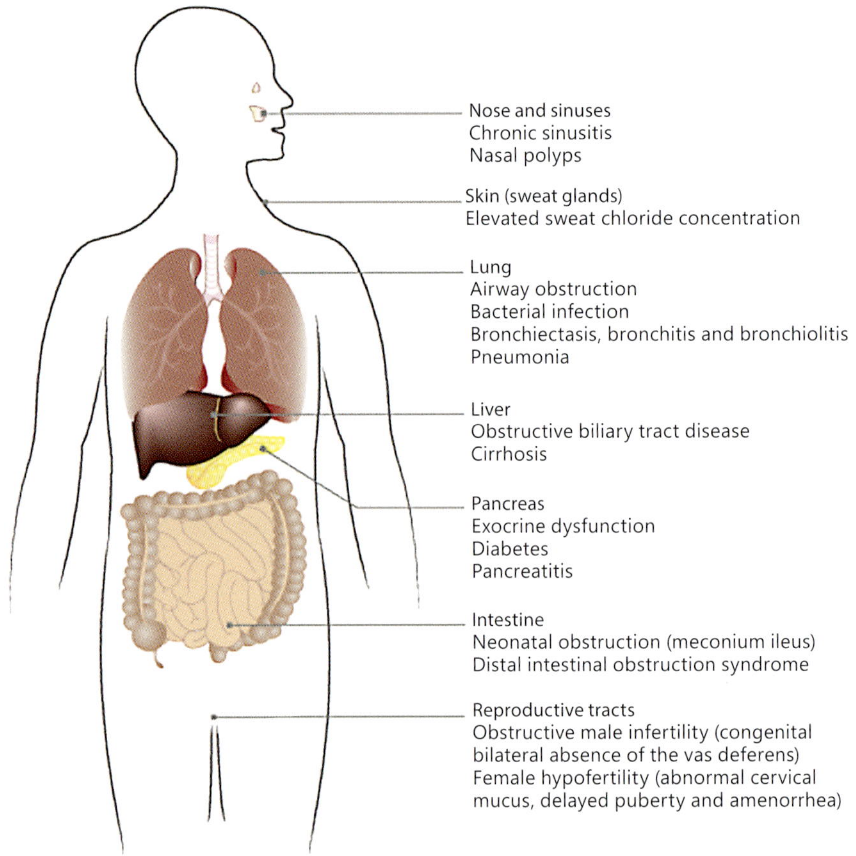

Fig. 2. CFTR tissue distribution and clinical symptoms in CF. CFTR is present at the surface of the epithelial cells in many organs, including the lung, liver, pancreas, digestive tract, reproductive tract, and skin. Disruption of CFTR function results in thickened, viscous secretions; mucus accumulation in the airways impairs mucociliary clearance, leading to chronic lung infections and inflammation. Abnormal secretion in the pancreas results in multiple digestive problems and nutrient malabsorption. In addition, male and female CF patients have reproductive symptoms: around 20% of CF females are hypofertile due to the thickening of the cervical mucus, malnutrition, delayed puberty and amenorrhea, and nearly all CF men are infertile due to obstructive infertility, namely CBAVD.

women and men. Approximately 20% of women with CF have fertility difficulties due to thickening of the cervical mucus and/or malnutrition [9], delayed puberty, and amenorrhea. Most importantly, nearly all CF men are infertile due to CBAVD [5].

More than 1,950 mutations, mostly corresponding to point mutations, have been identified in the CFTR gene since its discovery in 1989 and are deposited in the public CF databases (http://www.genet.sickkids.on.ca/cftr and http://cftr2.org) [10, 11]. Most of the mutations are very rare: less than 15 have a frequency above 1% (Table 1). The p.Phe508del mutation is the most frequent mutation worldwide and is found in nearly 70% of European CF patients [2–4]; this frequency varies between different populations in Europe. CFTR mutations have been classified

Table 1. Most common worldwide CFTR mutations

Mutation	Frequency, %	Population with the highest prevalence
F508del	66.0	–
G542X	2.4	Spanish
G551D	1.6	English
N1303K	1.3	Italian
W1282X	1.2	Jewish-Ashkenazi
Q359K/T360K	(87.5)	Jewish-Georgian
M1101K	(69)	Hutterite
Y122X	(48)	French, Reunion Island
1898+5G->T	~30	Chinese, Taiwanese
3120+1G->A	11	African-American
I148T	9.1	French-Canadian
3905insT	(6–17)	Swiss, Amish, Acadian
394delTT	(10–30)	Nordic, Finnish

More than 1,950 mutations, mostly corresponding to point mutations, have been identified in the *CFTR* gene, but less than 15 have a frequency above 1%. The data source is the CF Genetic Analysis Consortium (1994). The frequency is based on the screening of 43,849 CF chromosomes, although not all have been tested for the indicated mutations. The mutations were found in patients of Caucasian origin, except where otherwise indicated. The geographic location (or ethnic group) with the highest prevalence is indicated for some of the mutations. A rough relative frequency (in parentheses) is given for those mutations studied in relatively small samples or in the indicated populations only.

into 5 categories depending on the mechanisms by which they disrupt CFTR function [10] (Table 2), although the molecular consequences of only a subset of CFTR mutations are currently defined. Class I mutations affect protein synthesis; most of them, such as the p.Gly542X, p.Arg553X, and p.Trp1282X mutations, introduce a premature termination codon resulting in nonsense-mediated RNA decay and no CFTR protein production. Class II mutations affect protein processing or maturation; this class includes p.Phe508del, which is located in the NBD1 domain and results in the misfolding of CFTR and proteasomal degradation. Class III mutations are mostly located in the ATP-binding domains (NBD1 and NBD2) and lead to defective regulation of CFTR. Class IV mutations are predominantly located within the membrane-spanning domain and impair CFTR conductance. Finally, class V mutations mostly correspond to splice site mutations leading to smaller amounts of active CFTR protein; among them is the 5T allele, which leads to exon skipping and an inactive form of the CFTR protein.

CFTR mutations lead to various clinical consequences, resulting in a severe or mild form of the disease, a clinical spectrum which probably also depends on environmental and genetic modifiers [for a review, see 12]. Class I, II, and III mutations result in the total absence of CFTR protein from the plasma membrane of epithelial cells and are considered to be "severe" alleles, whereas class IV and V mutations are associated with residual protein amounts and/or function and constitute "mild" alleles. It is now recognized that 160 of the identified CFTR mutations account for 96–97% of CF alleles. Although numerous, all these mutations need to be further investigated; in particular, extensive genotype/phenotype correlation studies and in vitro analyses are required in order

Table 2. Classification of CFTR mutations based on their impact on CFTR function

	Class I	Class II	Class III	Class IV	Class V
CFTR defects	Synthesis	Processing Maturation	Regulation	Conductance	Function Synthesis
Mutation types	Nonsense, frameshift splice site genomic deletion	Missense indel	Missense (NBD1/2)	Missense (TMD1/2)	Splice site
Frequent mutations	G542X	F508del	G551D	R117H	IVS8-5T

CFTR mutations have been classified into 5 categories depending on the mechanisms by which they disrupt CFTR function. Class I mutations affect protein synthesis by introducing a premature termination codon, resulting in nonsense-mediated RNA decay and no CFTR protein production. Class II mutations affect protein processing or maturation; this class includes p.Phe508del, which is located in the NBD1 domain and results in the misfolding of CFTR and proteasomal degradation. Class III mutations are mostly located in the TMD domains and lead to defective regulation of CFTR. Class IV mutations impair CFTR conductance. Finally, class V mutations mostly correspond to splice site mutations, leading to smaller amounts of active CFTR protein; they include the 5T allele, which leads to exon skipping and an inactive form of the CFTR protein.

to understand the impact of the numerous mutations found in CF patients on CFTR protein/function. This information will be crucial for the development of genotype-specific therapies. Functional studies of these 160 mutations were prioritized in 2009 and are part of the Clinical and Functional Translation of CFTR project (CFTR2 database; http://www.cftr2.org/).

The Genetics and Function of CFTR in the Male Genital Tract

CBAVD, resulting in obstructive azoospermia, is diagnosed in at least 97% of CF patients [5]. It accounts for approximately 2% of all cases of male infertility and 25% of patients with excretory azoospermia [13]. The clinical symptoms of CBAVD are azoospermia with a low semen plasma volume (<1.5 mL) and bilateral atresia of the epididymis and vas deferens, which may be associated with the absence of seminal vesicles. Renal anomalies are also present in about 10–20% of the patients. Consistent with this phenotype, CFTR is expressed in the fetal and adult epididymis and vas deferens of rodents and humans [14–21]. In addition, a small conductance cAMP-activated Cl^- channel was identified in human fetal and adult rat epididymis [22–24]. More recently, combined microscopic morphological and CFTR expression studies of the male excretory duct in CF fetuses revealed the absence of excretory duct agenesis prior to 22 weeks of gestation, but suggested the presence of inflammatory- and mucinous-dependent disruptive mechanisms during the second trimester [25]. These observations confirm that the male genital tract is present during fetal life and that the mesonephric ducts develop normally, but that progressive secondary destruction of the vas deferens is induced by abnormal intraluminal secretion.

The presence of obstructive azoospermia in both CBAVD and CF patients has suggested that CBAVD may correspond to a mild/incomplete (genital) form of CF (i.e., CFTR-related disease). Indeed, the first genetic analysis of patients with isolated CBAVD revealed that they were heterozygous for the p.Phe508del allele at a much higher frequency than that of CF carriers in the general population (4–5%) [26]. Subsequent genetic analysis of CBAVD patients (extensively reviewed during the last decade [27–30]) identified the 3 following CFTR mutations as the most common causes of CBAVD: p.Phe508del (class II; 21.5% of alleles vs. 67% in the CF population), the 5T variant (class V; 19% of alleles vs. 5% in the CF population), and the p.R117H mutation (class IV; 6.4% of alleles vs. 0.5% in the CF population).

The most frequent CF mutation, p.Phe508del, has been well studied in vitro and in vivo. The p.Phe508del mutation leads to instability of the NBD1 domain due to improper local folding, resulting in the retention of the misfolded protein in the endoplasmic reticulum and its degradation by the ubiquitin/proteasome pathway [31, 32]. The 5T allele corresponds to a tract of 5 pyrimidines located upstream of the acceptor splice site of intron 8 (IVS-5T). The 5T allele promotes a high frequency of CFTR exon 9 skipping (75–90%), resulting in a nonfunctional, incomplete version of the CFTR protein. This is in contrast to the 7T and 9T alleles, which are more frequent in the general population (84 and 11%, respectively) but which are not deleterious because they induce much less exon skipping (25 and 15%, respectively) [33]. The p.Arg117His mutation is located in exon 4, encoding the transmembrane-spanning region; this mutation does not affect trafficking and localization of the protein at the plasma membrane, but results in a CFTR protein with reduced Cl^- transport [34].

Altogether, genetic analysis of men with CBAVD has revealed that 88% carry a combination of a severe (classes I–III) and mild (classes IV or V) mutation, and 12% a combination of 2 mild mutations; the 2 most common compound heterozygous genotypes are F508del/5T (28%) and F508del/R117H (6%). Of note, no CBAVD patients were found to be homozygous for the p. Phe508del mutation or a compound heterozygote for 2 severe mutations [27]. Until very recently, the genetic causes of the CBAVD for the remaining 22% of men negative for CFTR mutations was unknown. In 2016, Patat et al. [35] analyzed a cohort of 26 men with CBAVD without associated kidney anomalies, and identified 4 patients with maternally transmitted mutations in *ADGRG2* (MIM 300572), a gene located in the nonpseudoautosomal region of the X chromosome, encoding for the adhesion G protein-coupled receptor (GPCR) G2. *ADGRG2* (previously named GPR64 or HE6) is highly expressed within the efferent ducts [36, 37], which constitute the site of reabsorption of the testicular fluid carrying immature spermatozoa, and invalidation of the orthologous gene in the mouse was previously shown to induce obstructive infertility [38]. Interestingly, mutations in *ADGRG2* were found in men with a clinical description indistinguishable from that of CBAVD men carrying *CFTR* mutations, suggesting that the pathophysiological mechanisms resulting in the obstructive azoospermia might be similar. Hence, although ADGRG2 is an orphan receptor, and therefore its activation mechanisms and associated signal transduction pathways are still unknown, it might indirectly affect CFTR activity through conserved functions that have been described for GPCRs. This hypothesis is supported by the fact that: (i) fluid reabsorption has been shown to be tightly regulated by cAMP [39], (ii) cAMP can be produced by GPCRs upon activation, and (iii) CFTR activity is stimulated by phosphorylation of the R-domain by the cAMP-dependent protein kinase A. In the future, functional studies will be required in order to investigate a potential cooperation between CFTR and ADGRG2.

The Genetics and Function of CFTR in the Male Germline

Subsequent to the cloning of the *CFTR* gene in 1989, Trezise et al. [15, 40] rapidly undertook a detailed analysis of CFTR tissue and subcellular expression; CFTR mRNA was detected in the seminiferous tubules of adult rodents, particularly in the round spermatids of stages V–X. Thus, it was thought that CFTR could play a critical role during spermatogenesis and that CFTR deficiency in male haploid germ cells may contribute to CF male infertility. These results were confirmed in 2001 by Gong et al. [41], who detected CFTR protein and were able to measure a cAMP-activated chloride current in purified round spermatids.

While the above observations remained unexploited, an increasing number of conflicting studies were published suggesting a potential role for CFTR in sperm production and fertilization abilities. In 1996, van der Ven et al. [42] performed a genetic analysis on 127 unrelated healthy (non-CBAVD) American patients and showed that the frequency of *CFTR* mutations was significantly higher in healthy men with reduced sperm motility than the expected CF carrier frequency in the local population ($p = 0.00139$). In 1999, Pallares-Ruiz et al. [43] screened 50 men from southern France with reduced sperm quality using a panel of 850 *CFTR* mutations and 150 polymorphisms, but were unable to confirm the above results. Publications on this topic during the last decade are still in disagreement [44–50], but expression and functional studies of the CFTR channel in murine and human spermatozoa definitively confirmed its unexpected implication in the fertilizing capacity of sperm.

Ion fluxes play an essential role in the control of sperm motility and capacitation, a maturation event that occurs in the female genital tract and is required for fertilization (Fig. 3, 4). Capacitation involves substantial changes affecting the biochemical, electrophysiological, and functional properties of sperm. Cholesterol depletion induces the reorganization of membrane phospholipids and complex multiple ion movements lead to hyperpolarization of the sperm plasma membrane potential, intracellular alkalinization, and protein hyperphosphorylation [51]. Calcium (Ca^{2+}), chloride (Cl^-), and bicarbonate (HCO_3^-) ions are indispensable for this process. In particular, these 3 ions induce an increase in the intracellular cAMP concentration, leading to the activation of protein kinase A and phosphorylation cascades required for sperm motility and capacitation [52–54] (Fig. 3).

In 2007, detection of the CFTR protein in mature mouse and human sperm was concomitantly reported by 2 laboratories and shown to be restricted to the midpiece flagellar compartment and the equatorial segment of the head [55, 56]. Expression in guinea pigs was also documented, but shown to be restricted to the acrosome of the sperm head [57]. The requirement of CFTR for sperm motility and capacitation processes was demonstrated, in particular through the use of a specific activator and inhibitor of the CFTR channel (i.e., genistein and CFTR inh-172, respectively). CFTR was shown to be required for the rise in cAMP and intracellular pH upon the induction of sperm capacitation [56]. In addition, Cl^- influxes mediated by CFTR were shown to be required for the inhibition of the epithelial sodium channel (ENac) and sperm membrane hyperpolarization upon capacitation [55] (Fig. 4). More recently, electrophysiological evidence for the presence of CFTR on mouse sperm was also reported by Figueiras-Fierro et al. [58], and in human sperm, CFTR implication in protein hyperphosphorylation, a process mediated by the cAMP-dependent PKA activity during capacitation, was also demonstrated by work performed in the laboratory of P. Visconti [59]. Lastly, studies using a heterozygous mouse model of CF ($CFTR^{tm1Unc}$) showed that sperm from these mice have a low in vitro and in vivo fertilization capacity and impaired sperm motility and capacitation [56]. Taken together, the above data demonstrated the requirement of CFTR for sperm motility and capacitation in both humans and mice.

Recent studies have also revealed that CFTR knockout mice display impaired spermatogenesis with a reduced testicular weight and sperm count. In addition, in the mouse, CFTR was shown to be required for HCO_3^- influx in Sertoli cells and subsequent activation of the cAMP-CREB that is required for spermatogenesis [60].

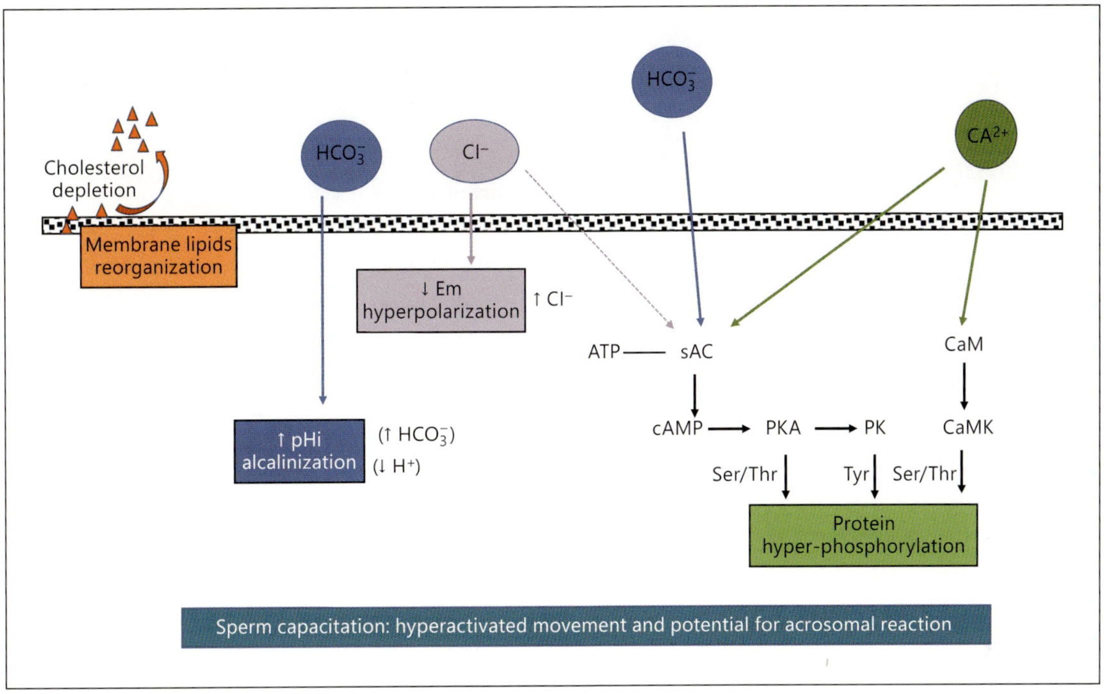

Fig. 3. Sperm modifications associated with capacitation. Capacitation is a maturation process occurring during sperm transit in the female genital tract, which is required for sperm to access and interact with the oocyte. Capacitation is associated with several changes affecting the biochemical, electrophysiological, and functional properties of the sperm. In particular, cholesterol depletion of the plasma membrane, which increase membrane fluidity, hyperpolarization, intracellular alkalinization and protein phosphorylation (hyperphosphorylation). Chloride influx contributes to hyperpolarization of the plasma membrane, which in turn activates voltage-dependent channels. Proton extrusion and bicarbonate influx contribute to intracellular alkalinization. The intracellular rises of calcium and bicarbonate are responsible for direct activation of the soluble adenylyl cyclase (sAC) and activation of PKA-dependent phosphorylation cascades. Calcium also binds to calmodulin and activates calmodulin-dependent phosphorylation cascades. Both cascades contribute to hyperphosphorylation on serine/threonine and tyrosine residues of proteins that are principally located on the flagellum. pHi, intracellular pH; Em, membrane potential; sAC, soluble adenylyl cyclase; cAMP, cyclic adenosine monophosphate; PKA, protein kinase A; PK, protein kinase; CaM, calmodulin; CaMK, calmodulin kinase.

If such function is conserved, CFTR deficiency may account for a reduced sperm count in humans, and therefore nonobstructive cases of human oligozoospermia.

Interestingly, coupling of CFTR with several members of the solute carrier 26 (SLC26) family of anion exchangers has been identified. SLC26 proteins are expressed throughout the body and are coexpressed with CFTR in various epithelia. During the last decade, crosstalk between CFTR and SLC26s has been well documented [61–65]. The physical interaction between CFTR and SLC26s is principally mediated by the conserved STAS domain of SLC26s and the R domain of CFTR, resulting in stimulation of the CFTR channel. Among the 10 members of the SLC26 family, SLC26 A3, A6, and A8 are expressed in sperm, colocalize with the CFTR channel, and stimulate CFTR activity [65, 66] (Fig. 4). In particular, SLC26A8 is uniquely expressed in the male germ line and its inactivation in the mouse leads to asthenozoospermia and male infertility.

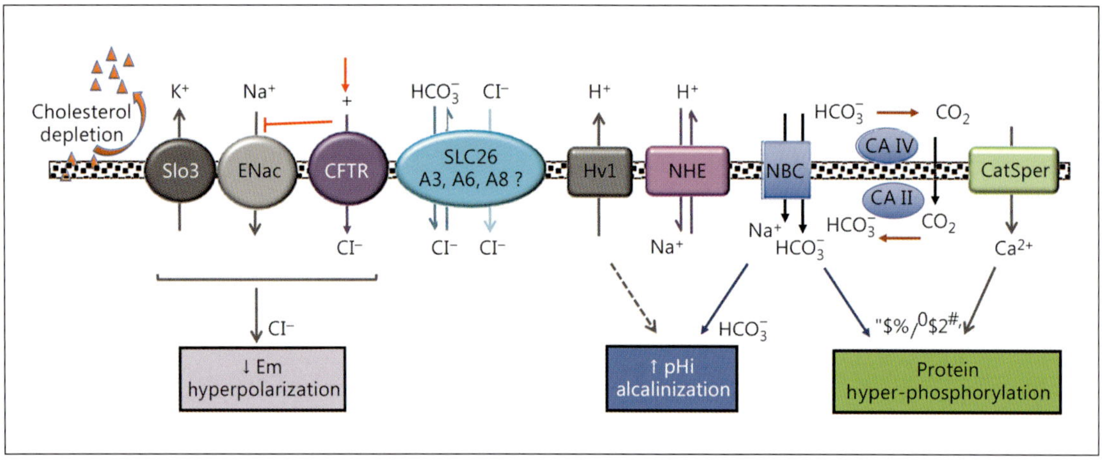

Fig. 4. Ion fluxes involved in sperm capacitation. A small number of channels known to be involved in anion exchanges during sperm capacitation are depicted in the scheme. We apologize to colleagues whose work is not referenced herein because of space limitations. Slo3, sperm-specific K^+ channel; ENaC, epithelial Na^+ channels; CFTR, cystic fibrosis transmembrane conductance channel; SLC26, solute carrier 26; Hv1, proton channel; NHE, Na^+/H^+ exchanger; NBC, sodium bicarbonate transporter; CA IV, carbonic anhydrase IV; CatSPER, sperm-specific Ca^{2+} channel.

Most importantly, mutations in the *SLC6A8* gene were identified and shown to induce proteasomal degradation of the CFTR/SLC26A8 complex in patients with asthenozoospermia, indicating the importance CFTR and SLC26A8 cooperation in the process of sperm maturation [67]. Of note, mutations in *SLC26A9*, which is mainly expressed in the lung, also abolish the stimulation of CFTR anion transport activity and have been reported in patients with idiopathic bronchiectasis [68]. These observations confirm the physiological relevance of CFTR/SLC26s coupling and its possible deregulation in CFTR-related diseases.

Altogether, specific, isolated, or combined CFTR mutations have not been clearly associated with reduced sperm quality in men without CF or CBAVD. However, current knowledge on CFTR expression and activity in the spermatozoa indicate that CFTR function is required for proper sperm motility, capacitation, and fertilization abilities, and that CFTR deficiency may lead to human sperm defects and male subfertility.

Patients Counselling and Infertility Treatment

Men with CBAVD are infertile due to obstructive azoospermia but can be helped to have children through assisted reproduction technology. Microepididymal sperm aspiration, in which a small amount of sperm is extracted from the epididymis, can be used for in vitro fertilization (intracytoplasmic sperm injection; ICSI); in this case the partner will have to follow a hormonal protocol in order to have oocytes harvested, fertilized with the extracted sperm, and reimplanted. Using this technology, the deleterious effects of CFTR mutations recently observed on sperm motility and capacitation might be circumvented as the epididymal extracted sperm will be directly injected in the cytoplasm of the oocytes. However, one cannot exclude that the lack of proper epididymal maturation of the sperm could have consequences on fertilization and embryo development in vitro; in relation to this issue, a recent report indicates that CFTR mutations in men with CBAVD are associated with a significantly increased risk of miscarriage and stillbirth following ICSI procedures [69].

In addition, while the success rates for this procedure have improved significantly over the years, it is time consuming and expensive. Lastly and most importantly, because of the high frequency of CFTR mutation in the general Caucasian population, genetic testing of the partner should be performed and, if they are shown to carry a CFTR mutation, a preimplantation genetic diagnosis should be considered to select embryos that do not carry the mutation.

Conclusion

While information about CFTR expression in male germ cells was available soon after the cloning of the CFTR gene in 1989, it took almost 20 years to discover the function of the CFTR channel in the maturation processes of spermatozoa, which are essential for fertilizing potential. CFTR participates in the network of complex cooperation and cross-regulation of ion channels and transporters involved in sperm function, as illustrated by the physical and functional interaction between CFTR and members of the SLC26 family and ENac transporters. One of the major reasons for this delay may have been the absence of strong genetic evidence for the association of CFTR mutations with reduced sperm quality and infertility/subfertility in non-CF, non-CBAVD patients, in contrast to CF-related diseases such as isolated CBAVD. Further genetic studies in larger cohorts of healthy and non-CBAVD men will be necessary to identify CFTR alleles that are formally associated with a reduced fertilizing capacity.

References

1 Quinton PM: Too much salt, too little soda: cystic fibrosis. Sheng Li Xue Bao 2007;59:397–415.

2 Lucotte G, Hazout S, de Braekeleer M: Complete map of cystic fibrosis mutation DF508 frequencies in Western Europe and correlation between mutation frequencies and incidence of disease. Hum Biol 1995;67:797–803.

3 Bobadilla JL, Macek M Jr, Fine JP, Farrell PM: Cystic fibrosis: a worldwide analysis of CFTR mutations – correlation with incidence data and application to screening. Hum Mutat 2002;19:575–606.

4 Castellani C, Picci L, Tamanini A, Girardi P, Rizzotti P, Assael BM: Association between carrier screening and incidence of cystic fibrosis. JAMA 2009;302:2573–2579.

5 Kaplan E, Shwachman H, Perlmutter AD, Rule A, Khaw KT, Holsclaw DS: Reproductive failure in males with cystic fibrosis. N Engl J Med 1968;279:65–69.

6 Riordan JR, Rommens JM, Kerem B, Alon N, Rozmahel R, Grzelczak Z, Zielenski J, Lok S, Plavsic N, Chou JL, et al: Identification of the cystic fibrosis gene: cloning and characterization of complementary DNA. Science 1989;245:1066–1073.

7 Wang Y, Wrennall JA, Cai Z, Li H, Sheppard DN: Understanding how cystic fibrosis mutations disrupt CFTR function: from single molecules to animal models. Int J Biochem Cell Biol 2014;52:47–57.

8 De Boeck K, Derichs N, Fajac I, de Jonge HR, Bronsveld I, Sermet I, Vermeulen F, Sheppard DN, Cuppens H, Hug M, Melotti P, Middleton PG, Wilschanski M: New clinical diagnostic procedures for cystic fibrosis in Europe. J Cyst Fibros 2011;10(suppl 2):S53–S66.

9 Gilljam M, Antoniou M, Shin J, Dupuis A, Corey M, Tullis DE: Pregnancy in cystic fibrosis: fetal and maternal outcome. Chest 2000;118:85–91.

10 Ferec C, Cutting GR: Assessing the disease-liability of mutations in CFTR. Cold Spring Harb Perspect Med 2012;2:a009480.

11 Fanen P, Wohlhuter-Haddad A, Hinzpeter A: Genetics of cystic fibrosis: CFTR mutation classifications toward genotype-based CF therapies. Int J Biochem Cell Biol 2014;52:94–102.

12 Cutting GR: Cystic fibrosis genetics: from molecular understanding to clinical application. Nat Rev Genet 2015;16:45–56.

13 Dubin L, Amelar RD: Etiologic factors in 1,294 consecutive cases of male infertility. Fertil Steril 1971;22:469–474.

14 Harris A, Chalkley G, Goodman S, Coleman L: Expression of the cystic fibrosis gene in human development. Development 1991;113:305–310.

15 Trezise AE, Linder CC, Grieger D, Thompson EW, Meunier H, Griswold MD, Buchwald M: CFTR expression is regulated during both the cycle of the seminiferous epithelium and the oestrous cycle of rodents. Nat Genet 1993;3:157–164.

16 Tizzano EF, Chitayat D, Buchwald M: Cell-specific localization of CFTR mRNA shows developmentally regulated expression in human fetal tissues. Hum Mol Genet 1993;2:219–224.

17 Patrizio P, Salameh WA: Expression of the cystic fibrosis transmembrane conductance regulator (CFTR) mRNA in normal and pathological adult human epididymis. J Reprod Fertil Suppl 1998;53:261–270.

18 Leung GP, Gong XD, Cheung KH, Cheng-Chew SB, Wong PY: Expression of cystic fibrosis transmembrane conductance regulator in rat efferent duct epithelium. Biol Reprod 2001;64:1509–1515.

19 Ruz R, Andonian S, Hermo L: Immunolocalization and regulation of cystic fibrosis transmembrane conductance regulator in the adult rat epididymis. J Androl 2004;25:265–273.
20 Hihnala S, Kujala M, Toppari J, Kere J, Holmberg C, Hoglund P: Expression of SLC26A3, CFTR and NHE3 in the human male reproductive tract: role in male subfertility caused by congenital chloride diarrhea. Mol Hum Reprod 2006;12:107–111.
21 Tizzano EF, Silver MM, Chitayat D, Benichou JC, Buchwald M: Differential cellular expression of cystic fibrosis transmembrane regulator in human reproductive tissues: clues for the infertility in patients with cystic fibrosis. Am J Pathol 1994;144:906–914.
22 Gong XD, Wong YL, Leung GP, Cheng CY, Silvestrini B, Wong PY: Lonidamine and analogue AF2785 block the cyclic adenosine 3′, 5′-monophosphate-activated chloride current and chloride secretion in the rat epididymis. Biol Reprod 2000;63:833–838.
23 Pollard CE, Harris A, Coleman L, Argent BE: Chloride channels on epithelial cells cultured from human fetal epididymis. J Membr Biol 1991;124:275–284.
24 Leung GP, Wong PY: Activation of cystic fibrosis transmembrane conductance regulator in rat epididymal epithelium by genistein. Biol Reprod 2000;62:143–149.
25 Marcorelles P, Gillet D, Friocourt G, Lede F, Samaison L, Huguen G, Ferec C: Cystic fibrosis transmembrane conductance regulator protein expression in the male excretory duct system during development. Hum Pathol 2012;43:390–397.
26 Dumur V, Gervais R, Rigot JM, Lafitte JJ, Manouvrier S, Biserte J, Mazeman E, Roussel P: Abnormal distribution of CF delta F508 allele in azoospermic men with congenital aplasia of epididymis and vas deferens. Lancet 1990;336:512.
27 Claustres M: Molecular pathology of the CFTR locus in male infertility. Reprod Biomed Online 2005;10:14–41.
28 Radpour R, Gourabi H, Dizaj AV, Holzgreve W, Zhong XY: Genetic investigations of CFTR mutations in congenital absence of vas deferens, uterus, and vagina as a cause of infertility. J Androl 2008;29:506–513.
29 Yu J, Chen Z, Ni Y, Li Z: CFTR mutations in men with congenital bilateral absence of the vas deferens (CBAVD): a systemic review and meta-analysis. Hum Reprod 2012;27:25–35.
30 Chen H, Ruan YC, Xu WM, Chen J, Chan HC: Regulation of male fertility by CFTR and implications in male infertility. Hum Reprod Update 2012;18:703–713.
31 Jensen TJ, Loo MA, Pind S, Williams DB, Goldberg AL, Riordan JR: Multiple proteolytic systems, including the proteasome, contribute to CFTR processing. Cell 1995;83:129–135.
32 Ward CL, Omura S, Kopito RR: Degradation of CFTR by the ubiquitin-proteasome pathway. Cell 1995;83:121–127.
33 Chillon M, Casals T, Mercier B, Bassas L, Lissens W, Silber S, Romey MC, Ruiz-Romero J, Verlingue C, Claustres M, et al: Mutations in the cystic fibrosis gene in patients with congenital absence of the vas deferens. N Engl J Med 1995;332:1475–1480.
34 Sheppard DN, Rich DP, Ostedgaard LS, Gregory RJ, Smith AE, Welsh MJ: Mutations in CFTR associated with mild-disease-form Cl^- channels with altered pore properties. Nature 1993;362:160–164.
35 Patat O, Pagin A, Siegfried A, Mitchell V, Chassaing N, Faguer S, Monteil L, Gaston V, Bujan L, Courtade-Saidi M, Marcelli F, Lalau G, Rigot JM, Mieusset R, Bieth E: Truncating mutations in the adhesion G protein-coupled receptor G2 gene *ADGRG2* cause an X-linked congenital bilateral absence of Vas deferens. Am J Hum Genet 2016;99:437–442.
36 Kirchhoff C: Osterhoff C, Samalecos A: HE6/GPR64 adhesion receptor co-localizes with apical and subapical F-actin scaffold in male excurrent duct epithelia. Reprod Suppl 2008;136:235–245.
37 Obermann H, Samalecos A, Osterhoff C, Schroder B, Heller R, Kirchhoff C: HE6, a two-subunit heptahelical receptor associated with apical membranes of efferent and epididymal duct epithelia. Mol Reprod Dev 2003;64:13–26.
38 Davies B, Baumann C, Kirchhoff C, Ivell R, Nubbemeyer R, Habenicht UF, Theuring F, Gottwald U: Targeted deletion of the epididymal receptor HE6 results in fluid dysregulation and male infertility. Mol Cell Biol 2004;24:8642–8648.
39 Man SY, Clulow J, Jones RC: Signal transduction in the ductuli efferentes testis of the rat: inhibition of fluid reabsorption by cyclic adenosine 3′, 5′-monophosphate. Biol Reprod 2003;69:1714–1718.
40 Trezise AE, Buchwald M: In vivo cell-specific expression of the cystic fibrosis transmembrane conductance regulator. Nature 1991;353:434–437.
41 Gong XD, Li JC, Cheung KH, Leung GP, Chew SB, Wong PY: Expression of the cystic fibrosis transmembrane conductance regulator in rat spermatids: implication for the site of action of antispermatogenic agents. Mol Hum Reprod 2001;7:705–713.
42 van der Ven K, Messer L, van der Ven H, Jeyendran RS, Ober C: Cystic fibrosis mutation screening in healthy men with reduced sperm quality. Hum Reprod 1996;11:513–517.
43 Pallares-Ruiz N, Carles S, Des Georges M, Guittard C, Arnal F, Humeau C, Claustres M: Complete mutational screening of the cystic fibrosis transmembrane conductance regulator gene: cystic fibrosis mutations are not involved in healthy men with reduced sperm quality. Hum Reprod 1999;14:3035–3040.
44 Ravnik-Glavac M, Svetina N, Zorn B, Peterlin B, Glavac D: Involvement of CFTR gene alterations in obstructive and non-obstructive infertility in men. Genet Test 2001;5:243–247.
45 Schulz S, Jakubiczka S, Kropf S, Nickel I, Muschke P, Kleinstein J: Increased frequency of cystic fibrosis transmembrane conductance regulator gene mutations in infertile males. Fertil Steril 2006;85:135–138.
46 Larriba S, Bonache S, Sarquella J, Ramos MD, Gimenez J, Bassas L, Casals T: Molecular evaluation of CFTR sequence variants in male infertility of testicular origin. Int J Androl 2005;28:284–290.
47 Ghorbel M, Baklouti-Gargouri S, Keskes R, Sellami-Ben Hamida A, Feki-Chakroun N, Bahloul A, Fakhfakh F, Ammar-Keskes L: Screening of ΔF508 mutation and IVS8-poly T polymorphism in *CFTR* gene in Tunisian infertile men without CBAVD. Andrologia 2012;44(suppl 1):376–382.
48 Jiang LY, Shan JJ, Tong XM, Zhu HY, Yang LY, Zheng Q, Luo Y, Shi QX, Zhang SY: Cystic fibrosis transmembrane conductance regulator is correlated closely with sperm progressive motility and normal morphology in healthy and fertile men with normal sperm parameters. Andrologia 2014;46:824–830.

49 Hering DM, Olenski K, Kaminski S: Genome-wide association study for poor sperm motility in Holstein-Friesian bulls. Anim Reprod Sci 2014;146:89–97.

50 Sharma H, Mavuduru RS, Singh SK, Prasad R: Increased frequency of CFTR gene mutations identified in Indian infertile men with non-CBAVD obstructive azoospermia and spermatogenic failure. Gene 2014;548:43–47.

51 Visconti PE, Westbrook VA, Chertihin O, Demarco I, Sleight S, Diekman AB: Novel signaling pathways involved in sperm acquisition of fertilizing capacity. J Reprod Immunol 2002;53:133–150.

52 Chen Y, Cann MJ, Litvin TN, Iourgenko V, Sinclair ML, Levin LR, Buck J: Soluble adenylyl cyclase as an evolutionarily conserved bicarbonate sensor. Science 2000;289:625–628.

53 Wertheimer EV, Salicioni AM, Liu W, Trevino CL, Chavez J, Hernandez-Gonzalez EO, Darszon A, Visconti PE: Chloride is essential for capacitation and for the capacitation-associated increase in tyrosine phosphorylation. J Biol Chem 2008;283:35539–35550.

54 Jaiswal BS, Conti M: Calcium regulation of the soluble adenylyl cyclase expressed in mammalian spermatozoa. Proc Natl Acad Sci USA 2003;100:10676–10681.

55 Hernandez-Gonzalez EO, Trevino CL, Castellano LE, de la Vega-Beltran JL, Ocampo AY, Wertheimer E, Visconti PE, Darszon A: Involvement of cystic fibrosis transmembrane conductance regulator in mouse sperm capacitation. J Biol Chem 2007;282:24397–24406.

56 Xu WM, Shi QX, Chen WY, Zhou CX, Ni Y, Rowlands DK, Yi Liu G, Zhu H, Ma ZG, Wang XF, Chen ZH, Zhou SC, Dong HS, Zhang XH, Chung YW, Yuan YY, Yang WX, Chan HC: Cystic fibrosis transmembrane conductance regulator is vital to sperm fertilizing capacity and male fertility. Proc Natl Acad Sci USA 2007;104:9816–9821.

57 Chen WY, Xu WM, Chen ZH, Ni Y, Yuan YY, Zhou SC, Zhou WW, Tsang LL, Chung YW, Hoglund P, Chan HC, Shi QX: Cl^- is required for HCO_3^- entry necessary for sperm capacitation in guinea pig: involvement of a Cl^-/HCO_3^- exchanger (SLC26A3) and CFTR. Biol Reprod 2009;80:115–123.

58 Figueiras-Fierro D, Acevedo JJ, Martinez-Lopez P, Escoffier J, Sepulveda FV, Balderas E, Orta G, Visconti PE, Darszon A: Electrophysiological evidence for the presence of cystic fibrosis transmembrane conductance regulator (CFTR) in mouse sperm. J Cell Physiol 2013;228:590–601.

59 Puga Molina LC, Pinto NA, Torres Rodriguez P, Romarowski A, Vicens Sanchez A, Visconti PE, Darszon A, Trevino CL, Buffone MG: Essential role of CFTR in PKA-dependent phosphorylation, alkalinization, and hyperpolarization during human sperm capacitation. J Cell Physiol 2017;232:1404–1414.

60 Xu WM, Chen J, Chen H, Diao RY, Fok KL, Dong JD, Sun TT, Chen WY, Yu MK, Zhang XH, Tsang LL, Lau A, Shi QX, Shi QH, Huang PB, Chan HC: Defective CFTR-dependent CREB activation results in impaired spermatogenesis and azoospermia. PLoS One 2011;6:e19120.

61 Ko SB, Shcheynikov N, Choi JY, Luo X, Ishibashi K, Thomas PJ, Kim JY, Kim KH, Lee MG, Naruse S, Muallem S: A molecular mechanism for aberrant CFTR-dependent HCO_3^- transport in cystic fibrosis. EMBO J 2002;21:5662–5672.

62 Bertrand CA, Zhang R, Pilewski JM, Frizzell RA: SLC26A9 is a constitutively active, CFTR-regulated anion conductance in human bronchial epithelia. J Gen Physiol 2009;133:421–438.

63 Chang MH, Plata C, Sindic A, Ranatunga WK, Chen AP, Zandi-Nejad K, Chan KW, Thompson J, Mount DB, Romero MF: Slc26a9 is inhibited by the R-region of the cystic fibrosis transmembrane conductance regulator via the STAS domain. J Biol Chem 2009;284:28306–28318.

64 Homma K, Miller KK, Anderson CT, Sengupta S, Du GG, Aguinaga S, Cheatham M, Dallos P, Zheng J: Interaction between CFTR and prestin (SLC26A5). Biochim Biophys Acta 2010;1798:1029–1040.

65 Rode B, Dirami T, Bakouh N, Rizk-Rabin M, Norez C, Lhuillier P, Lores P, Jollivet M, Melin P, Zvetkova I, Bienvenu T, Becq F, Planelles G, Edelman A, Gacon G, Toure A: The testis anion transporter TAT1 (SLC26A8) physically and functionally interacts with the cystic fibrosis transmembrane conductance regulator channel: a potential role during sperm capacitation. Hum Mol Genet 2012;21:1287–1298.

66 Chavez JC, Hernandez-Gonzalez EO, Wertheimer E, Visconti PE, Darszon A, Trevino CL: Participation of the Cl^-/HCO_3^- exchangers SLC26A3 and SLC26A6, the Cl^- channel CFTR, and the regulatory factor SLC9A3R1 in mouse sperm capacitation. Biol Reprod 2012;86:1–14.

67 Dirami T, Rode B, Jollivet M, Da Silva N, Escalier D, Gaitch N, Norez C, Tuffery P, Wolf JP, Becq F, Ray PF, Dulioust E, Gacon G, Bienvenu T, Toure A: Missense mutations in SLC26A8, encoding a sperm-specific activator of CFTR, are associated with human asthenozoospermia. Am J Hum Genet 2013;92:760–766.

68 Bakouh N, Bienvenu T, Thomas A, Ehrenfeld J, Liote H, Roussel D, Duquesnoy P, Farman N, Viel M, Cherif-Zahar B, Amselem S, Taam RA, Edelman A, Planelles G, Sermet-Gaudelus I: Characterization of SLC26A9 in patients with CF-like lung disease. Hum Mutat 2013;34:1404–1414.

69 Lu S, Cui Y, Li X, Zhang H, Liu J, Kong B, Cai F, Chen ZJ: Association of cystic fibrosis transmembrane-conductance regulator gene mutation with negative outcome of intracytoplasmic sperm injection pregnancy in cases of congenital bilateral absence of vas deferens. Fertil Steril 2014;101:1255–1260.

Aminata Touré
Institut Cochin
24, rue du Faubourg Saint Jacques
FR–75014 Paris (France)
E-Mail aminata.toure@inserm.fr

Vogt PH (ed): Genetics of Human Infertility. Monogr Hum Genet.
Basel, Karger, 2017, vol 21, pp 86–100 (DOI: 10.1159/000477280)

The Genetics of Androgen Receptor Signalling in Male Fertility

Laura O'Hara · Lee B. Smith

Medical Research Council Centre for Reproductive Health, University of Edinburgh, Edinburgh, UK

Abstract

The androgen testosterone has an essential trophic role in the development of male physiology and in adult spermatogenesis and fertility. Testosterone mainly exerts its effect through the androgen receptor (AR), a ligand-activated transcription factor that is activated by binding the androgens testosterone or dihydrotestosterone. Mutations in AR can result in the genetic disorder androgen insensitivity syndrome, which results in a feminised phenotype and developmental problems, including cryptorchidism and disrupted spermatogenesis, thus complicating the investigation of the role of AR in adulthood. Transgenic mouse models of conditional AR inactivation have helped to define cell-specific roles for AR in the testis and the wider male reproductive system, and revealed a complex paracrine signalling network that controls fertility through several cell types and differing mechanisms.

The androgen testosterone has an essential trophic role in the development of male physiology and in adult spermatogenesis and fertility. Disruption of testosterone production by hypophysectomy [1], Leydig cell ablation [2], or knockout of luteinising hormone receptor [3] demonstrates that spermatogenesis cannot proceed to completion in its absence. Testosterone mainly exerts its effect through the androgen receptor (AR), a ligand-activated transcription factor. Mutations in AR can result in the genetic disorder androgen insensitivity syndrome (AIS), in which androgen-dependent embryonic development of individuals with an XY genotype is disrupted. This results in a feminised phenotype and developmental problems, including cryptorchidism and disrupted spermatogenesis, complicating the investigation of the role of AR in adulthood [reviewed in 4]. Specific effects of AR in spermatogenesis have therefore been elucidated using animal models. Germ cells do not express AR despite requiring androgens for their survival and maturation [5–7]. However, AR is expressed in several somatic cell types of the mature testis [8] and it is widely accepted that the requirement of testosterone for spermatogenesis is mediated by these cell types. The specific roles of testosterone in spermatogenesis are summarised in Figure 1.

The Androgen Receptor

Structure of the Androgen Receptor

AR (alternative name NR3C4, nuclear receptor subfamily 3, group C, gene 4; OMIM entry: 313700) is a single copy gene present on the X chromosome at locus Xq11-Xq12 [9]. The length of the open reading frame of the human AR is 2,757 nucleotides over 8 coding exons, which produces a protein of 919 amino acids [10]. AR (like other members of the ligand-activated transcription factor superfamily) consists of 4 domains, the N-terminal domain (NTD), DNA-binding domain (DBD), hinge region, and ligand-binding domain (LBD) [10].

The NTD is coded for by exon 1 (amino acid residues 1–534), the DBD by exons 2 and 3 (residues 559–624), and the hinge (residues 625–663) and LBD (residues 664–919) by exons 4–8 [11]. The NTD of the AR comprises over half of the receptor protein. This region is poorly conserved both in length and sequence similarity among the members of the steroid receptor family [12]. Within this domain are 2 transcriptional "activation function" (AF) regions (commonly known as "AF1" and "AF5"), which can bind co-regulator proteins to increase or decrease the transcription of downstream genes [13, 14]. It also contains a variable polyglutamine (CAG) stretch that may be important in transcriptional regulation [15]. The AR DBD has the greatest sequence similarity with other steroid receptors: from 80% homology with progesterone receptor DBD down to 51% homology with oestrogen receptor α [16]. It is composed of 2 zinc finger motifs: the first is responsible for recognition of the target DNA sequence, while the second stabilises DNA-receptor interaction by contact with the DNA phosphate backbone [17, 18]. Between the 2 zinc fingers is an amino acid sequence that can recognise specific DNA response elements, thus making this domain vital for transcription of downstream genes [19]. At the overlap between the DNA binding and hinge regions is a nuclear targeting sequence

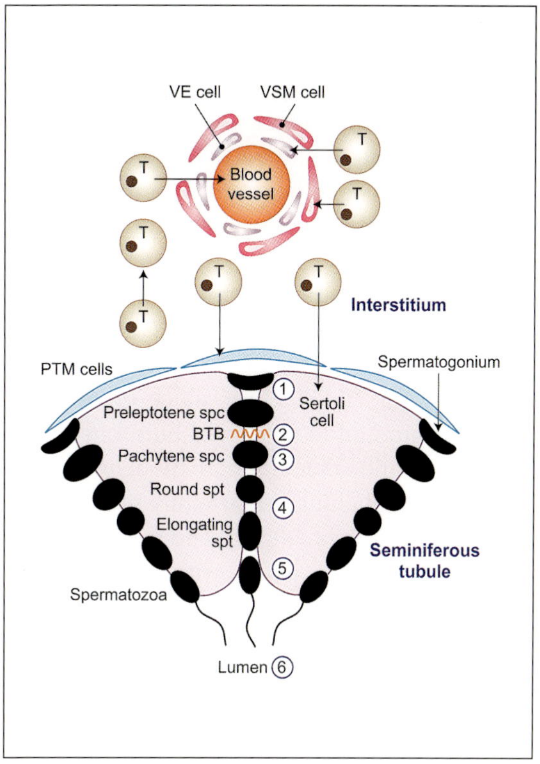

Fig. 1. The anatomy of the testis and control of spermatogenesis by androgens. The testis consists of seminiferous tubules embedded in an interstitial stroma. The stroma contains steroidogenic Leydig cells and blood vessels that are lined by vascular endothelial (VE) cells and surrounded by vascular smooth muscle (VSM) cells. PTM cells surround the seminiferous tubule. Sertoli cells extend into the tubules from the PTM cells to the lumen and support and contact the developing germ cells. Junctions between Sertoli cells form the BTB. Germ cells move toward the lumen as they mature during spermatogenesis: undifferentiated diploid spermatogonia are found on the basement membrane and spermatozoa are released from the apical surface of the Sertoli cell. During meiosis, spermatocytes transit the BTB. Testosterone produced by the Leydig cells has autocrine effects, as well as paracrine effects on VE, VSM, PTM, and Sertoli cells. It also diffuses into the testicular blood vessels to be transported to the wider body through the circulatory system. There are 6 critical processes in spermatogenesis regulated by testosterone: (1) maintenance of spermatogonial numbers, (2) maintenance of the BTB, (3) completion of meiosis by spermatocytes (spc), (4) adherence of elongated spermatids (spt) to Sertoli cells, (5) the release of mature spermatozoa, and (6) the formation of the seminiferous tubule lumen.

that is responsible for androgen-dependent translocation from the cytosol to the nucleus [20]. The hinge region is responsible for androgen-dependent conformational changes of the AR. The LBD is at the C-terminus of the AR. Its sequence is less conserved between other steroid hormone receptors to ensure the specific, high-affinity binding of androgens [21]. The LBD contains another transcription activation region (AF2) which can bind co-regulator proteins to increase or decrease transcription [19]. The LBD also contains a binding region for HSP90 (heat shock protein 90), which is common to all steroid hormone receptors: HSP90 and other HSPs are thought to be involved in maintaining the structure of the receptor in the absence of a ligand and preventing the receptor from associating with androgen response elements (AREs) on DNA in the absence of a ligand [20, 22].

The DNA, hinge, and LBDs of the mouse AR are virtually identical to the human AR, but there is approximately 15% variation in the NTD [23]. Despite this, mice with a transgenic knock-in of human AR show normal development and fertility [24].

Mechanisms of Androgen Receptor Signalling

Classical Mechanism of Androgen Receptor Signalling

The current model for genomic androgen signalling involves a multistep mechanism. Upon entry of testosterone into the androgen target cell, binding occurs to AR either directly or after its conversion to dihydrotestosterone by the enzyme 5α reductase. Binding to the receptor is followed by dissociation of the bound chaperone and HSPs [20]. This unmasks the DNA binding motifs and the nuclear localisation signal [25]. Androgen binding promotes AR hyperphosphorylation, which induces co-activator recruitment and transcriptional activation [26, 27]. The complex then translocates to the nucleus [28].

The receptor/ligand complex requires dimerisation to bind to AREs located in the regulatory regions of androgen-responsive genes [29]. Classical AREs are 15-bp sequences with 2 imperfect 6-bp repeats that are almost identical to glucocorticoid response elements, and therefore will also bind glucocorticoid receptors [30]. More recently, androgen-specific response elements have been discovered that will only bind activated AR. Reproductive homeobox on the X chromosome 5 (Rhox5) is a well-characterised androgen-responsive gene with 2 androgen-specific AREs in its promoter [31]. Rhox5 itself is a transcription factor found in Sertoli cells that is thought to direct some of the actions of AR in the testes [32]. In order to modify the transcription of genes with AREs, the AR/ligand homodimer complex further recruits additional proteins that together form a transcription activation/repression complex at discrete sites on the chromatin [33]. Co-factors are thought to be cell specific, so AR signalling can elicit particular responses in a wide variety of different tissues.

Non-Classical and Ligand-Independent Signalling of Androgens and Androgen Receptor

Androgens and AR can act in a rapid non-classical way without binding to genomic AREs. Non-classical effects of testosterone have now been demonstrated convincingly in several tissues, in particular in the reproductive, cardiovascular, immune, and musculoskeletal systems [reviewed in 34]. It is thought that non-classical signalling may explain the relative lack of genes discovered that contain AREs compared to the wide range of effects that testosterone can produce within a cell. AR can activate Src tyrosine kinase, which can induce phosphorylation of the CREB transcription factor, thus affecting the transcription of genes without binding to AREs [reviewed in 35]. In the reproductive system, evidence from both Sertoli cells and the prostate cancer LNCaP cell line show that testosterone can produce intracellular calcium influx via membrane depolarisation, leading to cytoskeletal rearrangement [36, 37]. AR can also act ligand independently. A set of constitutively active AR splice variants that lack the LBD have been discovered in hormone-refractory prostate cancer cells [38]. In the absence of ligand or in the presence of low androgenic concentrations, AR can also be stimulated by growth factors or proinflammatory cytokines, including interleukin-6 and insulin-like growth factor 1 [39, 40].

Clinical Disorders Resulting from Mutations in the Androgen Receptor

As of September 2014, more than 1,100 mutations in human AR have been identified [11]. Of these mutations, 90% lead to a decrease in AR signalling that results in the spectrum of AIS [41]. The remaining 10% are implicated in various cancers [reviewed in 11], premature ovarian failure [42], and Kennedy disease (X-linked spinal and bulbar muscular atrophy) [43], or are "silent" and do not have a phenotypic effect.

Androgen Insensitivity Syndrome

AIS is a condition that most often results from loss or reduction of AR function in a person with an XY karyotype. It has a spectrum of phenotypic severity. Complete AIS (CAIS) most often results from a complete loss-of-function mutation in the AR [reviewed in 4]. People with CAIS (historically known as testicular feminisation or Tfm) have an external female phenotype and are assigned a female gender at birth. However, due to an XY genotype they have small, undescended testes that do not undergo spermatogenesis, although they produce testosterone and anti-Müllerian hormone (AMH) like fully functional testes. The inability of the developing foetus to respond to testosterone results in underdevelopment of the Wolffian duct-derived epididymis, seminal vesicles, and vas deferens. The production of AMH results in a lack of uterus, oviducts, and the upper portion of the vagina. CAIS is often diagnosed in childhood due to hernias caused by the undescended testes, or with pubertal amenorrhoea. Normal spermatogenesis does not occur. Some tubules in the testis lack germ cells completely and the others contain a few spermatogonia, but no postmeiotic germ cells [44].

Partial AIS (PAIS; historically known as Reifenstein syndrome; OMIM database accession number: 312300) most often results from a partial loss-of-function mutation in AR. It is a spectrum of undervirilisation when the degree of androgen insensitivity is enough to partially prevent masculinisation, but is not enough to completely prevent masculinisation. The typical phenotype is a phallic structure that is intermediate between a clitoris and a penis with hypospadias and a bifid scrotum with or without cryptorchidism. Wolffian duct structures are typically partially or fully developed [45]. The testicular maturation of seminiferous tubules and Sertoli cells tends to be more advanced in patients with PAIS than those with CAIS [46], although the majority of patients with PAIS are still infertile. Mild AIS (MAIS) results from a mutation in AR that allows normal phenotypic masculinisation to take place but may affect spermatogenesis so the patient presents with infertility [47]. MAIS is correlated with a high luteinising hormone to testosterone ratio, known as the androgen sensitivity index.

The minimal incidence of CAIS (OMIM database accession number: 300068) is 1 in 99,000 [48] and the incidence of PAIS is estimated to be 1 in 130,000 [49]. The incidence of MAIS is not typically investigated except in the case of male infertility [50], thus its true prevalence is unknown [51].

The location of the mutation in the AR gene and the type of the mutation correlates with the resulting severity of the AIS phenotype [11]. Most premature termination mutations result in a truncated AR protein and CAIS. Single base substitutions can result in all grades of AIS, depending on what effect the substitution has on the amino acid sequence and 3-dimensional structure of the protein, and therefore how much of the function is retained. Mutations in AR that cause premature termination of transcription or large deletions generally result in CAIS due to a truncation of the protein and a completely non-functional AR. Both CAIS and PAIS can also be caused by single base substitutions that result in the complete transcription of AR protein that has reduced or ablated ligand-binding properties. Most of these occur in the LBD [11]. The most common functional AR defect results from the disruption of the hydrophobic ligand-binding pocket in the LBD, which disrupts ligand binding and prevents the binding of co-regulatory proteins [52]. Interestingly, a specific mutation does not always result in the same phenotype. Mutation of amino acid 840 from arginine to cysteine/histidine has a variety of phenotypic outcomes, even within the same family, and patients have been assigned both male and female gender identities [reviewed in 53].

MAIS is often associated with single-base substitution mutations in exon 1, which codes for the NTD that contains AF1 and AF5 [reviewed in 54], or in the region of the LBD that contains AF2 [55]. Missense mutations in this domain have a milder effect on AR function since the main role of the NTD is as a binding site for other transactivation proteins. Mutations may impair the binding or activity of these factors and result in a protein that may have reduced efficiency in specific cell types only. For example, in one patient, an adenine to guanine mutation in amino acid 886 of the AR gene (in the AF2 of the LBD) prevented its interaction with TIF2, a Sertoli cell-specific co-activator, thus impeding the genomic actions of AR only in Sertoli cells [56]. The frequency of AR mutations in patients with oligospermia or azoospermia under investigation for infertility is approximately 2–3% – a relatively small proportion of infertile men [47]. However, mutations of genes up or downstream of AR in its signalling pathway may also contribute to cases of infertility by reducing the efficiency of this pathway.

Association of Androgen Receptor Trinucleotide Repeats with Kennedy Disease and Infertility

Exon 1 of AR contains 2 variable trinucleotide repeats, one is a CAG polyglutamine (Q tract) and the other is a GGN polyglycine (G tract). The normal repeat number of the polyglutamine tract is between 8 and 31 repeats, and averages about 20 [57]. An expansion beyond 40 repeats causes Kennedy disease (X-linked spinal and bulbar muscular atrophy), with symptoms including progressive flaccid proximal paralysis and muscle atrophy, as well as endocrine disturbances including gynaecomastia and progressive infertility associated with mild androgen insensitivity [58]. A non-pathological increase in CAG repeat number has been shown to reduce AR transactivation [59] and levels of AR protein and messenger RNA (mRNA) [60] in vitro. Although longer polyglutamine tracts are associated with impaired sperm production in men [61], the association is disputed [reviewed in 62].

A polyglycine tract is further downstream of the polyglutamine tract in exon 1. The normal repeat number is between 10 and 30. Deletion of the polyglycine tract in vitro resulted in a 30% reduction in transactivation potential [59]. However, there is also conflicting evidence about whether the number of GGN repeats has an association with male infertility.

Use of Animal Models to Elucidate Roles of the Androgen Receptor in Male Fertility

The first animal model of androgen insensitivity was the Tfm ("testicular feminisation") mouse, described in 1970 by Lyon and Hawkes [63]. Tfm mice have an XY karyotype but small, inguinal testes, no Wolffian duct-derived organs, and feminised external genitalia, similar to the phenotype of CAIS patients. Some seminiferous tubules in the testis lack germ cells completely and the others contain a few spermatogonia, but postmeiotic germ cells are absent and normal spermatogenesis does not occur. This is analogous to the testicular histology seen in CAIS patients [44, 64]. It was subsequently discovered that Tfm is due to a single nucleotide deletion in exon 1 of the AR gene, and that the resulting frameshift introduces a premature termination codon [65]. Subsequently, mice with a total AR knockout (ARKO) which phenocopies the Tfm mouse have been produced by 4 groups using Cre/loxP technology. By mating a mouse line with the floxed region of the AR gene to one expressing Cre recombinase under the control of a constitutively active gene, genetic ablation of part of the AR resulting in loss of functional protein was achieved in all cells of the resulting offspring [64, 66–68].

Complete AR inactivation models such as the Tfm and ARKO have been vital in gaining information on the function of androgens during development, but since adult spermatogenesis is incomplete, Wolffian duct-derived structures (epididymis, vas deferens, and seminal vesicles) are absent and the mice have developmental problems, including cryptorchidism, and little knowledge can be gained about the postnatal role of androgens in these tissues. Cre-loxP transgenic mice are ideal for studying the postnatal actions of androgens and also for elucidating the specific roles of androgens in different cell types, as the promoter that drives Cre can be selected to be active postnatally, or in specific cell types. This system has been used to characterise the role of AR in fertility, both in the testis and wider male reproductive system.

Testicular Roles of the Androgen Receptor in Fertility

Various testicular cell-specific knockouts of AR have been produced. The Sertoli [66, 69, 70] and peritubular myoid (PTM) cell-specific [71] knockouts both have significant direct effects on fertility and will be discussed below. Other knockouts include a Leydig cell-specific knockout, which is fertile, but degeneration of seminiferous epithelium occurs with ageing and Leydig cells do not mature normally [72]. Spermatocyte [5, 73] and vascular endothelial knockouts are fertile, and a vascular smooth muscle knockout [74] is fertile but with impaired testicular vasomotion. The histology of the testis in the Sertoli, Leydig, and PTM cell ARKOs is summarised in Figure 2. Models of reduced testosterone have also been used to elucidate the roles of testicular AR signalling.

Role of Sertoli Cell Androgen Receptor Signalling in Fertility

Intratubular Sertoli cells are the somatic supporting cells of spermatogenesis. Each Sertoli cell spans the seminiferous tubule from the basement membrane to the lumen, and is tightly linked to a set of germ cells at specific stages by junction protein complexes [75]. AR is not present in the Sertoli cells of the mouse during embryonic and neonatal development. At postnatal day 4, a few Sertoli cells stain for AR, then a progressive increase in number and intensity is noted from day 5 [76]. This is analogous to humans, in which Sertoli cell AR is either weakly detected or not present up to 5 years, begins to be expressed at 8 years and is strongly expressed in adulthood [77–79]. After maturation, expression of AR in mouse Sertoli cells fluctuates in a seminiferous tubule stage-specific manner [8], appearing strongest at stages VI–VII. Expression is also cyclical in men, appearing strongest at stage III [80]. A model of AR overexpression in Sertoli cells beginning on day 2 induces a premature maturation of Sertoli cells and reduces final Sertoli cell numbers [81], suggesting it has a key role in Sertoli cell maturation. The final germ cell number is also reduced and germ cell development accelerated, illustrating the intimate dependence of germ cells on Sertoli cell AR signalling for their co-ordinated development.

Sertoli cell-specific ARKO (SCARKO) mouse lines have been created by 2 groups using the Cre-loxP system [66, 69], both using AMH-

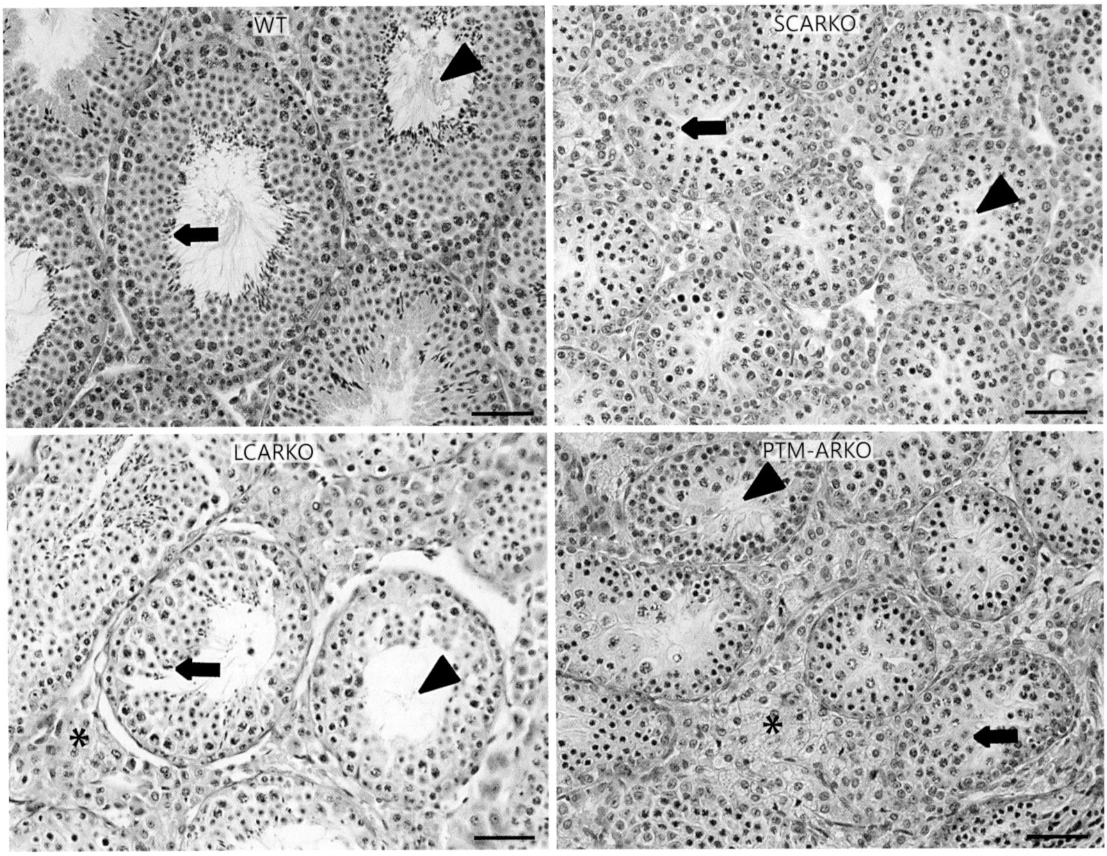

Fig. 2. The histological phenotype of 3 different testicular cell-specific ARKO lines. Wild-type (WT) control testicular histology shows seminiferous tubules with full spermatogenesis (arrows) up to mature spermatozoa. In Leydig cell (LC) ARKO testes spermatogenesis also results in mature spermatozoa, but there is a loss of germ cells with ageing, resulting in fewer spermatozoa. In both SCARKO and PTM-ARKO testes there are very few postmeiotic germ cells, although the PTM-ARKO also shows a loss of earlier germ cell stages, whereas the SCARKO has a meiotic block. Both WT control and LCARKO testes have patent seminiferous tubule lumens (arrowheads). In SCARKO and PTM-ARKO testes, the lumens are not patent. The interstitial Leydig cells (asterisks) appear visibly normal in WT and SCARKO mice, but exhibit hypertrophy in LCARKO and PTM-ARKO mice.

driven Cre recombinase. Unlike ARKO mice, SCARKO mice develop with an external phenotype similar to their control male littermates, with fully descended testes and intact Wolffian duct-derived structures [64]. However, histological analysis of their testes revealed a spermatogenic block at meiosis, a decrease in seminiferous tubule diameters, and abnormal seminiferous tubule lumens. Germ cell entry into meiosis appeared normal, but a progressive loss of pachytene primary spermatocytes occurs between stages VI and XII. The round spermatid number was 3% of controls and no elongating spermatids could be identified [66]. Mice with a Sertoli cell-specific ablation of the second zinc finger domain in the DBD (essential for DNA binding) display a similar postmeiotic block phenotype, which led investigators to initially conclude that progression of spermatocytes through meiosis is an event dependent on classical genomic signalling of AR

[82]. However, subsequent investigation into the non-classical Src-activated pathway proved that this was also affected in mice with an ablation of the AR DBD, and that mouse spermatogenesis could be disrupted by injection of inhibitors that disrupt either the classical or non-classical pathways [83]. An adult-onset SCARKO model also produces the same phenotype, thus proving that it is not due to a developmental effect [84].

The lack of post-meiotic germ cells has been postulated to be due to the lack of a functional blood-testis barrier (BTB) [85]. The BTB is the structure normally formed by tight junctions between adjacent Sertoli cells above the level of leptotene spermatocytes that partitions the adluminal compartment of the seminiferous tubule from the basal compartment so haploid germ cells can mature in an immunologically privileged microenvironment [86]. During maturation, sperm move along the Sertoli cell from the basement membrane to the lumen and traverse the BTB during meiosis. It is widely accepted that androgen signalling contributes to the maintenance of the BTB. Some studies on SCARKO mice show that the BTB is not present [87, 88], whereas others show that tight junctions in the SCARKO can form, but BTB formation is delayed and incomplete [85]. A number of genes encoding BTB proteins are downregulated or incorrectly expressed in SCARKO mice [88–90].

The lack of the seminiferous tubule lumen in SCARKO mice may be because of abnormal seminiferous tubule fluid secretion by Sertoli cells [66]. Seminiferous tubule fluid contains appropriate nutritional and hormonal factors necessary to support the adluminal stages of spermatogenesis that are unavailable from the circulation due to the presence of the BTB. It also acts as a transport mechanism for mature spermatozoa to exit the testis. Ligation of the efferent ducts of SCARKO mice does not cause an increase in testicular weight, contrary to controls, so SCARKO mice are likely to have reduced Sertoli cell fluid secretion [85]. It has been suggested that a seminiferous tubule lumen cannot be formed when the BTB is disrupted [91], and also that meiosis can only be completed after Sertoli cell fluid secretion has been established [reviewed in 92]. It is clear that AR influences BTB remodelling, meiosis, and the secretion of seminiferous tubule fluid by Sertoli cells, but it is currently unclear whether these processes are dependent on each other or just on AR signalling itself.

Because the SCARKO has a meiotic block, it is impossible to pinpoint any postmeiotic effects of androgen signalling in Sertoli cells. Before the advent of targeted knockouts, changes in spermatogenesis were identified in rodent models with reduced testosterone production such as the luteinising hormone receptor knockout (LuRKO) mouse [3], and rats implanted with low-dose testosterone and oestradiol (TE rats) to suppress luteinising hormone production at the pituitary [93]. Reduction in AR signalling in these models occurs in all cell types that express the receptor and, therefore, it is difficult to be certain that the effects are Sertoli cell specific. However, since Sertoli cells are the only cell type in intimate contact with postmeiotic germ cells on the apical side of the BTB, they are the most likely cell type to be affecting postmeiotic processes. Another study created a 'hypomorphic' SCARKO with a Sertoli cell-specific reduction but not ablation of AR signalling [70].

In rodent models with reduced testosterone, meiosis completes and spermatogenesis proceeds to the round spermatid stage, implying that meiosis itself is not as sensitive to a reduction in testosterone levels, although it is required [3]. A reduction in testosterone results in the premature detachment of spermatids from Sertoli cells at the round-to-elongating transition stage. Detached round spermatids accumulate in the cauda epididymis in both hypomorphic AR mice [70] and TE-implanted rats [94]. The detachment phenotype does not appear to be a problem with the expression of ectoplasmic specialisations, a type of adherens junction unique to the testis, as normal ectoplasmic specialisations were noted in TE rats when their testes were examined by electron microscopy [95]. Both hypomorphic AR mouse and TE rat models also show spermiation failure, characterised by elongating spermatid retention and subsequent phagocytosis by Sertoli cells [70, 96]. It has been shown that final disengagement of the spermatid from the Sertoli cell is affected by a reduction in testosterone [97] and that androgen signalling is necessary for the disengagement of a Sertoli cell complex containing $\alpha_6\beta_1$ integrin and phosphorylated focal adhesion kinase [98] from laminin $\alpha_3\beta_3\gamma_3$ on spermatids [99]. Control of both spermatid adhesion and spermiation is through a non-classical AR signalling pathway involving signalling of Src kinase [reviewed in 100], since administration of the c-Src inhibitor PP1 to adults can induce the loss of spermatocytes and round spermatids, but not elongating spermatids, from the seminiferous epithelium [101].

Since AR signalling appears to be required for both the attachment and disengagement of maturing germ cells at different stages of spermatogenesis, it may be that Src has different roles in each of these different junction complexes that are yet to be fully characterised. There is also evidence that fragments of laminin chains produced during spermiation induce remodelling of the BTB, thus co-ordinating these 2 androgen-dependent steps in spermatogenesis [102]. Studying BTB remodelling, spermatid adhesion, and spermiation as a co-ordinated process rather than isolated events may help to further elucidate the androgen-dependent co-ordination of the processes of spermatogenesis.

Array studies on the SCARKO model have produced data on gene expression changes [reviewed in 103], but have identified surprisingly few for a model with such a complex phenotype. This may be explained by the regulation of mRNAs involved in Sertoli and germ cell function by microRNAs (miRNAs) controlled by AR. Both Sertoli and germ cell expression of the miRNA-processing enzyme Dicer are essential for spermatogenesis [104, 105]. Many of these miRNAs are under the regulation of AR, as the expression of 28 miRNAs have been shown to change in an androgen deprivation model [106]. Most of these miRNAs are upregulated under androgen deprivation, resulting in the transcriptional downregulation of their targets. Pathway analysis suggested that testosterone-regulated miRNAs target genes involved in cell signalling and cell junction restructuring: both androgen-dependent processes required for normal spermatogenesis. Further analysis showed that the miR-471 miRNA binds to the 3′UTRs of Sertoli cell genes that are important for the process of spermatogenesis, including *Foxd1*, a forkhead/winged-helix transcription factor that is important in Sertoli metabolism, and desmocollin 1 (*Dsc1*), a demosomal cadherin that is required for Sertoli germ cell adhesion.

Role of Peritubular Myoid Cell Androgen Receptor Signalling in Fertility

A layer of PTM cells surrounds each seminiferous tubule. The contractility of PTM cells produces peristaltic waves that propel mature spermatozoa through the seminiferous tubules towards the rete testis [107]. Their other roles include the synthesis of basement membrane components [108, 109] and as a signalling interface between the seminiferous tubules and the interstitium. The mesenchymal precursors of PTM cells begin to express AR at or before e16.5 in the mouse [110], and 3 months of gestation in humans [78], and continue to express AR strongly throughout life.

Cell-specific PTM-ARKO mice have been produced using Cre-loxP transgenesis [71]. PTM-ARKO testes are 70% smaller than controls and have a progressive reduction of germ cell numbers at all stages (including spermatogonia) that is not seen in any other conditional ARKO model. Since spermatogonia are juxtaposed to the basement membrane they are in intimate contact with the PTM cells, meaning it is possible that the reduction in germ cell number results from the spermatogonia stage due to direct signalling between PTM cells and spermatogonia. PTM cells in the PTM-ARKO have a progressive loss of desmin and smooth muscle actin, indicating a degradation of the smooth muscle phenotype in PTM cells, and a disruption of laminin expression, which indicates problems with the seminiferous tubule basement membrane. These disruptions in PTM integrity may impair attachment and signalling to spermatogonia, and thus disrupt the spermatogonial stem cell niche [111]. The decrease in germ cell number in the PTM-ARKO is not due to a decrease in Sertoli cell number; however, levels of Sertoli cell-specific gene products, including Rhox5, Epp, and Tubb3, are reduced, showing that AR signalling in PTM cells has an effect on the transcriptome and function of Sertoli cells. It is likely that the effects of PTM cells on fertility is due to a combination of direct effects on spermatogonia and indirect effects through modulation of Sertoli cell function.

Extratesticular Roles of the Androgen Receptor in Fertility

Other than the specific testicular roles of AR that directly influence spermatogenesis, AR is also important in the development and function of other organs in the male reproductive system that contribute to male fertility. Conditional AR ablation lines have been created and investigated to elucidate its role in these varied cell types [112]. The roles of neuronal [113, 114] and epididymal [115–117] AR are essential for fertility and will be discussed below. Prostate epithelial ARKO mice have been shown to be fertile [118]. It is likely that the roles of AR in prostate smooth muscle, seminal vesicles, and vas deferens also contributes to fertility, but the knockout models analysed in these studies had testicular or epididymal knockouts that may have masked any contributions of AR in these organs [117, 119, 120].

Role of Epididymal Androgen Receptor Signalling in Fertility

The epididymis is a long, coiled single tube that receives sperm from the testis and transports it to the vas deferens. In rodents, sperm are stored in the epididymis prior to ejaculation. During transport, the sperm interact with the epididymal fluid and undergo the initial stages of extratesticular maturation that is essential for their ability to fertilise an oocyte. Expression of AR in the mesenchymal cells of the developing Wolffian duct is required for stabilisation of the duct during embryonic development and coiling of the proximal part of the duct that will develop into the epididymis. The absence of AR in the ARKO mouse prevents stabilisation of the Wolffian duct resulting in its degradation [121]. Treatment of embryonic rats with the AR antagonist flutamide after the stabilisation window prevents the coiling of the epididymis by birth [122]. Postnatally, the expression of AR in the epithelium of the epididymis also begins to influence its function. Two models of cell-specific ablation of AR in the proximal part of the epididymal epithelium result in infertility due to obstructive azoospermia [115, 123]. Another knockout of AR in the accessory glands and epididymis had a similar phenotype [117].

Role of Neuronal Androgen Receptor Signalling in Fertility

To determine whether AR-mediated signalling in the nervous system is essential for male sexual behaviour required for fertility, 2 groups made neuronal-specific knockouts of the AR using Nestin-Cre [113, 114]. Neuronal ARKO mice are hypofertile, with a significantly decreased epididymal sperm count, litter size, and total number of pups.

Neuronal ARKO mice are less likely to initiate mating behaviour (although once initiated, their display appears similar to that of WT males). Only 55% (compared to 100% of control males) exhibited mounting, intromissions, and thrusts within 10 h of housing with a control female in oestrus. They also spend less time fighting with intruder males and deposit fewer territorial urine marks in their cages.

Conclusion

AR is a ligand-activated transcription factor that is activated by binding the androgens testosterone or dihydrotestosterone. Androgen signalling through AR is vital for normal prenatal masculinisation, and also for male sexual maturation at puberty and adult spermatogenesis. Mutations in the AR cause AIS, a disorder with a spectrum of masculinisation effects. The severity of the disorder correlates with the position and type of the mutation in AR. At its mildest, androgen insensitivity allows normal physiological development but cause infertility so mutations in AR could potentially explain many cases of so-called idiopathic male infertility. Transgenic mouse models of conditional AR inactivation have helped to define cell-specific roles for AR in the testis and the wider male reproductive system and revealed a complex paracrine signalling network that controls fertility through several cell types and differing mechanisms. A significant task for future research is to focus on downstream targets of testosterone signalling if we are to fully understand and clinically support spermatogenesis in patients, an increasing number of whom are presenting with a low sperm count [124, 125].

References

1 Russell LD, Clermont Y: Degeneration of germ cells in normal, hypophysectomized and hormone treated hypophysectomized rats. Anat Rec 1977;187: 347–366.
2 Bartlett JM, Kerr JB, Sharpe RM: The effect of selective destruction and regeneration of rat Leydig cells on the intratesticular distribution of testosterone and morphology of the seminiferous epithelium. J Androl 1986;7:240–253.
3 Zhang FP, Poutanen M, Wilbertz J, Huhtaniemi I: Normal prenatal but arrested postnatal sexual development of luteinizing hormone receptor knockout (LuRKO) mice. Mol Endocrinol 2001;15: 172–183.
4 Mongan NP, Tadokoro-Cuccaro R, Bunch T, Hughes IA: Androgen insensitivity syndrome. Best Pract Res Clin Endocrinol Metab 2015;29:569–580.
5 Tsai MY, Yeh SD, Wang RS, Yeh S, Zhang C, Lin HY, Tzeng CR, Chang C: Differential effects of spermatogenesis and fertility in mice lacking androgen receptor in individual testis cells. Proc Natl Acad Sci USA 2006;103:18975–18980.
6 Johnston DS, Russell LD, Friel PJ, Griswold MD: Murine germ cells do not require functional androgen receptors to complete spermatogenesis following spermatogonial stem cell transplantation. Endocrinology 2001;142:2405–2408.
7 Lyon MF, Glenister PH, Lamoreux ML: Normal spermatozoa from androgen-resistant germ cells of chimaeric mice and the role of androgen in spermatogenesis. Nature 1975;258:620–622.
8 Zhou Q, Nie R, Prins GS, Saunders PT, Katzenellenbogen BS, Hess RA: Localization of androgen and estrogen receptors in adult male mouse reproductive tract. J Androl 2002;23:870–881.
9 Brown CJ, Goss SJ, Lubahn DB, Joseph DR, Wilson EM, French FS, Willard HF: Androgen receptor locus on the human X chromosome: regional localization to Xq11–12 and description of a DNA polymorphism. Am J Hum Genet 1989; 44:264–269.
10 Ribeiro RC, Kushner PJ, Baxter JD: The nuclear hormone receptor gene superfamily. Annu Rev Med 1995;46:443–453.
11 Gottlieb B, Beitel LK, Nadarajah A, Paliouras M, Trifiro M: The androgen receptor gene mutations database: 2012 update. Hum Mutat 2012;33:887–894.
12 Faber PW, Kuiper GG, van Rooij HC, van der Korput JA, Brinkmann AO, Trapman J: The N-terminal domain of the human androgen receptor is encoded by one, large exon. Mol Cell Endocrinol 1989;61:257–262.
13 Jenster G, van der Korput HA, Trapman J, Brinkmann AO: Identification of two transcription activation units in the N-terminal domain of the human androgen receptor. J Biol Chem 1995;270: 7341–7346.
14 McEwan IJ: Molecular mechanisms of androgen receptor-mediated gene regulation: structure-function analysis of the AF-1 domain. Endocr Relat Cancer 2004;11:281–293.
15 Lieberman AP, Harmison G, Strand AD, Olson JM, Fischbeck KH: Altered transcriptional regulation in cells expressing the expanded polyglutamine androgen receptor. Hum Mol Genet 2002;11: 1967–1976.

16 McEwan IJ, Brinkmann AO: Androgen physiology: receptor and metabolic disorders; in De Groot LJ, et al (eds): Endotext. Dartmouth, Endotext, 2009. http://www.endotext.org.
17 Berg JM: DNA binding specificity of steroid receptors. Cell 1989;57:1065–1068.
18 Freedman LP: Anatomy of the steroid receptor zinc finger region. Endocr Rev 1992;13:129–145.
19 Beato M, Truss M, Chavez S: Control of transcription by steroid hormones. Ann NY Acad Sci 1996;784:93–123.
20 Jenster G, Trapman J, Brinkmann AO: Nuclear import of the human androgen receptor. Biochem J 1993;293:761–768.
21 Mangelsdorf DJ, Thummel C, Beato M, Herrlich P, Schutz G, Umesono K, Blumberg B, Kastner P, Mark M, Chambon P, Evans RM: The nuclear receptor superfamily: the second decade. Cell 1995;83:835–839.
22 Picard D, Khursheed B, Garabedian MJ, Fortin MG, Lindquist S, Yamamoto KR: Reduced levels of hsp90 compromise steroid receptor action in vivo. Nature 1990;348:166–168.
23 Gaspar ML, Meo T, Tosi M: Structure and size distribution of the androgen receptor mRNA in wild-type and Tfm/Y mutant mice. Mol Endocrinol 1990;4:1600–1610.
24 Albertelli MA, Scheller A, Brogley M, Robins DM: Replacing the mouse androgen receptor with human alleles demonstrates glutamine tract length-dependent effects on physiology and tumorigenesis in mice. Mol Endocrinol 2006;20:1248–1260.
25 Kuil CW, Mulder E: Effects of androgens and antiandrogens on the conformation of the androgen receptor. Ann NY Acad Sci 1995;761:351–354.
26 Gioeli D, Ficarro SB, Kwiek JJ, Aaronson D, Hancock M, Catling AD, White FM, Christian RE, Settlage RE, Shabanowitz J, Hunt DF, Weber MJ: Androgen receptor phosphorylation: regulation and identification of the phosphorylation sites. J Biol Chem 2002;277:29304–29314.
27 Kuiper GG, Brinkmann AO: Phosphotryptic peptide analysis of the human androgen receptor: detection of a hormone-induced phosphopeptide. Biochemistry 1995;34:1851–1857.
28 Georget V, Lobaccaro JM, Terouanne B, Mangeat P, Nicolas JC, Sultan C: Trafficking of the androgen receptor in living cells with fused green fluorescent protein-androgen receptor. Mol Cell Endocrinol 1997;129:17–26.
29 Jones N: Transcriptional regulation by dimerization: two sides to an incestuous relationship. Cell 1990;61:9–11.
30 Roche PJ, Hoare SA, Parker MG: A consensus DNA-binding site for the androgen receptor. Mol Endocrinol 1992;6:2229–2235.
31 Barbulescu K, Geserick C, Schuttke I, Schleuning WD, Haendler B: New androgen response elements in the murine Pem promoter mediate selective transactivation. Mol Endocrinol 2001;15:1803–1816.
32 Hu ZY, Dandekar D, O'Shaughnessy PJ, De Gendt K, Verhoeven G, Wilkinson MF: Androgen-induced Rhox homeobox genes modulate the expression of AR-regulated Genes. Mol Endocrinol 2010;24:60–75.
33 McKenna NJ, Lanz RB, O'Malley BW: Nuclear receptor coregulators: cellular and molecular biology. Endocr Rev 1999;20:321–344.
34 Rahman F, Christian HC: Non-classical actions of testosterone: an update. Trends Endocrinol Metab 2007;18:371–378.
35 Walker WH: Testosterone signaling and the regulation of spermatogenesis. Spermatogenesis 2011;1:116–120.
36 Kampa M, Papakonstanti EA, Hatzoglou A, Stathopoulos EN, Stournaras C, Castanas E: The human prostate cancer cell line LNCaP bears functional membrane testosterone receptors that increase PSA secretion and modify actin cytoskeleton. FASEB J 2002;16:1429–1431.
37 Lyng FM, Jones GR, Rommerts FF: Rapid androgen actions on calcium signaling in rat sertoli cells and two human prostatic cell lines: similar biphasic responses between 1 picomolar and 100 nanomolar concentrations. Biol Reprod 2000;63:736–747.
38 Hu R, Dunn TA, Wei S, Isharwal S, Veltri RW, Humphreys E, Han M, Partin AW, Vessella RL, Isaacs WB, Bova GS, Luo J: Ligand-independent androgen receptor variants derived from splicing of cryptic exons signify hormone-refractory prostate cancer. Cancer Res 2009;69:16–22.
39 Malinowska K, Neuwirt H, Cavarretta IT, Bektic J, Steiner H, Dietrich H, Moser PL, Fuchs D, Hobisch A, Culig Z: Interleukin-6 stimulation of growth of prostate cancer in vitro and in vivo through activation of the androgen receptor. Endocr Relat Cancer 2009;16:155–169.
40 Kim HJ, Lee WJ: Ligand-independent activation of the androgen receptor by insulin-like growth factor-I and the role of the MAPK pathway in skeletal muscle cells. Mol Cells 2009;28:589–593.
41 Gottlieb B, Beitel LK, Trifiro MA: Androgen insensitivity syndrome; in Pagon RA, et al (eds): Gene Reviews. Seattle, University of Washington, 2014.
42 Panda B, Rao L, Tosh D, Dixit H, Padmalatha V, Kanakavalli M, Raseswari T, Deenadayal M, Gupta N, Chakrabarty B, Nallari P, Singh L: Germline study of AR gene of Indian women with ovarian failure. Gynecol Endocrinol 2011;27:572–578.
43 Lumbroso S, Lobaccaro JM, Vial C, Sassolas G, Ollagnon B, Belon C, Pouget J, Sultan C: Molecular analysis of the androgen receptor gene in Kennedy's disease: report of two families and review of the literature. Horm Res 1997;47:23–29.
44 Hannema SE, Scott IS, Rajpert-De Meyts E, Skakkebaek NE, Coleman N, Hughes IA: Testicular development in the complete androgen insensitivity syndrome. J Pathol 2006;208:518–527.
45 Brinkmann AO: Molecular basis of androgen insensitivity. Mol Cell Endocrinol 2001;179:105–109.
46 Muller J: Morphometry and histology of gonads from twelve children and adolescents with the androgen insensitivity (testicular feminization) syndrome. J Clin Endocrinol Metab 1984;59:785–789.
47 Hiort O, Holterhus PM, Horter T, Schulze W, Kremke B, Bals-Pratsch M, Sinnecker GH, Kruse K: Significance of mutations in the androgen receptor gene in males with idiopathic infertility. J Clin Endocrinol Metab 2000;85:2810–2815.
48 Boehmer AL, Brinkmann O, Bruggenwirth H, van Assendelft C, Otten BJ, Verleun-Mooijman MC, Niermeijer MF, Brunner HG, Rouwe CW, Waelkens JJ, Oostdijk W, Kleijer WJ, van der Kwast TH, de Vroede MA, Drop SL: Genotype versus phenotype in families with androgen insensitivity syndrome. J Clin Endocrinol Metab 2001;86:4151–4160.

49 Mazen I, El-Ruby M, Kamal R, El-Nekhely I, El-Ghandour M, Tantawy S, El-Gammal M: Screening of genital anomalies in newborns and infants in two Egyptian governorates. Horm Res Paediatr 2010;73:438–442.
50 Oakes MB, Eyvazzadeh AD, Quint E, Smith YR: Complete androgen insensitivity syndrome – a review. J Pediatr Adolesc Gynecol 2008;21:305–310.
51 Galani A, Kitsiou-Tzeli S, Sofokleous C, Kanavakis E, Kalpini-Mavrou A: Androgen insensitivity syndrome: clinical features and molecular defects. Hormones (Athens) 2008;7:17–29.
52 Hughes IA, Davies JD, Bunch TI, Pasterski V, Mastroyannopoulou K, MacDougall J: Androgen insensitivity syndrome. Lancet 2012;380:1419–1428.
53 Evans BA, Hughes IA, Bevan CL, Patterson MN, Gregory JW: Phenotypic diversity in siblings with partial androgen insensitivity syndrome. Arch Dis Child 1997;76:529–531.
54 Goglia U, Vinanzi C, Zuccarello D, Malpassi D, Ameri P, Casu M, Minuto F, Foresta C, Ferone D: Identification of a novel mutation in exon 1 of androgen receptor gene in an azoospermic patient with mild androgen insensitivity syndrome: case report and literature review. Fertil Steril 2011;96:1165–1169.
55 Zuccarello D, Ferlin A, Vinanzi C, Prana E, Garolla A, Callewaert L, Claessens F, Brinkmann AO, Foresta C: Detailed functional studies on androgen receptor mild mutations demonstrate their association with male infertility. Clin Endocrinol 2008;68:580–588.
56 Ghadessy FJ, Lim J, Abdullah AA, Panet-Raymond V, Choo CK, Lumbroso R, Tut TG, Gottlieb B, Pinsky L, Trifiro MA, Yong EL: Oligospermic infertility associated with an androgen receptor mutation that disrupts interdomain and coactivator (TIF2) interactions. J Clin Invest 1999;103:1517–1525.
57 Edwards A, Hammond HA, Jin L, Caskey CT, Chakraborty R: Genetic variation at five trimeric and tetrameric tandem repeat loci in four human population groups. Genomics 1992;12: 241–253.
58 La Spada AR, Wilson EM, Lubahn DB, Harding AE, Fischbeck KH: Androgen receptor gene mutations in X-linked spinal and bulbar muscular atrophy. Nature 1991;352:77–79.
59 Gao T, Marcelli M, McPhaul MJ: Transcriptional activation and transient expression of the human androgen receptor. J Steroid Biochem Mol Biol 1996;59: 9–20.
60 Choong CS, Kemppainen JA, Zhou ZX, Wilson EM: Reduced androgen receptor gene expression with first exon CAG repeat expansion. Mol Endocrinol 1996; 10:1527–1535.
61 Tut TG, Ghadessy FJ, Trifiro MA, Pinsky L, Yong EL: Long polyglutamine tracts in the androgen receptor are associated with reduced trans-activation, impaired sperm production, and male infertility. J Clin Endocrinol Metab 1997;82:3777–3782.
62 Jaaskelainen J: Molecular biology of androgen insensitivity. Mol Cell Endocrinol 2012;352:4–12.
63 Lyon MF, Hawkes SG: X-linked gene for testicular feminization in the mouse. Nature 1970;227:1217–1219.
64 Yeh S, Tsai MY, Xu Q, Mu XM, Lardy H, Huang KE, Lin H, Yeh SD, Altuwaijri S, Zhou X, Xing L, Boyce BF, Hung MC, Zhang S, Gan L, Chang C: Generation and characterization of androgen receptor knockout (ARKO) mice: an in vivo model for the study of androgen functions in selective tissues. Proc Natl Acad Sci USA 2002;99:13498–13503.
65 Gaspar ML, Meo T, Bourgarel P, Guenet JL, Tosi M: A single base deletion in the *Tfm* androgen receptor gene creates a short-lived messenger RNA that directs internal translation initiation. Proc Natl Acad Sci USA 1991;88:8606–8610.
66 De Gendt K, Swinnen JV, Saunders PT, Schoonjans L, Dewerchin M, Devos A, Tan K, Atanassova N, Claessens F, Lecureuil C, Heyns W, Carmeliet P, Guillou F, Sharpe RM, Verhoeven G: A Sertoli cell-selective knockout of the androgen receptor causes spermatogenic arrest in meiosis. Proc Natl Acad Sci USA 2004; 101:1327–1332.
67 Notini AJ, Davey RA, McManus JF, Bate KL, Zajac JD: Genomic actions of the androgen receptor are required for normal male sexual differentiation in a mouse model. J Mol Endocrinol 2005; 35:547–555.
68 Sato T, Matsumoto T, Kawano H, Watanabe T, Uematsu Y, Sekine K, Fukuda T, Aihara K, Krust A, Yamada T, Nakamichi Y, Yamamoto Y, Nakamura T, Yoshimura K, Yoshizawa T, Metzger D, Chambon P, Kato S: Brain masculinization requires androgen receptor function. Proc Natl Acad Sci USA 2004;101: 1673–1678.
69 Chang C, Chen YT, Yeh SD, Xu Q, Wang RS, Guillou F, Lardy H, Yeh S: Infertility with defective spermatogenesis and hypotestosteronemia in male mice lacking the androgen receptor in Sertoli cells. Proc Natl Acad Sci USA 2004;101:6876–6881.
70 Holdcraft RW, Braun RE, Androgen receptor function is required in Sertoli cells for the terminal differentiation of haploid spermatids. Development 2004; 131:459–467.
71 Welsh M, Saunders PT, Atanassova N, Sharpe RM, Smith LB: Androgen action via testicular peritubular myoid cells is essential for male fertility. FASEB J 2009;23:4218–4230.
72 O'Hara L, McInnes K, Simitsidellis I, Morgan S, Atanassova N, Slowikowska-Hilczer J, Kula K, Szarras-Czapnik M, Milne L, Mitchell RT, Smith LB: Autocrine androgen action is essential for Leydig cell maturation and function, and protects against late-onset Leydig cell apoptosis in both mice and men. FASEB J 2015;29:894–910.
73 O'Hara L, Smith LB: Androgen receptor signalling in vascular endothelial cells is dispensable for spermatogenesis and male fertility. BMC Res Notes 2012;5:16.
74 Welsh M, Sharpe RM, Moffat L, Atanassova N, Saunders PT, Kilter S, Bergh A, Smith LB: Androgen action via testicular arteriole smooth muscle cells is important for Leydig cell function, vasomotion and testicular fluid dynamics. PLoS One 2010;5:e13632.
75 Mruk DD, Cheng CY: Sertoli-Sertoli and Sertoli-Germ cell interactions and their significance in germ cell movement in the seminiferous epithelium during spermatogenesis. Endocr Rev 2004;25: 747–806.
76 Willems A, De Gendt K, Allemeersch J, Smith LB, Welsh M, Swinnen JV, Verhoeven G: Early effects of Sertoli cell-selective androgen receptor ablation on testicular gene expression. Int J Androl 2009;33: 507–517.

77 Berensztein EB, Baquedano MS, Gonzalez CR, Saraco NI, Rodriguez J, Ponzio R, Rivarola MA and Belgorosky A: Expression of aromatase, estrogen receptor α and β, androgen receptor, and cytochrome P-450_{scc} in the human early prepubertal testis. Pediatr Res 2006;60: 740–744.
78 Rey RA, Musse M, Venara M, Chemes HE: Ontogeny of the androgen receptor expression in the fetal and postnatal testis: its relevance on Sertoli cell maturation and the onset of adult spermatogenesis. Microsc Res Tech 2009;72:787–795.
79 Chemes HE, Rey RA, Nistal M, Regadera J, Musse M, Gonzalez-Peramato P, Serrano A: Physiological androgen insensitivity of the fetal, neonatal, and early infantile testis is explained by the ontogeny of the androgen receptor expression in Sertoli cells. J Clin Endocrinol Metab 2008;93:4408–4412.
80 Suarez-Quian CA, Martinez-Garcia F, Nistal M, Regadera J: Androgen receptor distribution in adult human testis. J Clin Endocrinol Metab 1999;84:350–358.
81 Hazra R, Corcoran L, Robson M, McTavish KJ, Upton D, Handelsman DJ, Allan CM: Temporal role of Sertoli cell androgen receptor expression in spermatogenic development. Mol Endocrinol 2013;27:12–24.
82 Lim P, Robson M, Spaliviero J, McTavish KJ, Jimenez M, Zajac JD, Handelsman DJ, Allan CM: Sertoli cell androgen receptor DNA binding domain is essential for the completion of spermatogenesis. Endocrinology 2009;150:4755–4765.
83 Toocheck C, Clister T, Shupe J, Crum C, Ravindranathan P, Lee TK, Ahn JM, Raj GV, Sukhwani M, Orwig KE, Walker WH: Mouse spermatogenesis requires classical and nonclassical testosterone signaling. Biol Reprod 2016;94:11.
84 Willems A, Roesl C, Mitchell RT, Milne L, Jeffery N, Smith S, Verhoeven G, Brown P, Smith LB: Sertoli cell androgen receptor signalling in adulthood is essential for post-meiotic germ cell development. Mol Reprod Dev 2015;82: 626–627.
85 Willems A, Batlouni SR, Esnal A, Swinnen JV, Saunders PT, Sharpe RM, Franca LR, De Gendt K, Verhoeven G: Selective ablation of the androgen receptor in mouse sertoli cells affects Sertoli cell maturation, barrier formation and cytoskeletal development. PLoS One 2010; 5:e14168.
86 Dym M, Fawcett DW: The blood-testis barrier in the rat and the physiological compartmentation of the seminiferous epithelium. Biol Reprod 1970;3:308–326.
87 Meng J, Holdcraft RW, Shima JE, Griswold MD, Braun RE: Androgens regulate the permeability of the blood-testis barrier. Proc Natl Acad Sci USA 2005; 102:16696–16700.
88 Wang RS, Yeh S, Chen LM, Lin HY, Zhang C, Ni J, Wu CC, di Sant'Agnese PA, deMesy-Bentley KL, Tzeng CR, Chang C: Androgen receptor in Sertoli cell is essential for germ cell nursery and junctional complex formation in mouse testes. Endocrinology 2006;147:5624–5633.
89 Denolet E, De Gendt K, Allemeersch J, Engelen K, Marchal K, Van Hummelen P, Tan KA, Sharpe RM, Saunders PT, Swinnen JV, Verhoeven G: The effect of a Sertoli cell-selective knockout of the androgen receptor on testicular gene expression in prepubertal mice. Mol Endocrinol 2006;20:321–334.
90 Eacker SM, Shima JE, Connolly CM, Sharma M, Holdcraft RW, Griswold MD, Braun RE: Transcriptional profiling of androgen receptor (AR) mutants suggests instructive and permissive roles of AR signaling in germ cell development. Mol Endocrinol 2007;21:895–907.
91 McCabe MJ, Allan CM, Foo CF, Nicholls PK, McTavish KJ, Stanton PG: Androgen initiates Sertoli cell tight junction formation in the hypogonadal (*hpg*) mouse. Biol Reprod 2012;87:38.
92 Rato L, Socorro S, Cavaco JE, Oliveira PF: Tubular fluid secretion in the seminiferous epithelium: ion transporters and aquaporins in Sertoli cells. J Membr Biol 2010;236:215–224.
93 McLachlan RI, O'Donnell L, Meachem SJ, Stanton PG, de Kretser DM, Pratis K, Robertson DM: Identification of specific sites of hormonal regulation in spermatogenesis in rats, monkeys, and man. Recent Prog Horm Res 2002;57:149–179.
94 O'Donnell L, McLachlan RI, Wreford NG, de Kretser DM, Robertson DM: Testosterone withdrawal promotes stage-specific detachment of round spermatids from the rat seminiferous epithelium. Biol Reprod 1996;55:895–901.
95 O'Donnell L, Stanton PG, Bartles JR, Robertson DM: Sertoli cell ectoplasmic specializations in the seminiferous epithelium of the testosterone-suppressed adult rat. Biol Reprod 2000;63: 99–108.
96 Saito K, O'Donnell L, McLachlan RI, Robertson DM: Spermiation failure is a major contributor to early spermatogenic suppression caused by hormone withdrawal in adult rats. Endocrinology 2000;141:2779–2785.
97 Beardsley A, O'Donnell L: Characterization of normal spermiation and spermiation failure induced by hormone suppression in adult rats. Biol Reprod 2003;68:1299–1307.
98 Beardsley A, Robertson DM, O'Donnell L: A complex containing $\alpha_6\beta_1$-integrin and phosphorylated focal adhesion kinase between Sertoli cells and elongated spermatids during spermatid release from the seminiferous epithelium. J Endocrinol 2006;190:759–770.
99 Yan HH, Cheng CY: Laminin α3 forms a complex with β3 and γ3 chains that serves as the ligand for α6β1-integrin at the apical ectoplasmic specialization in adult rat testes. J Biol Chem 2006; 281:17286–17303.
100 Chojnacka K, Mruk DD: The Src non-receptor tyrosine kinase paradigm: new insights into mammalian Sertoli cell biology. Mol Cell Endocrinol 2015; 415:133–142.
101 Lee NP, Cheng CY: Protein kinases and adherens junction dynamics in the seminiferous epithelium of the rat testis. J Cell Physiol 2005;202:344–360.
102 Cheng CY, Mruk DD: An intracellular trafficking pathway in the seminiferous epithelium regulating spermatogenesis: a biochemical and molecular perspective. Crit Rev Biochem Mol Biol 2009;44:245–263.
103 Verhoeven G, Willems A, Denolet E, Swinnen JV, De Gendt K: Androgens and spermatogenesis: lessons from transgenic mouse models. Philos Trans R Soc Lond B Biol Sci 2010;365:1537–1556.
104 Papaioannou MD, Pitetti JL, Ro S, Park C, Aubry F, Schaad O, Vejnar CE, Kuhne F, Descombes P, Zdobnov EM, McManus MT, Guillou F, Harfe BD, Yan W, Jegou B, Nef S: Sertoli cell Dicer is essential for spermatogenesis in mice. Dev Biol 2009;326:250–259.

105 Korhonen HM, Meikar O, Yadav RP, Papaioannou MD, Romero Y, Da Ros M, Herrera PL, Toppari J, Nef S, Kotaja N: Dicer is required for haploid male germ cell differentiation in mice. PLoS One 2011;6:e24821.
106 Panneerdoss S, Chang YF, Buddavarapu KC, Chen HI, Shetty G, Wang H, Chen Y, Kumar TR, Rao MK: Androgen-responsive microRNAs in mouse Sertoli cells. PLoS One 2012;7:e41146.
107 Farr CH, Ellis LC: In vitro contractility of rat seminiferous tubules in response to prostaglandins, cyclic GMP, testosterone and 2,4'-dibromoacetophenone. J Reprod Fertil 1980;58:37–42.
108 Skinner MK, Tung PS, Fritz IB: Cooperativity between Sertoli cells and testicular peritubular cells in the production and deposition of extracellular matrix components. J Cell Biol 1985; 100:1941–1947.
109 Richardson LL, Kleinman HK, Dym M: Basement membrane gene expression by Sertoli and peritubular myoid cells in vitro in the rat. Biol Reprod 1995;52: 320–330.
110 Drews U, Sulak O, Oppitz M: Immunohistochemical localisation of androgen receptor during sex-specific morphogenesis in the fetal mouse. Histochem Cell Biol 2001;116:427–439.
111 Mayerhofer A: Human testicular peritubular cells: more than meets the eye. Reproduction 2013;145:R107–R116.
112 De Gendt K, Verhoeven G: Tissue- and cell-specific functions of the androgen receptor revealed through conditional knockout models in mice. Mol Cell Endocrinol 2012;352:13–25.
113 Raskin K, de Gendt K, Duittoz A, Liere P, Verhoeven G, Tronche F, Mhaouty-Kodja S: Conditional inactivation of androgen receptor gene in the nervous system: effects on male behavioral and neuroendocrine responses. J Neurosci 2009;29:4461–4470.
114 Juntti SA, Tollkuhn J, Wu MV, Fraser EJ, Soderborg T, Tan S, Honda S, Harada N, Shah NM: The androgen receptor governs the execution, but not programming, of male sexual and territorial behaviors. Neuron 2010;66: 260–272.
115 O'Hara L, Welsh M, Saunders PT, Smith LB: Androgen receptor expression in the caput epididymal epithelium is essential for development of the initial segment and epididymal spermatozoa transit. Endocrinology 2011;152:718–729.
116 Krutskikh A, Poliandri A, Cabrera-Sharp V, Dacheux JL, Poutanen M, Huhtaniemi I: Epididymal protein Rnase10 is required for post-testicular sperm maturation and male fertility. FASEB J 2012;26:4198–4209.
117 Simanainen U, McNamara K, Davey RA, Zajac JD, Handelsman DJ: Severe subfertility in mice with AR inactivation in sex accessory organs, but not in testis. Endocrinology 2008;149:3330–3338.
118 Wu CT, Altuwaijri S, Ricke WA, Huang SP, Yeh S, Zhang C, Niu Y, Tsai MY, Chang C: Increased prostate cell proliferation and loss of cell differentiation in mice lacking prostate epithelial androgen receptor. Proc Natl Acad Sci USA 2007;104:12679–12684.
119 Welsh M, Moffat L, Jack L, McNeilly A, Brownstein D, Saunders PT, Sharpe RM, Smith LB: Deletion of androgen receptor in the smooth muscle of the seminal vesicles impairs secretory function and alters its responsiveness to exogenous testosterone and estradiol. Endocrinology 2010;151:3374–3385.
120 Welsh M, Moffat L, McNeilly A, Brownstein D, Saunders PT, Sharpe RM, Smith LB: Smooth muscle cell-specific knockout of androgen receptor: a new model for prostatic disease. Endocrinology 2011;152:3541–3551.
121 Welsh M, Sharpe RM, Walker M, Smith LB, Saunders PT: New insights into the role of androgens in wolffian duct stabilization in male and female rodents. Endocrinology 2009;150: 2472–2480.
122 Welsh M, Saunders PT, Sharpe RM: The critical time window for androgen-dependent development of the Wolffian duct in the rat. Endocrinology 2007;148:3185–3195.
123 Krutskikh A, De Gendt K, Sharp V, Verhoeven G, Poutanen M, Huhtaniemi I: Targeted inactivation of the androgen receptor gene in murine proximal epididymis causes epithelial hypotrophy and obstructive azoospermia. Endocrinology 2011;152:689–696.
124 Jorgensen N, Joensen UN, Jensen TK, Jensen MB, Almstrup K, Olesen IA, Juul A, Andersson AM, Carlsen E, Petersen JH, Toppari J, Skakkebaek NE: Human semen quality in the new millennium: a prospective cross-sectional population-based study of 4,867 men. BMJ Open 2012;2:e000990.
125 Sharpe RM: Sperm counts and fertility in men: a rocky road ahead. EMBO Rep 2012;13:398–403.

Lee B. Smith
Medical Research Council Centre for Reproductive Health
University of Edinburgh, 47 Little France Crescent
Edinburgh EH16 4TJ (UK)
E-Mail lee.smith@ed.ac.uk

Vogt PH (ed): Genetics of Human Infertility. Monogr Hum Genet.
Basel, Karger, 2017, vol 21, pp 101–115 (DOI: 10.1159/000477281)

The Genetics of Postmeiotic Male Germ Cell Differentiation from Round Spermatids to Mature Sperm

Tiina Lehtiniemi · Noora Kotaja
Institute of Biomedicine, University of Turku, Turku, Finland

Abstract
After meiotic divisions, postmeiotic haploid spermatids are faced with the challenge of undergoing a dramatic morphological transformation to form mature, highly specialized spermatozoa. The main processes required for the development of functional spermatozoa include the formation of an acrosome and a flagellum, and compaction of sperm chromatin and nuclear shaping. The haploid differentiation program (spermiogenesis) is governed by the well-coordinated expression of a wide variety of genes required for the morphological and metabolic changes. It is clear that disturbances at any given point of spermiogenesis lead to a reduced ability to conceive offspring due to either a reduced number or abnormal morphology and function of spermatozoa. Defective spermatozoa are often observed in infertile males, including sperm with an abnormal morphology (teratozoospermia), defective motility (asthenozoospermia), or lowered number of sperm in the semen (oligozoospermia). Male infertility is often a multifactorial disorder, which hinders our understanding of the causal factors. However, genetic studies have revealed several genes affected in infertile males with spermiogenic defects. Furthermore, genetically modified mouse models have provided valuable information about the important genes required for haploid germ cell-specific processes.

Male Germ Differentiation-Associated Male Infertility

Gamete differentiation is a unique process with unique mechanisms, one of the most critical being meiosis that results in haploid cells and generates genomic diversity. Meiosis is a key process for both female and male gametogenesis. The difference between these 2 developmental programs is the haploid differentiation phase (spermiogenesis) specific for male gametogenesis. Spermiogenesis encompasses dramatic morphological transformation of round spermatids into mature spermatozoa equipped with specialized structures that enable their independent movement and fertilization of an egg in the female reproductive tract [1]. Three major morphological changes

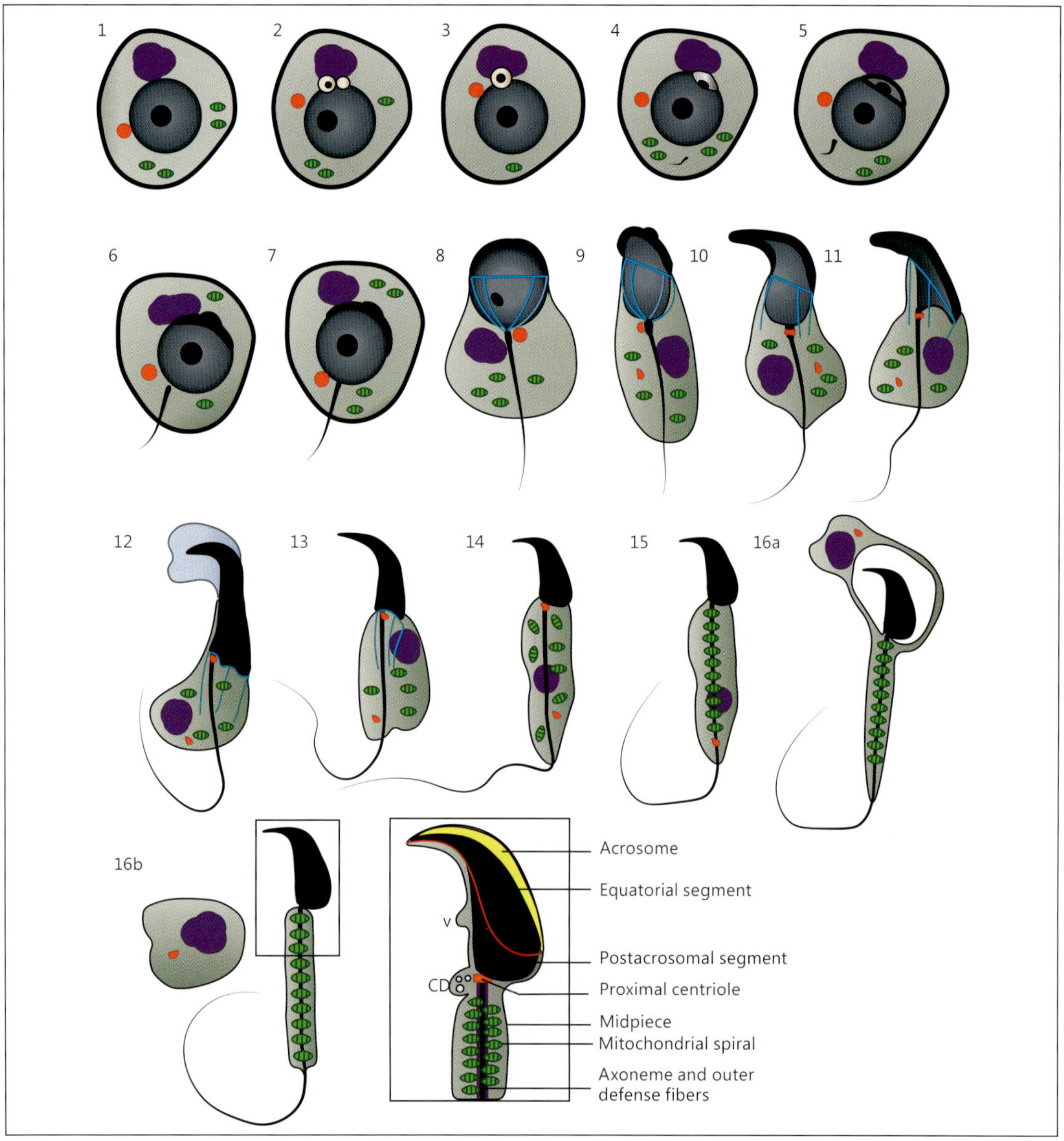

Fig. 1. Schematic diagram of haploid male germ cell differentiation in mice. Haploid differentiation, also known as spermiogenesis, consists of 16 steps. The acrosome and flagellum already start forming in round spermatids (steps 1–8) while elongation (steps 9–16) and nuclear condensation (steps 11–16) take place later on. The acrosome starts forming as the juxtanuclear Golgi complex (purple) provides vesicles for it. Proacrosomal vesicles are seen in step 2 spermatids, while a single rounded acrosomal vesicle emerges by step 3 spermatids. The developing acrosome then expands over the anterior nucleus in the following steps and makes contact with the cell surface in step 8 spermatids. Spermatids subsequently elongate, the nucleus flattens, and usually by step 12 nuclear condensation has taken place. The sperm head then shortens and mitochondria (green) become aligned to form a prominent midpiece. Excess cytoplasm is finally shed off and spermatozoa are released into the lumen. The chromatoid body (orange) is a haploid-specific germ granule particularly prominent in round spermatids. The manchette (blue) is a transient microtubule structure, which has a role in sculpting the nucleus shape. CD, cytoplasmic droplet; V, ventral spur.

in this process are the formation of an acrosome, chromatin compaction with head shaping, and development of a flagellum (Fig. 1).

Both the acrosome and flagellum start developing in haploid round spermatids. Acrosome formation begins in very early round spermatids and it gradually expands and spreads over the entire anterior half of the sperm head. Simultaneously, on the opposite site of the nucleus, the construction of the flagellum begins with the formation of an axoneme and continues later in development by the addition of the accessory structures such as outer dense fibers, fibrous sheath, and mitochondrial sheath. At the end of the round spermatid phase, the cell polarizes and enters the nuclear elongation/condensing phase. During elongation, the nuclear size is reduced as a result of chromatin compaction, and the nucleus obtains its typical ovoid shape. Finally, at spermiation, when the fully developed sperm is released into the lumen, the cytoplasm is shed off and sperm moves to the epididymis for further maturation.

Disturbances at any given point of spermiogenesis lead to a reduced ability to conceive offspring due to either a reduced number of spermatozoa or abnormal morphology and function of spermatozoa [2]. Oligoasthenoteratozoospermia is a condition where a combination of qualitative and quantitative sperm defects occur. These defects include a low number of sperm (oligozoospermia), poor sperm movement (asthenozoospermia), and abnormalities in the sperm shape (teratozoospermia). Teratozoospermia represents a heterogeneous group including a wide range of abnormal sperm phenotypes affecting, solely or simultaneously, the head, neck, midpiece, and tail. Teratozoospermia is defined as a percentage of morphologically abnormal spermatozoa above the lower reference limit, which was set by the World Health Organization (WHO) to 4% at the last evaluation [3, 4]. A complete lack of sperm in the ejaculate may be caused by abnormal spermatogenesis (nonobstructive azoospermia; NOA) or normal sperm production in the presence of obstruction (obstructive azoospermia).

Quantitative or qualitative changes in the semen are observed in half the cases of infertile couples. In approximately 30–50% of male infertility cases, the cause of sperm defects remains unknown (idiopathic) and could be congenital or acquired. Genetic factors are frequently involved and it has been estimated that male infertility of a genetic origin affects about 1 in 40 adult men [5]. The known genetic causes of male infertility include chromosomal abnormalities, mitochondrial DNA mutations, and monogenic mutations affecting sperm production or morphology, as well as endocrine disorders of genetic origin. Deletions in the long arm of the Y chromosome (Yq) are among the best-known mutations to associate with defects in sperm production, and 5–20% of infertile men have been reported to have the microdeletion in the azoospermic factor regions (AZFa, AZFb, and AZFc) of the Y chromosome [6]. A complete deletion of the AZFa region results in an SCO (Sertoli cell-only) pathology, while complete AZFb deletions cause meiotic arrest. Complete AZFc deletion leads to variable seminal (azoospermia to severe oligozoospermia) and testicular phenotypes (SCO to hypospermatogenesis in distinct testicular tubules) [7, 8].

Several studies have shown that reactive oxygen species and free radicals can cause oxidative stress that causes mitochondrial DNA mutations with adverse consequences in fertility [9]. The midpiece of the mammalian sperm contains around 70–80 mitochondria, each containing only 1 copy of mtDNA. Apart from a few nuclear genes, mitochondria have their own genome that encodes for numerous proteins involved in the energy production needed for sperm motility. In humans, around 85% of sperm samples contain large-scale mtDNA deletions of variable sizes, and most spermatozoa have 2–7 mtDNA deletions. An age-related increase in oxidative stress

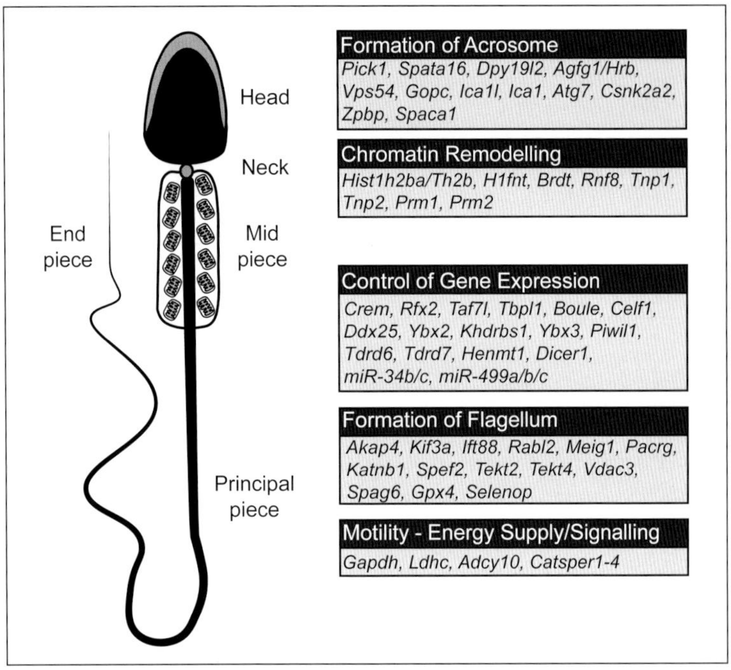

Fig. 2. Genes involved in the development of spermatozoa. Spermatozoa consist of the head, neck, midpiece, and tail. The head contains highly condensed chromatin and the acrosome. The shape of the sperm head is a species-specific feature. The proximal centriole is located at the neck, which separates the head from the tail. Divided into 3 parts, the tail consists of the midpiece (mitochondria), principal piece (fibrous sheath), and end piece (only axoneme and outer dense fibers). Mutations in several genes have been indicated to affect fertility by disrupting the developmental process of these structures. Examples of these genes that are further discussed in the text are grouped here by the process that their disruption primarily affects.

and mutated mtDNA has been associated with male infertility [10, 11].

Monogenic disorders occur as a direct consequence of a single gene being defective. It is likely that the majority of the genetic causes of male infertility are still uncharacterized, likely due to the multifactorial nature of the disorder and large number of genes involved. However, progress has been made and, for example, the genetic investigations of severe teratozoospermias have identified recurrent mutations with 3 specific phenotypes: macrozoospermia, characterized by a large sperm head and several flagella; globozoospermia, with a round-shaped sperm head and an absence of mitochondria in the midpiece, and multiple morphological abnormalities of the flagella [12].

Genetically modified mouse models have greatly extended our knowledge of genes that play a role in haploid male germ cell differentiation, and enabled the identification of several candidate genes potentially involved in human sperm defects (Fig. 2). Here, selected genes involved in the critical processes during spermiogenesis, namely control of haploid gene expression, acrosome formation, development of flagellum and motility, and chromatin remodeling will be discussed, taking into account the data received from model organisms with an emphasis on mice. It has to be noted that even though these processes are discussed separately, they are closely interconnected and interdependent, as exemplified by the phenotypes of many knockout mouse models that show various defects in several processes.

Control of Haploid Gene Expression

The testis expresses hundreds of protein-coding genes that are not expressed anywhere else in the body, and the transcriptional profiles alter from one cell type to another during spermatogenesis [13]. Furthermore, male germ cells, particularly premeiotic spermatocytes and postmeiotic round spermatids, have exceptionally diverse transcriptomes, encompassing a great variety of small

RNAs, long noncoding RNAs, and poorly conserved intergenic sequences in addition to protein-coding RNAs [14]. Therefore, the control of gene expression is of fundamental importance during spermatogenesis.

A few transcription factors have been shown to be critical regulators of haploid cell gene expression. One of the best known examples is the cyclic AMP response element (CRE) modulator (CREM) that exists in multiple isoforms and binds to consensus palindromic CRE to regulate the transcription of its target genes [15]. Deletion of the *Crem* gene in mice leads to a block in spermatogenesis at the round spermatid phase and therefore male infertility [16]. The CREMτ activator isoform is specifically accumulated in postmeiotic round spermatids, where it acts together with germ cell-specific coactivators such as ACT (activator of CREM in the testis) [17, 18]. Moreover, the function of ACT depends on a kinesin KIF17b [19], and sperm-associated antigen 8 (SPAG8) has also been suggested to take part in the CREMτ-ACT complex [20]. In humans, a study of 361 NOA patients and 368 controls in the Chinese population revealed that none of the candidate SNPs of ACT, KIF17b, and SPAG8 showed a significant association with the risk of NOA. However, the results demonstrated that 2 CREM gene SNPs, rs4934540 and rs2295415, led to a decreased NOA risk, indicating they might be protective factors for spermatogenesis [21].

Another important transcription factor for haploid male germ cell differentiation is regulatory factor X2 (RFX2). Similar to *Crem* knockout mice, spermatogenesis in *Rfx2* knockout mice is arrested at the round spermatid phase; however, the target genes of CREM and RFX2 are largely nonoverlapping [22]. Interestingly, testis-specific paralogs of somatically expressed components of general transcription machinery have also important regulatory roles in spermiogenic gene expression, as exemplified by TAF7L, a testis-specific paralog of TBP-associate factor 7 (TAF7) and TBP-related factor 2 (TRF2). *Trf2* knockout males are sterile with almost a complete arrest of spermiogenesis and apoptosis of round spermatids, whereas deletion of the *Taf7l* gene leads to a reduced sperm count, abnormal sperm morphology, and reduced motility [23].

Due to the chromatin compaction caused by histone-protamine transition (see below), transcription is mostly silenced in condensing spermatids. Therefore, mRNAs for many spermiogenic proteins are synthesized earlier in spermatogenesis and are kept temporarily stored until later steps. The storage and release of RNAs are mainly controlled by RNA-binding proteins (RBPs) that bind their targets either nonspecifically or through specific motifs to form RNP (ribonucleoprotein) complexes. Considering the large number of transcripts present in germ cells, it is not surprising that testes also harbor testis-specific RBPs, the largest group of tissue-specific RBPs in humans [24]. Knockout mouse models have revealed the critical role for many of these RBPs, such as BOULE, CELF1, DDX25, MSY2, SAM68, MSY4, and PIWIL1/MIWI, in haploid differentiation and spermatid elongation [25].

In germ cells, many RNA species and RBPs accumulate in germ cell-specific RNP granules, commonly known as germ granules. Postmeiotic haploid round spermatids are characterized by an unusually large germ granule, the chromatoid body, which appears to have a central role in the PIWI-interacting RNA (piRNA) pathway [26]. piRNAs form a large and complex group of small RNAs that bind to PIWI proteins (MIWI, MILI, and MIWI2 in mice). The functions of piRNAs are diverse [27]. During early phases of male germ cell development, they play an important role in transposon silencing. However, postnatal pachytene piRNAs also direct meiotic and postmeiotic mRNAs and long noncoding RNAs for degradation. When the main round spermatid-expressed PIWI protein, MIWI, is removed or catalytically inactivated in mice, spermatogenesis is arrested at the round spermatid phase [28, 29]. Furthermore, many other chromatoid body components that are also implicated in piRNA pathways, such as the Tudor domain-containing proteins TDRD6 and TDRD7, are required for normal haploid differentiation in mice [26]. In addition, loss-of-function of methyltransferase HENMT1 in mice results in the loss of 2′-O-methylation of piRNAs, piRNA instability, and a germ cell arrest at the elongation phase [30]. Altogether, these studies highlight the essential role of piRNA-targeted regulation in spermiogenesis.

MicroRNAs (miRNAs) are also expressed in a cell type-specific manner during spermatogenesis. Several conditional knockout mouse models for the gene encoding for the miRNA processing enzyme DICER have been generated. While deletion of the *Dicer1* gene in late embryonic germ cells causes severe meiotic defects, later deletion of *Dicer1* in postnatal spermatogonia results in major defects in haploid differentiation [31]. Interestingly, the deletion of the 2 main miRNA clusters expressed in round spermatids, miR-34b/c and miR-499a/b/c, result in oligoasthenoteratozoospermia and infertility, which signifies their importance for spermiogenesis [32]. However, the independent deletion of either one of these clusters does not affect spermatogenesis or male fertility [31, 32].

Chromatin Remodeling during Spermiogenesis

Epigenetic regulation refers to semipermanent changes in gene expression resulting from modifications of chromatin structure, rather than changes in DNA sequence. The main mechanisms of epigenetic regulation include DNA methylation primarily within CpG dinucleotides and covalent modifications of histone tails. Male germ cells undergo drastic epigenetic remodeling during development, beginning with near-to-complete erasure of epigenetic marks in primordial germ cells and the reestablishment of novel, sex-specific marks [33]. Postnatal spermatogenesis is also characterized by major epigenetic transitions, particularly during meiosis (synapsis, recombination, and sex chromosome inactivation) and haploid differentiation. Haploid spermatids undergo the most remarkable chromatin remodeling that includes almost genome-wide removal of histones and their replacement by small basic proteins, protamines, which enables the extreme compaction of male germ cell nuclei [34]. Several mouse and human studies have demonstrated the importance of proper nuclear condensation and chromatin compaction for fertility.

Prior to histone-protamine transition, various histone variants are incorporated into the chromatin in a temporally regulated manner. Up to 46 different histones and histone variants have been detected in the human sperm nuclear proteome [35]. Histone variants, such as testis-specific histones H3T, TH2B, H2AL2 and H2Abbd, are suggested to create less stable nucleosomes, therefore facilitating nucleosome disassembly and histone displacement [34]. Mouse models with depleted or C-terminally modified TH2B revealed that TH2B controls the final transformation of nucleosomes into protamine-packed structures; without functional TH2B, spermatogenesis is arrested in condensing spermatids and no mature spermatozoa are produced [36]. Testis-specific linker histone variants, such as H1t, HILS, and H1T2, are also involved in the regulation of haploid chromatin condensation. Mice deficient in H1T2 that associates with chromatin domains localized at the apical pole of the nucleus of late round and elongating spermatids, show impaired spermatid chromatin compaction resulting in reduced fertility [37].

In addition to the incorporation of histone variants, a large-scale histone hyperacetylation is required to further loosen the nucleosome architecture to enable histone-protamine transition [34]. Hyperacetylated histones are selectively recognized and bound by the first bromodomain (BD1) of BRDT, a testis-specific BET (bromo- and extraterminal domain) protein [38]. Mice expressing BRDT lacking BD1 show dramatic defects observed in elongating spermatids caused by defective histone replacement [39, 40]. Interestingly, in addition to its critical role in histone-protamine transition, BRDT was shown to drive a specific histone acetylation-guided gene expression program during spermatogenesis [40]. Due to the critical role of BRDT in spermatogenesis, a small molecule inhibitor (JQ1) that can cross the blood-testis barrier and selectively and reversibly inhibit BET subfamily proteins has been suggested as a potential compound for male contraception [41]. Ubiquitination of H2A and H2B by the E3 ubiquitin ligase RNF8 has been revealed as an important signal for promoting H4 hyperacetylation. In addition, mutation of the *Rnf8* gene in mice disrupts hyperacetylation and global nucleosome removal [42].

The replacement of almost all canonical histones by protamines occurs in a stepwise fashion. First, so-called transition proteins (TP1 and TP2) are incorporated and transition proteins are subsequently replaced by 2 protamines (P1 and P2) that stably bind the paternal genome. Mice deficient of either TP1 or TP2 are subfertile due to fewer condensed sperm nuclei. Double *Tnp1/Tnp2* knockout mice are completely infertile, which confirms their importance for haploid chromatin compaction [43]. P1 and P2 have been suggested to have distinct roles in spermatogenesis due to biochemical differences in their structure. In different mammals, the ratio of the 2 protamines varies. In humans, the P1:P2 ratio is normally equal, or falls between a narrow range of 0.8–1.2. An abnormal P1:P2 ratio leads to reduced fertility, and may also affect the transmission of epigenetic information via paternal DNA [44]. In mice, mutation of 1 allele of either of the protamine genes leads to infertility due to disrupted nuclear condensation and sperm function [45, 46].

Protamines are essential for nuclear condensation and may therefore facilitate the hydrodynamic shape of the sperm head and protect the paternal genome from physical and chemical damage. Protamines can also play a role in epigenetic processes. Interestingly, although the histone-protamine transition takes place in a genome-wide comprehensive manner, it is not complete. In the end, about 15% of human sperm chromatin [47] and 1% of mouse sperm chromatin contains nucleosomes [48]. In recent years, several studies aiming to characterize the distribution of the retained nucleosomes in mammalian spermatozoa have been published, with partially conflicting results. For example, several studies showed that histones are not randomly distributed but that retained nucleosomes are frequently in loci enriched in the regulatory regions of genes important for embryogenesis [49–51]. On the other hand, other studies failed to show enrichment of nucleosomes in promoters of genes for developmental regulators and reported that nucleosomes are retained predominantly on distal gene-poor regions [52, 53]. In any case, retained nucleosomes could have an important role in the sperm chromatin reorganization in the oocyte, for example, and perhaps in the selective activation of paternal genes in the early embryo.

It is clear that the dynamic changes in the epigenome and chromatin remodeling are required for the normal development of spermatozoa, and any defects in epigenetic modifications may have detrimental effects on fertility. Importantly, alterations in the sperm chromatin and epimutations may not only affect spermatogenesis, but also result in epigenetic errors contributing to failed postfertilization development [54]. Sperm DNA methylation is one of the epigenetic processes that is associated with abnormal sperm parameters and male infertility, but also affects the clinical results of assisted reproductive techniques and is linked with embryonic development [55]. Oligozoospermic patients have been shown to often undergo aberrant DNA methylation in sperm (e.g., imprinted loci). Interestingly, spermatozoa with normal morphology and motility may also have defects in DNA methylation that lead to unexplained infertility, recurrent abortions, or developmental defects [55, 56]. It has also been shown that spermatozoa from normozoospermic (semen with normal characteristics in a seminogram) men able to perform IVF but whose female partners did not achieve pregnancy have altered levels of proteins compared to spermatozoa from men with similar semen parameters but with successful pregnancy outcomes. These include proteins involved in chromatin assembly (e.g., histone variants), suggesting that these epigenetic defects could prevent embryonic development [57, 58]. Due to the possibility of transmission of abnormal epigenetic information carried by spermatozoa to the next generation, the use of sperm with aberrant chromatin for intracytoplasmic sperm injection (ICSI) may have severe consequences on the progeny, which highlights the necessity of careful evaluation and diagnosis of male infertility before proceeding to ICSI.

Formation of the Acrosome

The acrosome is a large vesicle at the anterior half of the sperm head. It contains various hydrolytic enzymes that are released as the sperm comes into contact with the egg. This facilitates the penetrance of sperm through the zona pellucida and allows it to fuse with the egg. Therefore, the acrosome plays a crucial role during fertilization. In round spermatids, acrosome biogenesis first starts by budding vesicles from the trans-Golgi network that then fuse to form a preacrosomal vesicle. The acroplaxome is a specific cytoskeletal structure formed under it that helps to anchor the developing acrosome to the nuclear envelope. The acrosomal vesicle eventually grows as additional vesicles fuse with it, allowing it to stretch and spread over the anterior nuclear pole [59].

If the process of the acrosome formation is disrupted, a malformed acrosome may arise or, in the most extreme cases, the acrosome may be lacking altogether. Globozoospermia, characterized by acrosomeless round-headed sperm, is a condition that causes primary infertility due to the inability of globozoospermic sperm to adhere and penetrate the zona pellucida. Complete globozoospermia (type 1) is a rare (<0.1% incidence) condition characterized by 100% acrosomeless spermatozoa in the ejaculate. A larger group of men have a milder phenotype, partial globozoospermia (type 2), with an increased amount of round-headed sperm and acrosome malformations [60].

In humans, mutations in *PICK1*, *SPATA16*, and *DPY19L2* have been identified in globozoospermia patients [61–65]. Furthermore, in several genetically modified mouse models, globozoospermia-like phenotypes have been observed, and thus potential target genes such as *Ck2α'*, *Zpbp*, *Hsp90b1*, *Vps54*, *Dpy19l2*, *Atg7*, *Ica1l*, *Pick1*, *Gopc*, *Spaca1*, and *Hrb* have been discovered. Deletions and point mutations of the *DPY19L2* gene constitute a major cause of complete globozoospermia in humans and are found in more than 70% of patients. DPY19L2 belongs to a family of transmembrane proteins present in the nuclear envelope. It is predominantly expressed in spermatids and localizes in the inner nuclear membrane where it is needed to anchor the acrosome to the nucleus. In *Dpy19l2* knockout mice, the acrosome starts to form but it soon separates from the nucleus and is subsequently removed from the sperm with cytoplasm, thus producing a phenotype of complete globozoospermia with round-headed spermatozoa [66].

HRB, VPS54, PICK1, and GOPC1 proteins have been shown to be involved in Golgi-derived vesicle trafficking and fusion necessary for acrosome biogenesis. HRB (HIV Rev-binding protein) is associated with the cytosolic surface of proacrosomic vesicles. In HRB-deficient mice, proacrosomic vesicles form but they remain unable to fuse, therefore blocking the acrosomal development [67]. A similar phenotype is seen in the wobbler mouse, where the vesicular sorting protein VPS54 is mutated. The recessive Vps54 (L967Q) mutation in the mouse results in motor neuron degeneration and male infertility caused by the lack of proper acrosome formation and a disorganized tail midpiece [68].

Protein interacting with C-kinase 1 (PICK1) is a peripheral membrane protein crucial for vesicle trafficking from the Golgi to the acrosome. PICK1-deficient mice are infertile due to defects in acrosome development [69]. This defect can be rescued by testes-specific reexpression of PICK1 [70]. Expression of PICK1 in testes has also been shown to be reduced in Islet cell autoantigen 1-like (ICA1L)-deficient mice. ICA1L associates with PICK1 in spermatids where they are both highly expressed and trafficked together. *Ica1l* knockout mice are subfertile and have characteristics of partial globozoospermia (some of the spermatozoa have detectable acrosomes). Double knockout of *Ica1l* and its homolog islet cell autoantigen 69 kDa (*Ica1*) leads to complete male sterility [71]. Therefore, ICA1L, ICA69, and PICK1 all appear to participate in acrosome formation, but so far only PICK1 mutation has been linked to globozoospermia in humans [63].

In Golgi-associated PDZ- and coiled-coil motif-containing protein (GOPC)-deficient mice, only poorly formed proacrosomic granules are detected instead of a normal acrosomal vesicle [72]. Furthermore, in ATG7-deficient mice that also have a globozoospermia-like phenotype, GOPC fails to be recruited to the acrosome. It has therefore been suggested that ATG7 regulates GOPC and they are both involved in vesicle transport from the Golgi to the preacrosome [73]. Casein kinase II alpha' (CK2α') subunit is preferentially expressed in the testis, and *Csnk2a2* knockout males are infertile and display acrosomal defects, a 30% reduced sperm count, and abnormal motility [74]. Interestingly, SPATA16, which contains 6 CK2 phosphorylation sites, was found to be mutated in 3 brothers with globozoospermia [62]. The localization of SPATA16 in the Golgi apparatus and in proacrosomal vesicles in mice suggests its direct involvement in acrosome biogenesis [75].

Zona pellucida binding protein (ZPBP1/sp38) and sperm acrosome associated 1 (SPACA1) are proteins specifically expressed in haploid cells that are involved in the formation and function of the acrosome. ZPBP1 localizes to the acrosomal membrane and it is important for the acrosomal reaction with zona pellucida [76]. ZPBP1-deficient mice are sterile due to a lack of forward sperm motility and defects in acrosome compaction [77]. Interestingly, in both the GOPC- and ZPBP1-deficient mice, SPACA1 is also defective, which may contribute to the phenotypes of these mutants discussed earlier. SPACA1 is a transmembrane protein located in the equatorial segment of spermatozoa. In SPACA1-deficient mice, acrosomal expansion is inhibited, which leads to the disappearance of the acrosome from mature spermatozoa and therefore infertility [78].

Development of Flagellum and Motility

Motility powered by the sperm flagellum is essential for the sperm to reach the egg [79]. Flagellar motility is driven by a core structure of the sperm tail known as an axoneme, which is composed of 9 microtubule doublets surrounding a central microtubule pair (9 + 2). The axoneme is enclosed and protected by accessory structures including dense fibers, a mitochondrial sheath, and a fibrous sheath. Together, the flagellar structural elements and motor proteins work in a coordinated and regulated fashion to generate waveforms and to produce progressive movement. Defective flagellum is the principal cause of sperm motility disorders [2].

Anomalies of the flagella include a large variety of possible morphological defects such as absent, short, bent, angulated, irregular, or detached flagella or, as in most cases, a heterogenous mix of multiple morphological anomalies. Anomalies can be secondarily caused by various andrological conditions, but several primary flagellar anomalies, most likely of genetic origin, have also been described. These genetic disorders include primary ciliary dyskinesia (PCD) and the dysplasia of the fibrous sheath (DFS). PCD is a rare genetic disease of childhood characterized by motile ciliary dysfunction that leads to neonatal respiratory distress, chronic sinopulmonary disease causing sinusitis, bronchiectasis, recurrent ear infections, and infertility due to the defects in sperm flagellum. PCD usually originates from a lack of dynein arms in the axonemal microtubules of cilia and flagella, and it is the result of recessive mutations in one of many genes. During the past decade, advances in DNA sequencing, genomics, and proteomics have driven the identification of mutations in several genes that are causative of motile cilia defects in PCD. In humans, mutations in *DNAH5*, *DNAAF1* (*LRRC50*), *DNAI1*, and *HYDIN* cause severe asthenozoospermia [80–83]. Furthermore, infertility has been reported in men carrying a mutation in such genes as *DNAI2*, *RSPH9*, *RSPH4A*, or *HEATR2* [84–86]. However, not all PCDs are associated with an infertility phenotype and, for example, men with *CCDC114* and *DNAH11* mutations can procreate spontaneously [87, 88]. This highlights the fact that despite close structural similarities, sperm flagella have unique characteristics in their biogenesis compared to cilia.

In DFS, spermatozoa have short, thick, and irregular tails because of the overabundance and disorganization of the fibrous sheath [89]. A-kinase anchoring proteins (AKAPs) are primary components of the fibrous sheath, which surrounds the outer dense fibers and the axoneme in the flagellum. AKAPs are scaffold proteins for kinases and phosphatases which can form macromolecular complexes with other proteins involved in signal transduction [90]. AKAP4-depleted male mice have normal sperm counts but are infertile due to their DFS-like phenotype; however, mutations in AKAP genes are not frequently found in affected human individuals [89, 91]. The genetic origin of DFS is still obscure, and the potential candidate genes might be found among genes encoding for the structural proteins of the flagellum, regulators of flagellar assembly, or signaling pathways. For example, genetically modified mouse models with a disrupted intraflagellar transport (IFT) system often manifest the DFS-like phenotype (see below).

In mice, defects in axoneme formation lead to either a lack of flagellum, abnormalities in flagellar structure, or motility defects. The axonemal development begins in early round spermatids with the maturation of the mother centriole into a basal body that serves as a nucleation site for the axoneme. The extension is dependent on the IFT system which transports molecules along the inner axonemal microtubules by 2 motor proteins: kinesin II and dynein1b [92]. Several mouse models deficient in an IFT component have been reported to present flagellar defects. Mice with germ cell-specific knockout of the motor unit of kinesin II, KIF3A, are infertile with severe impairments of axonemal formation [93]. Interestingly, *Kif3a*-null male mice also have defects in the organization of another microtubular structure in elongating spermatids, the manchette, resulting in malformed sperm heads. The manchette is a transient microtubular and F-actin-containing structure at the caudal site of the spermatid nucleus that is required for head shaping and protein delivery during elongation [94]. Mice with mutated IFT-B complex protein IFT88 also display defects in sperm tail development as well as abnormal head shaping [95]. Furthermore, mutation in the gene encoding RABL2, which binds IFT-B complex proteins, causes a reduction in sperm tail length and decreases sperm motility in mice [96].

Meiosis-expressed gene 1 (MEIG1) has been shown to form a complex with parkin coregulated gene (PACRG) in the manchette and this complex has been suggested to transport cargo needed for flagella formation along the microtubules [97]. Both MEIG1- and PACRG-deficient mice have abnormal sperm flagellar structures combined with disrupted manchette structures. The critical role of microtubule dynamics in male fertility is further demonstrated by a mouse model with a mutation in the p80 regulatory subunit of katanin, a microtubule-severing enzyme, which localizes in the manchette in elongating spermatids [98]. Katanin p80 mutation in mice results in defective head shaping due to the problems in the manchette and defective flagellar structures [98]. Interestingly, a mutation of sperm flagellar protein 2 (SPEF2) was identified as a cause for the immotile short-tail sperm defect in the Finnish Yorkshire pig population [99]. The analysis of a mouse line with *Spef2* mutation revealed a similar short-tail phenotype [100]. The involvement of SPEF2 in IFT has been suggested, but the exact function in SPEF2 in sperm tail formation remains unclear.

Tektin family members (TEKT1–5) are microtubule-associated proteins that are preferentially expressed in spermatids and thought to be important for progressive sperm motility. *Tekt2*-null male mice are infertile, while *Tekt4*-null male mice are subfertile with normal epididymal sperm counts. They both display a reduced forward velocity of spermatozoa, the former due to flagellar bending and the latter due to uncoordinated waveform propagation along the flagellum [101, 102]. *Tekt3*-null male mice are fertile although they produce sperm with reduced progressive motility and forward progression [103]. Other proteins required for the formation and function of the flagellum are voltage-dependent anion channels (VDAC proteins; metabolite channel proteins located at the mitochondrial outer membrane) [104], sperm-associated antigen 6 (SPAG6) [105], and selenoproteins (selenoprotein P and GPx4) [106].

Motility defects do not always originate form structural defects, but disrupted energy supply and signaling transduction are also required for the flagellar movement. When released from the seminiferous epithelium in the testis, mammalian sperm display minimal or no motility and are unable to fertilize an oocyte. During the transit along the epididymal tubule, spermatozoa gain their fertilization ability. The progressive motility is gained only upon ejaculation, and the hyperactivation of spermatozoa takes place in the female reproductive tract. ATP that provides energy essential for coordinated movement is provided by oxidative phosphorylation in the midpiece of the spermatozoon where the mitochondria are localized, and glycolysis in the principal piece [107]. Mammalian sperm contains several unique isozymes of glycolysis, including glyceraldehyde 3-phosphate dehydrogenase-S (GAPDHS), phosphoglycerate kinase-2 (PGK2), and lactate dehydrogenase-C4 (LDHC4). *Gapdhs*-null males are infertile and display sluggish movement without forward progression [108]. *Ldhc* knockout males produce morphologically normal spermatozoa, but they do not acquire hyperactivated motility and have compromised capacitation [109].

Other spermatozoal genes involved in capacitation, which is induced by bicarbonate and dependent on cAMP, include bicarbonate- and calcium-responsive sAC (soluble adenylyl cyclase), which is the major source of cAMP in sperm. Targeted disruption of sAC causes male infertility due to the lack of sperm motility despite normal sperm morphology and counts [110]. Furthermore, cation channel-like (CATSPER) proteins localize to the midpiece and principal piece of the sperm tail, and a lack of any of the 4 proteins results in male infertility due to a failure to produce hyperactivated motility. Mutations in CATSPER1 and 2 have also been identified in infertile male patients [111].

References

1 Yan W: Male infertility caused by spermiogenic defects: lessons from gene knockouts. Mol Cell Endocrinol 2009; 306:24–32.

2 Chemes EH, Rawe YV: Sperm pathology: a step beyond descriptive morphology: origin, characterization and fertility potential of abnormal sperm phenotypes in infertile men. Hum Reprod Update 2003;9:405–428.

3 Ombelet W, Menkveld R, Kruger TF, Steeno O: Sperm morphology assessment: historical review in relation to fertility. Hum Reprod Update 1995;1: 543–557.

4 Cooper TG, Noonan E, von Eckardstein S, Auger J, Baker HW, Behre HM, Haugen TB, Kruger T, Wang C, Mbizvo MT, Vogelsong KM: World Health Organization reference values for human semen characteristics. Hum Reprod Update 2010;16:231–245.

5 Tüttelmann F, Simoni M, Kliesch S, Ledig S, Dworniczak B, Wieacker P, Röpke A: Copy number variants in patients with severe oligozoospermia and Sertoli-cell-only syndrome. PLoS One 2011;6:e19426.

6 Vogt PH: Genomic heterogeneity and instability of the AZF locus on the human Y chromosome. Mol Cell Endocrinol 2004;224:1–9.

7 Vogt PH, Falcao CL, Hanstein R, Zimmer J: The AZF proteins. Int J Androl 2008;31:383–394.

8 Yu X-W, Wei Z-T, Jiang Y-T, Zhang S-L: Y chromosome azoospermia factor region microdeletions and transmission characteristics in azoospermic and severe oligozoospermic patients. Int J Clin Exp Med 2015;8:14634–14646.

9 Benkhalifa M, Ferreira YJ, Chahine H, Louanjli N, Miron P, Merviel P, Copin H: Mitochondria: participation to infertility as source of energy and cause of senescence. Int J Biochem Cell Biol 2014;55:60–64.

10 Kumar DP, Sangeetha N: Mitochondrial DNA mutations and male infertility. Indian J Hum Genet 2009;15:93–97.

11 Amaral S, Amaral A, Ramalho-Santos J: Aging and male reproductive function: a mitochondrial perspective. Front Biosci (Schol Ed) 2013;5:181–197.

12 Coutton C, Escoffier J, Martinez G, Arnoult C, Ray PF: Teratozoospermia: spotlight on the main genetic actors in the human. Hum Reprod Update 21: 455–485.

13 Chalmel F, Rolland AD: Linking transcriptomics and proteomics in spermatogenesis. Reproduction 2015; 150:R149–R157.

14 Soumillon M, Necsulea A, Weier M, Brawand D, Zhang X, Gu H, Barthès P, Kokkinaki M, Nef S, Gnirke A, Dym M, de Massy B, et al: Cellular source and mechanisms of high transcriptome complexity in the mammalian testis. Cell Rep 2013;3:2179–2190.

15 Kimmins S, Kotaja N, Davidson I, Sassone-Corsi P: Testis-specific transcription mechanisms promoting male germcell differentiation. Reproduction 2004; 128:5–12.

16 Nantel F, Monaco L, Foulkes NS, Masquilier D, LeMeur M, Henriksen K, Dierich A, Parvinen M, Sassone-Corsi P: Spermiogenesis deficiency and germcell apoptosis in CREM-mutant mice. Nature 1996;380:159–162.

17 Fimia GM, De Cesare D, Sassone-Corsi P: CBP-independent activation of CREM and CREB by the LIM-only protein ACT. Nature 1999;398:165–169.

18 Kotaja N, De Cesare D, Macho B, Monaco L, Brancorsini S, Goossens E, Tournaye H, Gansmuller A, Sassone-Corsi P: Abnormal sperm in mice with targeted deletion of the act (activator of cAMP-responsive element modulator in testis) gene. Proc Natl Acad Sci USA 2004;101:10620–10625.

19 Macho B, Brancorsini S, Fimia GM, Setou M, Hirokawa N, Sassone-Corsi P: CREM-dependent transcription in male germ cells controlled by a kinesin. Science 2002;298:2388–2390.

20 Wu H, Chen Y, Miao S, Zhang C, Zong S, Koide SS, Wang L: Sperm associated antigen 8 (SPAG8), a novel regulator of activator of CREM in testis during spermatogenesis. FEBS Lett 2010;584:2807–2815.

21 He X-J, Song B, Du W-D, Cao Y-X, Zhang Y, Ruan J, Tian H, Zhou F-S, Zuo X-B, Wu H, Zha X, Xie X-S, et al: CREM variants rs4934540 and rs2295415 conferred susceptibility to nonobstructive azoospermia risk in the Chinese population. Biol Reprod 2014;91:52.

22 Kistler WS, Baas D, Lemeille S, Paschaki M, Seguin-Estevez Q, Barras E, Ma W, Duteyrat J-L, Morlé L, Durand B, Reith W: RFX2 is a major transcriptional regulator of spermiogenesis. PLoS Genet 2015;11:e1005368.

23 White-Cooper H, Davidson I: Unique aspects of transcription regulation in male germ cells. Cold Spring Harb Perspect Biol 2011;3:a002626.

24 Gerstberger S, Hafner M, Tuschl T: A census of human RNA-binding proteins. Nat Rev Genet 2014;15:829–845.

25 Idler RK, Yan W: Control of messenger RNA fate by RNA-binding proteins: an emphasis on mammalian spermatogenesis. J Androl 2012;33:309–337.

26 Meikar O, Da Ros M, Korhonen H, Kotaja N: Chromatoid body and small RNAs in male germ cells. Reproduction 2011;142:195–209.

27 Weick E-M, Miska EA: piRNAs: from biogenesis to function. Development 2014;141:3458–3471.

28 Deng W, Lin H: miwi, a murine homolog of piwi, encodes a cytoplasmic protein essential for spermatogenesis. Dev Cell 2002;2:819–830.

29 Reuter M, Berninger P, Chuma S, Shah H, Hosokawa M, Funaya C, Antony C, Sachidanandam R, Pillai RS: Miwi catalysis is required for piRNA amplification-independent LINE1 transposon silencing. Nature 2011;480:264–267.

30 Lim SL, Qu ZP, Kortschak RD, Lawrence DM, Geoghegan J, Hempfling A-L, Bergmann M, Goodnow CC, Ormandy CJ, Wong L, Mann J, Scott HS, et al: HENMT1 and piRNA stability are required for adult male germ cell transposon repression and to define the spermatogenic program in the mouse. PLoS Genet 2015;11:e1005620.

31 Kotaja N: MicroRNAs and spermatogenesis. Fertil Steril 2014;101:1552–1562.

32 Giacomo M, Rasmussen KD, Much C, Azzi C, Perlas E, Morgan M, O'Carroll D: Oligoasthenoteratozoospermia and infertility in mice deficient for miR-34b/c and miR-449 loci. PLoS Genet 2014;10:e1004597.

33 Meikar O, Da Ros M, Kotaja N: Epigenetic regulation of male germ cell differentiation. Subcell Biochem 2012;61: 119–138.

34 Goudarzi A, Shiota H, Rousseaux S, Khochbin S: Genome-scale acetylation-dependent histone eviction during spermatogenesis. J Mol Biol 2014;426:3342–3349.
35 Castillo J, Amaral A, Oliva R: Sperm nuclear proteome and its epigenetic potential. Andrology 2014;2:326–338.
36 Montellier E, Boussouar F, Rousseaux S, Zhang K, Buchou T, Fenaille F, Shiota H, Debernardi A, Héry P, Curtet S, Jamshidikia M, Barral S, et al: Chromatin-to-nucleoprotamine transition is controlled by the histone H2B variant TH2B. Genes Dev 2013;27:1680–1692.
37 Martianov I, Brancorsini S, Catena R, Gansmuller A, Kotaja N, Parvinen M, Sassone-Corsi P, Davidson I: Polar nuclear localization of H1T2, a histone H1 variant, required for spermatid elongation and DNA condensation during spermiogenesis. Proc Natl Acad Sci USA 2005;102:2808–2813.
38 Morinière J, Rousseaux S, Steuerwald U, Soler-López M, Curtet S, Vitte A-L, Govin J, Gaucher J, Sadoul K, Hart DJ, Krijgsveld J, Khochbin S, et al: Cooperative binding of two acetylation marks on a histone tail by a single bromodomain. Nature 2009;461:664–668.
39 Shang E, Nickerson HD, Wen D, Wang X, Wolgemuth DJ: The first bromodomain of Brdt, a testis-specific member of the BET sub-family of double-bromodomain-containing proteins, is essential for male germ cell differentiation. Development 2007;134:3507–3515.
40 Gaucher J, Boussouar F, Montellier E, Curtet S, Buchou T, Bertrand S, Hery P, Jounier S, Depaux A, Vitte A-L, Guardiola P, Pernet K, et al: Bromodomain-dependent stage-specific male genome programming by Brdt. EMBO J 2012;31:3809–3820.
41 Matzuk MM, McKeown MR, Filippakopoulos P, Li Q, Ma L, Agno JE, Lemieux ME, Picaud S, Yu RN, Qi J, Knapp S, Bradner JE: Small-molecule inhibition of BRDT for male contraception. Cell 2012;150:673–684.
42 Lu LY, Wu J, Ye L, Gavrilina GB, Saunders TL, Yu X: RNF8-dependent histone modifications regulate nucleosome removal during spermatogenesis. Dev Cell 2010;18:371–384.
43 Zhao M, Shirley CR, Hayashi S, Marcon L, Mohapatra B, Suganuma R, Behringer RR, Boissonneault G, Yanagimachi R, Meistrich ML: Transition nuclear proteins are required for normal chromatin condensation and functional sperm development. Genes (New York) 2004;38:200–213.
44 Francis S, Yelumalai S, Jones C, Coward K: Aberrant protamine content in sperm and consequential implications for infertility treatment. Hum Fertil 2014;17:80–89.
45 Cho C, Willis WD, Goulding EH, Jung-Ha H, Choi YC, Hecht NB, Eddy EM: Haploinsufficiency of protamine-1 or -2 causes infertility in mice. Nat Genet 2001;28:82–86.
46 Cho C: Protamine 2 deficiency leads to sperm DNA damage and embryo death in mice. Biol Reprod 2003;69:211–217.
47 Gatewood JM, Cook GR, Balhorn R, Bradbury EM, Schmid CW: Sequence-specific packaging of DNA in human sperm chromatin. Science 1987;236:962–964.
48 Balhorn R, Gledhill BL, Wyrobek AJ: Mouse sperm chromatin proteins: quantitative isolation and partial characterization. Biochemistry 1977;16:4074–4080.
49 Hammoud SS, Nix DA, Zhang H, Purwar J, Carrell DT, Cairns BR: Distinctive chromatin in human sperm packages genes for embryo development. Nature 2009;460:473–478.
50 Erkek S, Hisano M, Liang C-Y, Gill M, Murr R, Dieker J, Schübeler D, van der Vlag J, Stadler MB, Peters AHFM: Molecular determinants of nucleosome retention at CpG-rich sequences in mouse spermatozoa. Nat Struct Mol Biol 2013;20:868–875.
51 Brykczynska U, Hisano M, Erkek S, Ramos L, Oakeley EJ, Roloff TC, Beisel C, Schubeler D, Stadler MB, Peters AH: Repressive and active histone methylation mark distinct promoters in human and mouse spermatozoa. Nat Struct Mol Biol 2010;17:679–687.
52 Samans B, Yang Y, Krebs S, Sarode GV, Blum H, Reichenbach M, Wolf E, Steger K, Dansranjavin T, Schagdarsurengin U: Uniformity of nucleosome preservation pattern in mammalian sperm and its connection to repetitive DNA elements. Dev Cell 2014;30:23–35.
53 Carone BR, Hung J-H, Hainer SJ, Chou M-T, Carone DM, Weng Z, Fazzio TG, Rando OJ: High-resolution mapping of chromatin packaging in mouse embryonic stem cells and sperm. Dev Cell 2014;30:11–22.
54 Lane M, Robker RL, Robertson SA: Parenting from before conception. Science 2014;345:756–760.
55 Boissonnas CC, Jouannet P, Jammes H: Epigenetic disorders and male subfertility. Fertil Steril 2013;99:624–631.
56 Urdinguio RG, Bayon GF, Dmitrijeva M, Torano EG, Bravo C, Fraga MF, Bassas L, Larriba S, Fernandez AF: Aberrant DNA methylation patterns of spermatozoa in men with unexplained infertility. Hum Reprod 2015;30:1014–1028.
57 Carrell DT, Aston KI, Oliva R, Emery BR, De Jonge CJ: The "omics" of human male infertility: integrating big data in a systems biology approach. Cell Tissue Res 2015;363:295–312.
58 Azpiazu R, Amaral A, Castillo J, Estanyol JM, Guimerà M, Ballescà JL, Balasch J, Oliva R: High-throughput sperm differential proteomics suggests that epigenetic alterations contribute to failed assisted reproduction. Hum Reprod 2014;29:1225–1237.
59 Abou-Haila A, Tulsiani DR: Mammalian sperm acrosome: formation, contents, and function. Arch Biochem Biophys 2000;379:173–182.
60 Dam AH, Pijnenburg AJ, Hendriks JC, Westphal H, Ramos L, Kremer JA: Intracytoplasmic sperm injection in partial globozoospermia. Fertil Steril 2012;97:60–66.
61 Koscinski I, Elinati E, Fossard C, Redin C, Muller J, Velez de la Calle J, Schmitt F, Ben Khelifa M, Ray P, Kilani Z, Barratt CLR, Viville S: DPY19L2 deletion as a major cause of globozoospermia. Am J Hum Genet 2011;88:344–350.
62 Dam AH, Koscinski I, Kremer JA, Moutou C, Jaeger A-S, Oudakker AR, Tournaye H, Charlet N, Lagier-Tourenne C, van Bokhoven H, Viville S: Homozygous mutation in SPATA16 is associated with male infertility in human globozoospermia. Am J Hum Genet 2007;81:813–820.
63 Liu G, Shi Q-W, Lu G-X: A newly discovered mutation in PICK1 in a human with globozoospermia. Asian J Androl 2010;12:556–560.

64 Zhu F, Gong F, Lin G, Lu G: *DPY19L2* gene mutations are a major cause of globozoospermia: identification of three novel point mutations. Mol Hum Reprod 2013;19:395–404.

65 Ghédir H, Ibala-Romdhane S, Okutman O, Viot G, Saad A, Viville S: Identification of a new *DPY19L2* mutation and a better definition of *DPY19L2* deletion breakpoints leading to globozoospermia. Mol Hum Reprod 2016;22:35–45.

66 Pierre V, Martinez G, Coutton C, Delaroche J, Yassine S, Novella C, Pernet-Gallay K, Hennebicq S, Ray PF, Arnoult C: Absence of Dpy19l2, a new inner nuclear membrane protein, causes globozoospermia in mice by preventing the anchoring of the acrosome to the nucleus. Development 2012;139:2955–2965.

67 Kang-Decker N, Mantchev GT, Juneja SC, McNiven MA, van Deursen JM: Lack of acrosome formation in Hrb-deficient mice. Science 2001;294:1531–1533.

68 Paiardi C, Pasini ME, Gioria M, Berruti G: Failure of acrosome formation and globozoospermia in the wobbler mouse, a Vps54 spontaneous recessive mutant. Spermatogenesis 2011;1:52–62.

69 Xiao N, Kam C, Shen C, Jin W, Wang J, Lee KM, Jiang L, Xia J: PICK1 deficiency causes male infertility in mice by disrupting acrosome formation. J Clin Invest 2009;119:802–812.

70 Li X, Mao Z, Wu M, Xia J: Rescuing infertility of *Pick1* knockout mice by generating testis-specific transgenic mice via testicular infection. Sci Rep 2013;3: 2842.

71 He J, Xia M, Tsang WH, Chow KL, Xia J: ICA1L forms BAR-domain complexes with PICK1 and is crucial for acrosome formation in spermiogenesis. J Cell Sci 2015;128:3822–3836.

72 Yao R, Ito C, Natsume Y, Sugitani Y, Yamanaka H, Kuretake S, Yanagida K, Sato A, Toshimori K, Noda T: Lack of acrosome formation in mice lacking a Golgi protein, GOPC. Proc Natl Acad Sci USA 2002;99:11211–11216.

73 Wang H, Wan H, Li X, Liu W, Chen Q, Wang Y, Yang L, Tang H, Zhang X, Duan E, Zhao X, Gao F, et al: Atg7 is required for acrosome biogenesis during spermatogenesis in mice. Cell Res 2014; 24:852–869.

74 Xu X, Toselli PA, Russell LD, Seldin DC: Globozoospermia in mice lacking the casein kinase II alpha' catalytic subunit. Nat Genet 1999;23:118–121.

75 Lu L, Lin M, Xu M, Zhou Z-M, Sha J-H: Gene functional research using polyethylenimine-mediated in vivo gene transfection into mouse spermatogenic cells. Asian J Androl 2006;8:53–59.

76 Yatsenko AN, O'Neil DS, Roy A, Arias-Mendoza PA, Chen R, Murthy LJ, Lamb DJ, Matzuk MM: Association of mutations in the zona pellucida binding protein 1 (*ZPBP1*) gene with abnormal sperm head morphology in infertile men. Mol Hum Reprod 2012;18:14–21.

77 Lin Y-N, Roy A, Yan W, Burns KH, Matzuk MM: Loss of zona pellucida binding proteins in the acrosomal matrix disrupts acrosome biogenesis and sperm morphogenesis. Mol Cell Biol 2007;27: 6794–6805.

78 Fujihara Y, Satouh Y, Inoue N, Isotani A, Ikawa M, Okabe M: SPACA1-deficient male mice are infertile with abnormally shaped sperm heads reminiscent of globozoospermia. Development 2012; 139:3583–3589.

79 Turner RM: Tales from the tail: what do we really know about sperm motility? J Androl 2003;24:790–803.

80 Fliegauf M, Olbrich H, Horvath J, Wildhaber JH, Zariwala MA, Kennedy M, Knowles MR, Omran H: Mislocalization of DNAH5 and DNAH9 in respiratory cells from patients with primary ciliary dyskinesia. Am J Respir Crit Care Med 2005;171:1343–1349.

81 Loges NT, Olbrich H, Becker-Heck A, Häffner K, Heer A, Reinhard C, Schmidts M, Kispert A, Zariwala MA, Leigh MW, Knowles MR, Zentgraf H, et al: Deletions and point mutations of LRRC50 cause primary ciliary dyskinesia due to dynein arm defects. Am J Hum Genet 2009;85:883–889.

82 Guichard C, Harricane M-C, Lafitte J-J, Godard P, Zaegel M, Tack V, Lalau G, Bouvagnet P: Axonemal dynein intermediate-chain gene (DNAI1) mutations result in situs inversus and primary ciliary dyskinesia (Kartagener Syndrome). Am J Hum Genet 2001;68:1030–1035.

83 Olbrich H, Schmidts M, Werner C, Onoufriadis A, Loges NT, Raidt J, Banki NF, Shoemark A, Burgoyne T, Al Turki S, Hurles ME, Köhler G, et al: Recessive HYDIN mutations cause primary ciliary dyskinesia without randomization of left-right body asymmetry. Am J Hum Genet 2012;91:672–684.

84 Loges NT, Olbrich H, Fenske L, Mussaffi H, Horvath J, Fliegauf M, Kuhl H, Baktai G, Peterffy E, Chodhari R, Chung EMK, Rutman A, et al: DNAI2 mutations cause primary ciliary dyskinesia with defects in the outer dynein arm. Am J Hum Genet 2008;83:547–558.

85 Castleman VH, Romio L, Chodhari R, Hirst RA, de Castro SCP, Parker KA, Ybot-Gonzalez P, Emes RD, Wilson SW, Wallis C, Johnson CA, Herrera RJ, et al: Mutations in radial spoke head protein genes *RSPH9* and *RSPH4A* cause primary ciliary dyskinesia with central-microtubular-pair abnormalities. Am J Hum Genet 2009;84:197–209.

86 Horani A, Druley TE, Zariwala MA, Patel AC, Levinson BT, Van Arendonk LG, Thornton KC, Giacalone JC, Albee AJ, Wilson KS, Turner EH, Nickerson DA, et al: Whole-exome capture and sequencing identifies HEATR2 mutation as a cause of primary ciliary dyskinesia. Am J Hum Genet 2012;91;685–693.

87 Onoufriadis A, Paff T, Antony D, Shoemark A, Micha D, Kuyt B, Schmidts M, Petridi S, Dankert-Roelse JE, Haarman EG, Daniels JMA, Emes RD, et al: Splice-site mutations in the axonemal outer dynein arm docking complex gene CCDC114 cause primary ciliary dyskinesia. Am J Hum Genet 2013;92:88–98.

88 Schwabe GC, Hoffmann K, Loges NT, Birker D, Rossier C, de Santi MM, Olbrich H, Fliegauf M, Failly M, Liebers U, Collura M, Gaedicke G, et al: Primary ciliary dyskinesia associated with normal axoneme ultrastructure is caused by DNAH11 mutations. Hum Mutat 2008; 29:289–298.

89 Chemes HE, Rawe VY: The making of abnormal spermatozoa: cellular and molecular mechanisms underlying pathological spermiogenesis. Cell Tissue Res 2010;341:349–357.

90 Edwards AS, Scott JD: A-kinase anchoring proteins: protein kinase A and beyond. Curr Opin Cell Biol 2000;12:217–221.

91 Miki K, Willis WD, Brown PR, Goulding EH, Fulcher KD, Eddy EM: Targeted disruption of the *Akap4* gene causes defects in sperm flagellum and motility. Dev Biol 2002;248:331–342.

92 Rosenbaum JL, Witman GB: Intraflagellar transport. Nat Rev Mol Cell Biol 2002;3:813–825.

93 Lehti MS, Kotaja N, Sironen A: KIF3A is essential for sperm tail formation and manchette function. Mol Cell Endocrinol 2013;377:44–55.

94 Kierszenbaum AL, Tres LL: The acrosome-acroplaxome-manchette complex and the shaping of the spermatid head. Arch Histol Cytol 2004;67:271–284.

95 Kierszenbaum AL, Rivkin E, Tres LL, Yoder BK, Haycraft CJ, Bornens M, Rios RM: GMAP210 and IFT88 are present in the spermatid golgi apparatus and participate in the development of the acrosome-acroplaxome complex, head-tail coupling apparatus and tail. Dev Dyn 2011;240:723–736.

96 Lo JCY, Jamsai D, O'Connor AE, Borg C, Clark BJ, Whisstock JC, Field MC, Adams V, Ishikawa T, Aitken RJ, Whittle B, Goodnow CC, et al: RAB-like 2 has an essential role in male fertility, sperm intra-flagellar transport, and tail assembly. PLoS Genet 2012;8:e1002969.

97 Li W, Tang W, Teves ME, Zhang Z, Zhang L, Li H, Archer KJ, Peterson DL, Williams DC, Strauss JF, Zhang Z: A MEIG1/PACRG complex in the manchette is essential for building the sperm flagella. Development 2015;142:921–930.

98 O'Donnell L, Rhodes D, Smith SJ, Merriner DJ, Clark BJ, Borg C, Whittle B, O'Connor AE, Smith LB, McNally FJ, de Kretser DM, Goodnow CC, et al: An essential role for katanin p80 and microtubule severing in male gamete production. PLoS Genet 2012;8:e1002698.

99 Sironen A, Thomsen B, Andersson M, Ahola V, Vilkki J: An intronic insertion in KPL2 results in aberrant splicing and causes the immotile short-tail sperm defect in the pig. Proc Natl Acad Sci USA 2006;103:5006–5011.

100 Sironen A, Kotaja N, Mulhern H, Wyatt TA, Sisson JH, Pavlik JA, Miiluniemi M, Fleming MD, Lee L: Loss of SPEF2 function in mice results in spermatogenesis defects and primary ciliary dyskinesia. Biol Reprod 2011;85:690–701.

101 Tanaka H, Iguchi N, Toyama Y, Kitamura K, Takahashi T, Kaseda K, Maekawa M, Nishimune Y: Mice deficient in the axonemal protein Tektin-t exhibit male infertility and immotile-cilium syndrome due to impaired inner arm dynein function. Mol Cell Biol 2004;24:7958–7964.

102 Roy A, Lin Y-N, Agno JE, DeMayo FJ, Matzuk MM: Absence of tektin 4 causes asthenozoospermia and subfertility in male mice. FASEB J 2007;21:1013–1025.

103 Roy A, Lin Y-N, Agno JE, DeMayo FJ, Matzuk MM: Tektin 3 is required for progressive sperm motility in mice. Mol Reprod Dev 2009;76:453–459.

104 Sampson MJ, Decker WK, Beaudet AL, Ruitenbeek W, Armstrong D, Hicks MJ, Craigen WJ: Immotile sperm and infertility in mice lacking mitochondrial voltage-dependent anion channel type 3. J Biol Chem 2001;276:39206–39212.

105 Sapiro R, Kostetskii I, Olds-Clarke P, Gerton GL, Radice GL, Strauss III JF: Male infertility, impaired sperm motility, and hydrocephalus in mice deficient in sperm-associated antigen 6. Mol Cell Biol 2002;22:6298–6305.

106 Ahsan U, Kamran Z, Raza I, Ahmad S, Babar W, Riaz MH, Iqbal Z: Role of selenium in male reproduction – a review. Anim Reprod Sci 2014;146:55–62.

107 du Plessis SS, Agarwal A, Mohanty G, van der Linde M: Oxidative phosphorylation versus glycolysis: what fuel do spermatozoa use? Asian J Androl 2015;17:230–235.

108 Miki K, Qu W, Goulding EH, Willis WD, Bunch DO, Strader LF, Perreault SD, Eddy EM, O'Brien DA: Glyceraldehyde 3-phosphate dehydrogenase-S, a sperm-specific glycolytic enzyme, is required for sperm motility and male fertility. Proc Natl Acad Sci USA 2004;101:16501–16506.

109 Odet F, Duan C, Willis WD, Goulding EH, Kung A, Eddy EM, Goldberg E: Expression of the gene for mouse lactate dehydrogenase C (*Ldhc*) is required for male fertility. Biol Reprod 2008;79:26–34.

110 Esposito G, Jaiswal BS, Xie F, Krajnc-Franken MAM, Robben TJAA, Strik AM, Kuil C, Philipsen RLA, van Duin M, Conti M, Gossen JA, Jaiswal BS: Mice deficient for soluble adenylyl cyclase are infertile because of a severe sperm-motility defect. Proc Natl Acad Sci USA 2004;101:2993–2998.

111 Singh AP, Rajender S: CatSper channel, sperm function and male fertility. Reprod Biomed Online 2015;30:28–38.

Noora Kotaja
Institute of Biomedicine
University of Turku
Kiinamyllynkatu 10
FI–20520 Turku (Finland)
E-Mail noora.kotaja@utu.fi

Vogt PH (ed): Genetics of Human Infertility. Monogr Hum Genet.
Basel, Karger, 2017, vol 21, pp 116–127 (DOI: 10.1159/000477282)

The Epigenetics of Sperm Chromatin

Monis B. Shamsi[a] · Luke Simon[a] · Douglas T. Carrell[a–c]

[a]Andrology and IVF Laboratory, Department of Surgery (Urology), [b]Department of Obstetrics and Gynecology, and [c]Department of Human Genetics, University of Utah, Salt Lake City, UT, USA

Abstract

The development of spermatozoa from primordial germ cells (PGCs) involves the transition of the genome through a program of sequential epigenetic events, resulting in the genome-wide erasure and subsequent reestablishment of DNA methylation at most loci, along with reprogramming of histone modification profiles and the chromatin remodeling. Following successful fertilization, the epigenetic signatures of the paternal genome are altered during the early embryonic stages compatible with the embryonic developmental program that begins a new life cycle. We highlight the remodeling of the sperm epigenome, beginning from PGCs to the early embryonic stages, preparing for a normal embryonic growth. Additionally, recent studies have shown a significant association between aberrant DNA epigenetic signatures in spermatozoa with idiopathic male infertility and an increased frequency of spontaneous abortions and imprinting disorders. Here we present an overview of the important epigenetic changes that occur to male PGCs until the reprogramming of the preimplantation embryo. In addition, we also highlight the errors in the epigenetic signatures and their consequences.

The term "epigenetics" encompasses heritable, regulatory mechanisms of gene expression that are not associated with the DNA coding sequence, but complement the information of genetic code [1]. The epigenome contributes to the cellular potential, which gives rise to different cell types. The precursors for cellular differentiation are stringently regulated processes, which are driven by an array of inputs and are synchronized with epigenetic changes reinforcing the commitment decisions. These epigenetic modifications are stable and heritable, allowing a faithful and directed differentiation process over numerous cell divisions. However, the reprogramming event in primordial germ cells (PGCs) that reverses epigenetic barriers to plasticity and resets the genomic potential is an important aspect of this unidirectional process [1]. The epigenetic barriers reenforced during cellular differentiation must accommodate the needs of sexual reproduction, wherein preparation for the next generation requires a reset of the epigenome to a basic and totipotent state.

Sperm are highly differentiated cells, entrusted to transfer accurate paternal information to the oocyte. During development from PGCs to the fully mature sperm, the stringent epigenetic signals are critical for its function [2] and any error in the epigenetic regulation or reprogramming may reduce its function and impair reproductive potential. Furthermore, precise epigenetic reprogramming during the preimplantation period is also important for proper embryonic and postembryonic development, as it controls the expression of early developmental genes, cell cleavage, and cell determination. In adult tissues, the early embryonic genes are repressed when tissue-specific genes are activated. Imprinted genes maintain their methylation marks established during the gamete stage and are not affected by the general (de)methylation process during the preimplantation stage [2].

The epigenetic preparation for sexual reproduction is classified into a 3-step process consisting of: (1) erasure of somatic signatures in the PGCs via a comprehensive reprogramming process, (2) establishment of sex-specific and germ cell-specific epigenetic signatures, and (3) the postfertilization removal of these signatures to trigger the embryonic developmental program, which results in the beginning of a new life cycle. These epigenetic mechanisms are important for ensuring the meiosis and terminal differentiation program during gametogenesis, reliable retention of epigenetic information in the gametes for the next generation, and for the erasure of erroneous inheritable epimutations before the beginning of the next generation [3].

Although the basic principles of epigenetic reprogramming in embryos and germ cells have been studied for many years, findings of recent epigenetic studies, combined with improved next-generation sequencing technology, have led to a greater understanding of previously elusive reprogramming mechanisms. Here, we present the important epigenetic events that take place from the PGC stage until the reprogramming events in the preimplantation embryo. We also highlight some of the potential causative and contributory epigenetic factors/events that are related to diseases, particularly related to infertility.

Epigenetic Events from Primordial Germ Cells to a Mature Differentiated Sperm

Mammalian germ cells arise relatively late during embryonic development. They originate from a small population of extraembryonic mesoderm cells of the epiblast. Germ cell development and meiotic division eventually lead to the conversion of diploid cells to haploid gametes, which give rise to a new diploid organism that is different from that of the parents. During these stages of germ cell differentiation, genome-wide changes in DNA methylation, covalent modifications of histones (methylation and acetylation), and remodeling of chromatin-associated complexes contribute to cells that acquire the capacity to support postfertilization development.

DNA Methylation

Cells from the PGC founder population proliferate and migrate toward the genital ridges, where they colonize, before the formation of the gonads. During and after migration, PGCs undergo global epigenetic changes (Fig. 1). The de novo DNA methyltransferases (DNMTs) are silenced during this time interval when PGCs are reacquiring totipotency on their way to the genital ridge. This silencing facilitates DNA demethylation. Although genome-wide loss of DNA methylation appears to initiate in migrating PGCs, it mainly occurs after colonization of the genital ridges and affects about 80–90% of the genome [1]. The process includes the loss of methylation marks that control somatic gene expression and also removes DNA methylation imprints from imprinted gene loci. Different isozymes of the DNMT family of enzymes are involved in DNA methylation. DNMT1 ensures the maintenance of methylation, while DNMT3A,

3B, and 3L specifically regulate the methylation process in germ cells. DNMT3A and 3B are known for their catalytic activity, whereas DNMT3L lacks such catalytic activity and acts as a cofactor to DNMT3A [2].

The genome-wide DNA methylation patterns are reestablished during prophase I in the type A spermatogonial stage, in spermatogonia, and in spermatocytes prior to meiotic cell division [3]. DNA methylation occurs in a sequence-specific manner and is complete prior to the termination of the pachytene spermatocyte stage [3]. The main targets of methylation are non-CpG island sequences in both distinct loci and repetitive sequences, in addition to CpG islands [3]. These regions can either be within known genes or between genes [3]. The methylation status of certain genes may vary as the germ cell passes through the various stages of spermatogenesis and may or may not correspond to their gene's expression pattern. Pioneering work by Gkountela et al. [4] suggests that overall DNA demethylation, and imprinting and histone modification reprogramming, occurs separately in human PGCs; however, they occur much earlier and concurrently in mouse models.

Histone Modifications

Histone modification, and changes in PGCs and spermatogonia do play an important role in chromatin reorganization and are required for normal meiotic process for the maturation of gametes (Fig. 1). During the methylation of histones, H3 or H4 lysine methylation promote gene activation or repression and is regulated by histone methyltransferase and demethylase families [5]. H3K4 methylation is generally associated with gene expression, whereas H3K9 and H3K27 methylation is linked to gene silencing. The timing of the establishment and removal of methylation markers is essential to spermatogenesis: mono-, di-, and trimethylation modifications of H3K4, H3K9, and H3K27 are essential for their progression through spermatogenesis [6]. The methylation level of H3K4 peaks in spermatogonial stem cells and is required for stem cells to begin differentiation and in order to become spermatocytes. It then diminishes during meiosis. In contrast, the methylation levels of H3K9 and H3K27 are increased during meiosis, but the removal of H3K-9me at the end of meiosis is essential to the onset of spermiogenesis.

Hyperacetylation of histone H4 is responsible for the replacement of histones with protamines in haploid spermatids. The HI1s1-binding histone variant (histone-1-like protein in spermatids 1) is expressed in the elongated spermatids [7]. These 2 epigenetic regulatory mechanisms, i.e., DNA methylation and histone modification, are closely related to each other during the process of gene expression. Successful regulation and control of gene expression requires close cooperation and interaction between these 2 mechanisms.

Histone-Protamine Transition

Protamination is an epigenetic regulatory process specific to sperm cells. Prior to fertilization, the paternal haploid genome carried by mature sperm is packaged tightly by protamines, making the chromatin organization more compact than the somatic cell (Fig. 1). Protamination not only facilitates compaction of the nucleus, but is also required for sperm motility. Indirectly, such organization protects the sperm genome from oxidative-mediated damage in the male and female reproductive tract. The compaction obtained by the exchange of histones to protamines is estimated to be one-sixth of its original volume. Such compaction is only possible due to the unique basic nature of the protamines binding to negatively charged chromatin. During the process of histone-protamine exchange, histones are first replaced by transition proteins (TPs), and the TPs are then replaced to protamines in a sequence-specific manner.

Histone acetylation is known to play an important role during the early stages of spermatogenesis. When histones are hyperacetylat-

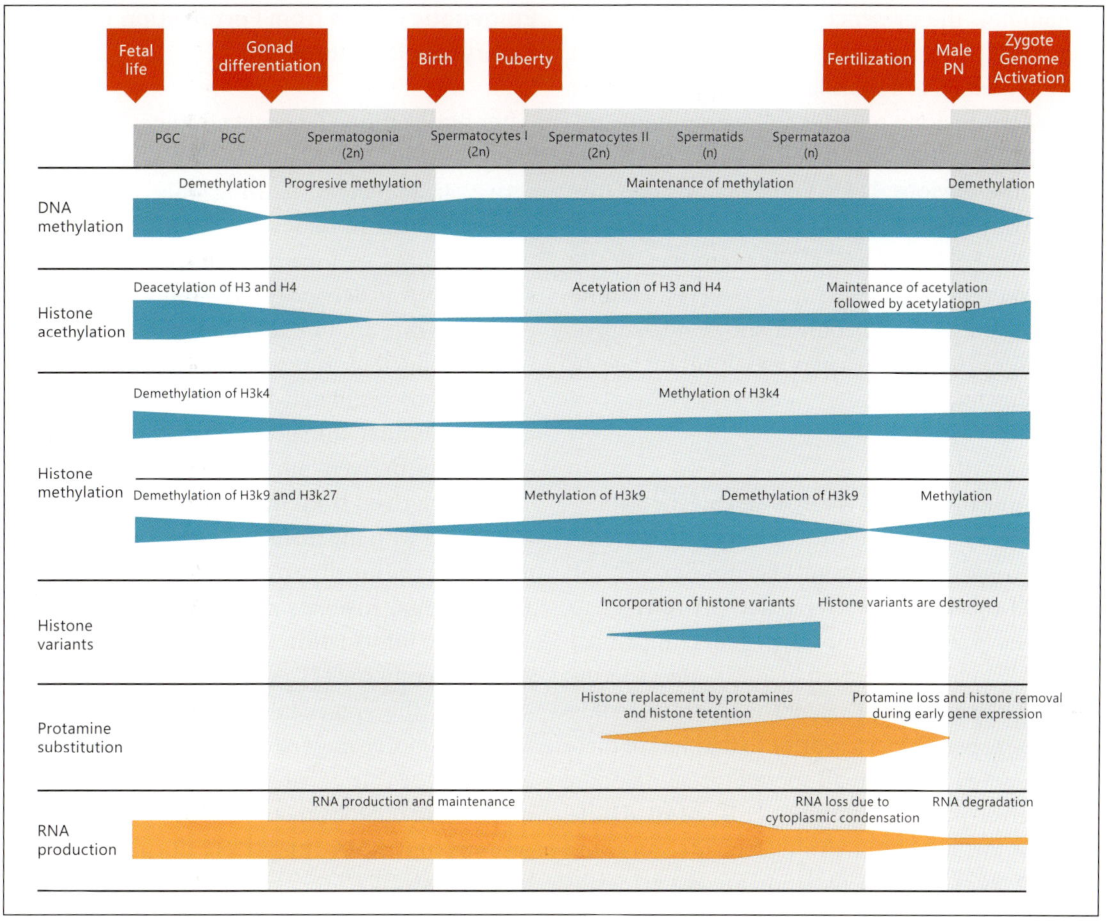

Fig. 1. Epigenetic transitions in the development of sperm. This timeline highlights the varied epigenetic modifications to DNA methylation, histone modifications, and RNA production from fetal development through zygotic genome activation. Of note is the extensive remodeling completed before the spermatocyte stage of spermatogenesis, followed by protamination in late spermiogenesis. PN, pronucleus.

ed, its affinity to DNA is decreased by the loss of their positive charge, leading to a more relaxed configuration of the chromatin structure, enabling transcription to occur. Such loose protein-DNA configuration stimulates DNA strand breaks caused by topoisomerase enzyme, and facilitates the removal of histones and their subsequent replacement with TPs [8, 9]. TPs 1 and 2 are moderate, basic nonhistone-like proteins. These proteins bind to DNA, and thus play critical roles in the separation of histone variants, and are later replaced by protamine. Two protamines (P1 and P2) are nearly equally expressed in normal fertile human males. TP- and protamine-expressing genes are known to considerably overlap. They also have a unique transitional regulatory mechanism. Their posttranslational mechanism involves phosphorylation required for appropriate chromatin condensation [10].

Even though spermatogenesis is characterized by events such as the exchange of histones for protamines, the presence of histones in mature sperm still plays a critical role in the development and maintenance of spermatozoa. Approximately 15% of the histone remains following the incorporation of protamines, much of which lies in the pericentric regions [11]. Four major core histones, H2A, H2B, H3, and H4 [12], and their variants H2AL1, H2AL2 and H2BL1, are specifically retained in the mature spermatozoa [11]. Despite their low frequency in comparison to nucleoprotamines, nucleohistones play an important role in male gametogenesis.

Imprinting of Genes

Imprinting of paternal genes is an epigenetic phenomenon that mediates the monoallelic parent-of-origin-specific expression of genes. Sex-specific epigenetic patterns on discrete loci are referred to as genetic imprints or imprinted genes. Imprinted epigenetic marks are erased in PGCs and a sperm-specific remethylation occurs in spermatogonia and type I spermatocytes, prior to the start of meiosis, in a way in which all spermatozoa maintain the correct paternal imprints [13]. Most of the methylation is acquired during fetal life, but complete levels of DNA methylation are not achieved until the pachytene spermatocyte stage [3].

Allele-specific paternal epigenetic modifications are established during gametogenesis and are maintained throughout somatic development. The allelic methylation originates from the germline, hence the differentially methylated regions (DMRs) are often referred to as germline DMRs. These germline-derived DMRs retain the methylation on the maternally or paternally derived alleles resulting in 1 copy being heavily methylated and the other unmethylated [14]. Only a small number of genes have been reported to have paternal imprinting, including the IGF2/H19, RASGRF1, and GTL2 loci. Imprinted genes have been shown to influence early embryonic development, placental function, and also have an impact on behavior and metabolic adaptation during the later part of life [15, 16].

Epigenetic Events from Fertilization to Early Embryonic Development

After fertilization, the oocyte initiates the remodeling of sperm chromatin into a transcriptionally active arrangement. During this process, the sperm chromatin undergoes extensive structural modifications to form a male pronucleus. The sperm DNA is decondensed from a highly compact structure to an expanded state making the male pronucleus transcriptionally active. Such changes are facilitated by the removal of protamines bound to the sperm DNA and replaced by maternally derived nucleosomes. However, the histones derived from the sperm seem to remain associated with the male pronucleus and contribute transcriptionally to the developing embryo. The paternal histones could potentially deliver epigenetic information to the oocyte and the developing embryo [17]. Although the mechanisms involving the epigenetic contribution of sperm remains poorly understood, recent studies have analyzed the role of paternal epigenetic dynamics in the form of DNA methylation, histone modifications, and RNA transcripts during early embryogenesis.

Role of the Paternal Epigenome in Postfertilization Events

The transfer of nucleohistones enriched during the development of specific genes of human sperm suggests a specific role of paternal epigenome during early embryogenesis. The remnant histones play a fundamental role during postfertilization development as they carry important modifications like methylation, acetylation, phosphorylation, and ubiquitination, represented as "histone code" [18]. The histone code is established in sperm for specific functions. Histone methylation and ubiquitination can promote or suppress gene expression. Acetylation of histones relaxes the sperm chromatin and facilitates gene transcription. The phosphorylation of histones is associated with gene activation [19].

Protamines do not play an important role during embryo development; however, in the sperm their presence is required to protect the DNA from oxidative-mediated damage. In a mature sperm, the establishment of inter- and intra-protamine disulfide bonds helps package the paternal genome and lock the chromatin into a virtual crystalline state. The paternal genome is inactive until it reaches the ooplasm, where the maternal factors rapidly access the paternal chromatin and begin the replacement of protamines with maternal histones before the formation of the paternal pronucleus (Fig. 1). The establishment and maintenance of DNA methylation during the dynamic process of chromatin modeling is poorly understood. However, the imprinting of paternal genes is already established in the sperm at the time of fertilization. Interestingly, the global demethylation process that occurs throughout the paternal genome prior to syngamy does not affect imprinted genes. The imprinting of differentially methylated regions facilitates either the transcription or suppression of genes, ensuring the expression of paternal or maternal alleles during early embryogenesis, but not both [20].

Until a decade ago, it was thought that the solo function of sperm was to successfully transfer a haploid paternal genome to the oocyte. In 2004, Ostermeier et al. [21] demonstrated the effective transfer of paternal RNA to the oocyte along with the sperm chromatin. Human sperm was shown to contain a complex composition of RNA and they appear to be fully processed by having 3′-poly-A-tails and lack intron sequences [21].

Two years later, Zhao et al. [22] reported that about 4,000–5,000 different RNA transcripts were detected in a mature sperm population. It is notable that half of the RNA population present in sperm is unique to some individuals or to an ejaculate. Recent studies have shown that the paternal epigenetic information in the form of histone modifications, DNA methylations, organization of sperm chromatin and sperm RNAs plays an essential role during early embryogenesis [23, 24]. Considering the important role of the paternal epigenome in early embryonic development, any abnormality in the paternal epigenetic landscape can lead to altered sperm function [25], reduced fertilization capacity [26], abnormal embryo development [27], and a detrimental pregnancy outcome [28].

Postfertilization of Paternal Histones

In somatic cells, histones play an important role in the folding of chromatin structures that facilitates gene expression. To perform such functions, the amino terminal tails protrude from the histones and are modified by the addition of small groups such as methyl, acetyl, and phosphoryl groups. Increasing evidence suggests that these modifications of histone provide a platform that is recognized by signaling molecules, which can give rise to downstream events that lead to transcription and cell signaling [29]. Similarly, the histone-based epigenome in sperm includes these modifications at specific regions of the sperm genome that are important for early embryonic development [23]. These modifications to histones are observed to exist in singlets, pairs, and/or triplets. For example, acetylation of lysine 5 on H4 results in H4K5ac, while methylation of lysine 4 or 36 on H3 results in H3K4me3 and H3K36me3, respectively (Fig. 1). The histones are classified into canonical variants (H2A, H2B, H3, H4) and a testes-specific histone (tH2B) variant [12].

For many years, the role of sperm-specific histones was unknown. It was thought that they were remnant histones left behind following incomplete histone to protamine exchange. The level of paternal histones retained seemed to be too low to induce a significant effect on gene regulation during embryogenesis. However, the findings of Hammoud et al. [23] challenged the widely held assumption of histone retention, where the epigenetic contribution of sperm is not only confined to paternally imprinted genes and paternal

RNA, but also associated with histone code. For example, when modified histones were localized on chromatin immunoprecipitation-based array analysis, 3K4me2 was enriched at many promoters required for developmental transcription factors [23]. Similarly, high levels of H3K4me3 were exhibited and localized proximal to several transcription and signaling factors (including *EVX1/2*, *ID1*, *STAT3*, *KLF5*, *FGF9*, *SOX7/9*, certain *HOX* genes, and certain noncoding RNAs) important for embryo development [23]. H3K27me3 is another histone variant that is commonly observed in embryonic stem cells and is also identified in sperm at promoters of developmental genes and pericentric regions.

The modification, enrichment, and organization of histones at regulatory regions of genes are considered as promising contributions of histone code to early embryonic development. Experiments using animal models suggest that a 1-cell embryo is transcriptionally active, and RNA polymerase I, II, and III are functional at this stage [30]. Studies using BrUTP, which is a substrate for RNA polymerase II, suggests that endogenous gene expression in the male pronucleus is 4–5 times higher than the female pronucleus [31]. There is evidence suggesting that DNA replication and transcription are linked with each other, where inhibiting of zygotic DNA replication results in an approximate 40% reduction in transcription in the 1-cell embryo [32]. The histone code may be the key to providing access to the male pronucleus for the maternally derived transcriptional mechanism.

Postfertilization of Sperm Methylome

In mammalian species, DNA methylation is removed and reestablished in a sequence-specific manner during gametogenesis [13]. As a result, a sperm-specific DNA methylation profile is established which is markedly different from the somatic cells, but resembles the embryonic stem cells. For example, most of the promoters in sperm and embryonic stem cells are hypomethylated; however, the hypomethylated promoter regions in sperm are bound to histones [23] while the hypomethylated promoters are associated with transcriptional factions like OCT4, SOX2, and KLF4, etc. in human embryonic stem cells [33]. The association of developmentally important regions with histones along with hypomethylation of these regions ensures transcriptional competence and paternal gene activation during early embryonic development.

It is notable that the paternal imprinted genes are reorganized immediately following fertilization [13]. As observed in mammalian species, in the paternal pronucleus erasure of global DNA methylation occurs where most of the sperm-derived methylation marks are removed [34]. However, this process is not complete throughout the male pronucleus, and some regions of the paternal genome, such as the imprinted genes and retrotransposons, are not demethylated [34]. The process of demethylation is accompanied by the simultaneous exchange of protamine by oocyte-derived histones and these changes to the paternal genome are complete prior to activation of the zygotic genome [34].

Postfertilization of Sperm-Derived RNAs

In addition to the transfer of haploid genome, sperm also delivers a small volume of paternally derived RNA to the oocyte (Fig. 1). The paternally derived RNA is fully processed, lacks intronic sequences, and contains 3′-poly-A-tails. It was believed that paternal RNA is nonfunctional as they are remnants of gene expression during the spermatic stage. The importance of paternal RNA was brought to light when it was revealed to potentially impact early embryonic development. Later, Ostermeier et al. [21] confirmed the importance of new sperm-derived RNA after fertilization. The same group showed that the paternally derived RNA remains intact 3 h after fertilization and some of the RNAs present in the sperm are absent in the oocyte postfertilization. Several types of RNA have been observed in sperm, namely mRNA, tRNA, rRNA, miRNAs, PIWI-interacting piRNAs, and repeat-associated small RNAs.

The paternally derived mRNAs are classified into 3 types based on their function: mRNA without function, mRNA with function, and foreign mRNA. An example of mRNA without function is protamine 2-encoding mRNA, where such mRNAs are rapidly degenerated postfertilization. Some mRNAs are taken up by the sperm and do not originate from the testis; such mRNAs are termed foreign mRNA. An example of foreign mRNA is clusterin, which is expressed in the epididymis and prostate. A well-known example of mRNA with postfertilization functions is mRNA translated for AKAP-4 protein, which is involved in signal transduction required for the activation of oocyte immediately after fertilization. FOXG1B and heat shock-binding protein 1 are some important paternally derived mRNAs required for cellular differentiation and embryo patterning during early embryogenesis. In addition, a number of recent studies have suggested the possible function of sperm-derived mRNAs, which could modulate transcription from the male pronucleus [35]. Although a large volume of paternally derived mRNA will be degraded in the oocyte, a small quantity of functionally intact mRNA is required for the activation of the embryonic genome. The function of many stable paternal mRNAs is yet to be established.

Postfertilization of Sperm Nuclear Matrix Organization

The sperm nuclear matrix is the structural component of the sperm nucleus. It consists of a protein structure to which the DNA molecule is attached in a well-organized 3-dimensional loop-like structure. Such a structure is important in somatic cells, where the matrix serves as a scaffold for replication and transcription. The nuclear matrix and organization of the DNA loop domain are unlikely to serve their function in mature sperm because replication and translation is absent in sperm; however, their importance for early embryonic development was first suggested by Ward and Coffey [36]. Using a mouse model, the same group demonstrated that the organization of DNA in the sperm nuclear matrix is essential for replication [37]. The sperm nuclear matrix expands in the embryo following the replacement of protamine by maternal histones resulting in a functional skeletal framework essential for DNA replication. A notable difference between the sperm nuclear matrix and that of the somatic cell is the length of loop domain. The sperm matrix generally accommodates approximately 50 kb of DNA compared to the 25- to 100-kb loop of an active somatic cell. Despite the crystalline nature of sperm DNA, the sperm nuclear matrix has more openly accessible regions that could help the maternal factors to target sperm DNA postfertilization. Histone modifications and the sperm nuclear matrix together play an important role in the dynamics of gene expression, as this structural organization is important for the access of genes required for early embryonic development. The functional importance of the sperm nuclear matrix is yet to be fully understood; however, abnormalities in sperm nuclear packing have been shown to result in male infertility.

Sperm Epigenetic Abnormalities and Their Clinical Aspects

The precise transfer of information through genetic code in the sperm chromatin is essential for the efficient reproductive potential of the sperm, to maintain a successful pregnancy, and for the postnatal health of the offspring. A genetic or epigenetic abnormality may cause infertility or even diseases in the offspring. An important character that distinguishes epigenetic modifications from genetic modifications or mutations is their reversibility. Epigenetic modifications are normally erased in the germ line. Incomplete erasure is known to result in epigenetic inheritance.

Epigenetic modifications can also be transmitted to the offspring when they occur after fertilization and prior to the specification of the germ line.

Methylation defects may not only arise by genetic mutations in the methylation machinery, but also by epigenetic mechanistic alterations in their target genes. Several recent studies have shown a strong association of aberrant DNA methylation or epimutations of some imprinted genes in spermatozoa in patients with idiopathic infertility [38, 39]. Men with moderate or severe oligospermia often display abnormalities in both maternal and paternal imprints. It has been reported that nearly 50% of patients from an oligozoospermic cohort had defective DNA methylation in the paternally imprinted gene *H19* and/or the maternally imprinted gene *MEST* [40]. Decreased progressive sperm motility and poor sperm morphology has also been associated with DNA methylation errors of *MEST* [41]. A meta-analysis of studies describing associations of male infertility with spermatozoal DNA methylation of *H19* and/or *MEST* demonstrated that it is more likely for infertile patients to have aberrant *MEST* (odds ratio 3.4, 95% confidence interval 1.98–5.84, $p < 0.0001$) or *H19* (odds ratio 14.62, 95% confidence interval 7.34–29.12, $p < 0.0001$) DNA methylation in spermatozoa compared to fertile men [42]. DNA methylation aberrations of *H19* and the *MTHFR* promoter in paternal spermatozoa were also found in cases of spontaneous abortions, suggesting an impact of spermatozoal DNA methylation on pregnancy outcome [43]. Recent studies have also reported associations between the aberrant DNA methylation of nonimprinted genes and CpG loci with oligozoospermia, abnormal sperm morphology, and reduced sperm motility [44, 45].

The paternal histones retained after fertilization also play an essential role in the association of aberrant DNA methylation and male infertility. The 10–15% of retained histones, which mark genes and loci, play an important role during early embryonic development [23]. Failures in histone retention and modification or aberrations in protamine distribution have been shown to cause male infertility [46, 47]. Aberrant spermatozoal DNA methylation in men with abnormal protamine replacement has also been reported [48].

In fertile men, P1 and P2 exist in equal proportions. A derangement of the P1/P2 ratio has also been reported in patients with male infertility [26]. Erroneous processing of protamine transcript leads to an increase in the production of immature P2 precursors associated with subfertility [46, 49]. Contradictory findings have been reported for the association of an abnormal protamine ratio with decreased sperm count, sperm function, and poor embryonic quality [46, 50, 51]. The average P1/P12 ratio has also been reported to vary with time within the same individual [52]. Abnormal replacement of histones by protamines is also associated with reduced semen quality, and decreased success rates of IVF and pregnancy [10, 26, 53].

Findings from different studies suggest that epigenetic abnormalities impact embryo development [24, 54] and could be the cause of miscarriages [43, 55]. These findings have led to the concept that spermatozoal DNA methylation has some potential predictive power for pregnancy outcome [43, 55–57]. A significantly higher ($p < 0.001$) *ALU* DNA methylation was reported in sperm from individuals with pregnancy and live birth, whereas in the same study significantly lower ($p = 0.027$) *ALU* DNA methylation levels were found in spontaneous abortions [56]. Another study reported that global DNA methylation of human spermatozoa is associated with the pregnancy rate but not fertilization rate or quality of embryos [57].

Aberrant imprinting is involved in human syndromes such as Silver-Russell, Albright, Prader-Willi, Angelman, Beckwith-Wiedemann and Wilms' tumor [58]. Although the prevalence of these disorders is extremely low, these imprinting disorders occur more frequently after assisted reproductive techniques when compared to children conceived through natural conception. Imprinted abnormalities play a critical role in disorders during embryonic growth and behavioral development, and also in carcinogenesis. The role of imprinting abnormalities has been shown to induce neurobehavioral disorders, such as autism, bipolar affective disorder, and schizophrenia [59]. Aberrant imprinting during the preimplantation developmental process may lead to severe consequences, such as cancer. Imprinted genes play a crucial role and any error in them may lead to a higher chance of embryo developmental arrest and death, fetal growth retardation, or overgrowth.

Conclusion

Germ cells have the unique task of carrying information from one generation to another; it is critical for them to "remember" the "appropriate and benefitting" but "forget" the "detrimental and harmful" information that could be passed to the offspring. Therefore, gametogenesis not only transforms the genomic content into a state that readily supports pre- and postnatal development, but also acts as a barrier in the transfer of information that could be lethal to the next generation. To accomplish this task, the epigenetic machinery at different levels of germ cell development involves mechanisms that act on different target molecules within the genome.

The prominent mechanisms of epigenetic programming that have been discussed here are the removal and reacquisition of DNA methylation in the germ cell stage and in the preimplantation window, the histone-protamine substitution during spermatogenesis and replacement by maternal histones during zygote genome activation, histone modifications, the role of paternal RNAs, and sex-specific gene imprinting. Although many of the epigenetic transitions have been elucidated, there are still many questions to be answered.

With advancements in technology, we anticipate that in the next few years a more comprehensive and much more detailed picture of epigenetic modifications in the sperm chromatin will be revealed. Furthermore, the significant associations of epigenetic abnormalities with male infertility, increased frequency of spontaneous abortions, and imprinting disorders are very strong, as shown by the studies discussed above. Although it is not a practical option in the current scenario, considering the pace at which our understanding of the epigenetic events in sperm chromatin is increasing, analysis of the sperm epigenome may become a new valuable diagnostic marker in clinical reproductive biology.

References

1 Kota SK, Feil R: Epigenetic transitions in germ cell development and meiosis. Dev Cell 2010;19:675–686.

2 Suetake I, Shinozaki F, Miyagawa J, Takeshima H, Tajima S: DNMT3L stimulates the DNA methylation activity of Dnmt3a and Dnmt3b through a direct interaction. J Biol Chem 2004;279:27816–27823.

3 Oakes CC, La Salle S, Smiraglia DJ, Robaire B, Trasler JM: Developmental acquisition of genome-wide DNA methylation occurs prior to meiosis in male germ cells. Dev Biol 2007;307:368–379.

4 Gkountela S, Li Z, Vincent JJ, Zhang KX, Chen A, Pellegrini M, Clark AT: The ontogeny of cKIT+ human primordial germ cells proves to be a resource for human germ line reprogramming, imprint erasure and in vitro differentiation. Nat Cell Biol 2013;15:113–122.

5 Lachner M, Jenuwein T: The many faces of histone lysine methylation. Curr Opin Cell Biol 2002;14:286–298.

6 Godmann M, Auger V, Ferraroni-Aguiar V, Di Sauro A, Sette C, Behr R, Kimmins S: Dynamic regulation of histone H3 methylation at lysine 4 in mammalian spermatogenesis. Biol Reprod 2007;77:754–764.

7 Sonnack V, Failing K, Bergmann M, Steger K: Expression of hyperacetylated histone H4 during normal and impaired human spermatogenesis. Andrologia 2002;34:384–390.

8 Song N, Liu J, An S, Nishino T, Hishikawa Y, Koji T: Immunohistochemical analysis of histone H3 modifications in germ cells during mouse spermatogenesis. Acta Histochem Cytochem 2011;44:183–190.

9 Rousseaux S, Gaucher J, Thevenon J, Caron C, Vitte AL, Curtet S, Derobertis C, Faure AK, Levy R, Aknin-Seifer I, Ravel C, Siffroi JP, Mc Elreavey K, Lejeune H, Jimenez C, Hennebicq S, Khochbin S: Spermiogenesis: histone acetylation triggers male genome reprogramming. Gynecol Obstet Fertil 2009; 37:519–522.
10 Aoki VW, Carrell DT: Human protamines and the developing spermatid: their structure, function, expression and relationship with male infertility. Asian J Androl 2003;5:315–324.
11 Govin J, Escoffier E, Rousseaux S, Kuhn L, Ferro M, Thevenon J, Catena R, Davidson I, Garin J, Khochbin S, Caron C: Pericentric heterochromatin reprogramming by new histone variants during mouse spermiogenesis. J Cell Biol 2007;176:283–294.
12 Gatewood JM, Cook GR, Balhorn R, Schmid CW, Bradbury EM: Isolation of four core histones from human sperm chromatin representing a minor subset of somatic histones. J Biol Chem 1990; 265:20662–20666.
13 Reik W, Dean W, Walter J: Epigenetic reprogramming in mammalian development. Science 2001;293:1089–1093.
14 Kobayashi H, Sakurai T, Imai M, Takahashi N, Fukuda A, Yayoi O, Sato S, Nakabayashi K, Hata K, Sotomaru Y, Suzuki Y, Kono T: Contribution of intragenic DNA methylation in mouse gametic DNA methylomes to establish oocyte-specific heritable marks. PLoS Genet 2012;8:e1002440.
15 Dent CL, Isles AR: Brain-expressed imprinted genes and adult behaviour: the example of Nesp and Grb10. Mamm Genome 2014;25:87–93.
16 Madon-Simon M, Cowley M, Garfield AS, Moorwood K, Bauer SR, Ward A: Antagonistic roles in fetal development and adult physiology for the oppositely imprinted *Grb10* and *Dlk1* genes. BMC Biol 2014;12:771.
17 Brunner AM, Nanni P, Mansuy IM: Epigenetic marking of sperm by post-translational modification of histones and protamines. Epigenetics Chromatin 2014;7:2.
18 Carrell DT: Epigenetics of the male gamete. Fertil Steril 2012;97:267–274.
19 Berger SL: Histone modifications in transcriptional regulation. Curr Opin Genet Dev 2002;12:142–148.
20 Chong S, Whitelaw E: Epigenetic germline inheritance. Curr Opin Genet Dev 2004;14:692–696.
21 Ostermeier GC, Miller D, Huntriss JD, Diamond MP, Krawetz SA: Reproductive biology: delivering spermatozoan RNA to the oocyte. Nature 2004;429: 154.
22 Zhao Y, Li Q, Yao C, Wang Z, Zhou Y, Wang Y, Wang L, Qiao Z: Characterization and quantification of mRNA transcripts in ejaculated spermatozoa of fertile men by serial analysis of gene expression. Hum Reprod 2006;21:1583–1590.
23 Hammoud SS, Nix DA, Zhang H, Purwar J, Carrell DT, Cairns BR: Distinctive chromatin in human sperm packages genes for embryo development. Nature 2009;460:473–478.
24 Jenkins TG, Carrell DT: The paternal epigenome and embryogenesis: poising mechanisms for development. Asian J Androl 2011;13:76–80.
25 Oakes CC, Kelly TL, Robaire B, Trasler JM: Adverse effects of 5-aza-2′-deoxycytidine on spermatogenesis include reduced sperm function and selective inhibition of de novo DNA methylation. J Pharmacol Exp Ther 2007;322:1171–1180.
26 Aoki VW, Liu L, Jones KP, Hatasaka HH, Gibson M, Peterson CM, Carrell DT: Sperm protamine 1/protamine 2 ratios are related to in vitro fertilization pregnancy rates and predictive of fertilization ability. Fertil Steril 2006;86: 1408–1415.
27 Doerksen T, Trasler JM: Developmental exposure of male germ cells to 5-azacytidine results in abnormal preimplantation development in rats. Biol Reprod 1996;55:1155–1162.
28 Kelly TL, Li E, Trasler JM: 5-aza-2′-deoxycytidine induces alterations in murine spermatogenesis and pregnancy outcome. J Androl 2003;24:822–830.
29 Sims RJ III, Reinberg D: Is there a code embedded in proteins that is based on post-translational modifications? Nat Rev Mol Cell Biol 2008;9:815–820.
30 Ram PT, Schultz RM: Reporter gene expression in G2 of the 1-cell mouse embryo. Dev Biol 1993;156:552–556.
31 Bouniol C, Nguyen E, Debey P: Endogenous transcription occurs at the 1-cell stage in the mouse embryo. Exp Cell Res 1995;218:57–62.
32 Aoki F, Worrad DM, Schultz RM: Regulation of transcriptional activity during the first and second cell cycles in the preimplanation mouse embryo. Dev Biol 1997;181:296–307.
33 Boyer LA, Lee TI, Cole MF, Johnstone SE, Levine SS, Zucker JP, Guenther MG, Kumar RM, Murray HL, Jenner RG, Gifford DK, Melton DA, Jaenisch R, Young RA: Core transcriptional regulatory circuitry in human embryonic stem cells. Cell 2005;122:947–956.
34 Abdalla H, Hirabayashi M, Hochi S: Demethylation dynamics of the paternal genome in pronuclear-stage bovine zygotes produced by in vitro fertilization and ooplasmic injection of freeze-thawed or freeze-dried spermatozoa. J Reprod Dev 2009;55:433–439.
35 Miller D, Ostermeier GC: Towards a better understanding of RNA carriage by ejaculate spermatozoa. Hum Reprod Update 2006;12:757–767.
36 Ward WS, Coffey DS: DNA packaging and organization in mammalian spermatozoa: comparison with somatic cells. Biol Reprod 1991;44:569–574.
37 Shaman JA, Yamauchi Y, Ward WS: The sperm nuclear matrix is required for paternal DNA replication. J Cell Biochem 2007;102:680–688.
38 Kobayashi H, Sato A, Otsu E, Hiura H, Tomatsu C, Utsunomiya T, Sasaki H, Yaegashi N, Arima T: Aberrant DNA methylation of imprinted loci in sperm from oligospermic patients. Hum Mol Genet 2007;16:2542–2551.
39 Camprubí C, Pladevall M, Grossmann M, Garrido N, Pons MC, Blanco J: Semen samples showing an increased rate of spermatozoa with imprinting errors have a negligible effect in the outcome of assisted reproduction techniques. Epigenetics 2012;7:1115–1124.
40 Marques CJ, Costa P, Vaz B, Carvalho F, Fernandes S, Barros A, Sousa M: Abnormal methylation of imprinted genes in human sperm is associated with oligozoospermia. Mol Hum Reprod 2008;14: 67–74.
41 Poplinski A, Tüttelmann F, Kanber D, Horsthemke B, Gromoll J: Idiopathic male infertility is strongly associated with aberrant methylation of MEST and IGF2/H19 ICR1. Int J Androl 2010;33: 642–649.

42 Kläver R, Gromoll J: Bringing epigenetics into the diagnostics of the andrology laboratory: challenges and perspectives. Asian J Androl 2014;16: 669–674.

43 Rotondo JC, Bosi S, Bazzan E, Di Domenico M, De Mattei M, Selvatici R, Patella A, Marci R, Tognon M, Martini F: Methylenetetrahydrofolate reductase gene promoter hypermethylation in semen samples of infertile couples correlates with recurrent spontaneous abortion. Hum Reprod 2012;27:3632–3638.

44 Houshdaran S, Cortessis VK, Siegmund K, Yang A, Laird PW, Sokol RZ: Widespread epigenetic abnormalities suggest a broad DNA methylation erasure defect in abnormal human sperm. PLoS One 2007;2:e1289.

45 Nanassy L, Carrell DT: Abnormal methylation of the promoter of CREM is broadly associated with male factor infertility and poor sperm quality but is improved in sperm selected by density gradient centrifugation. Fertil Steril 2011;95:2310–2314.

46 Carrell DT, Liu L: Altered protamine 2 expression is uncommon in donors of known fertility, but common among men with poor fertilizing capacity, and may reflect other abnormalities of spermiogenesis. J Androl 2001;22:604–610.

47 Hammoud SS, Nix DA, Hammoud AO, Gibson M, Cairns BR, Carrell DT: Genome-wide analysis identifies changes in histone retention and epigenetic modifications at developmental and imprinted gene loci in the sperm of infertile men. Hum Reprod 2011;26:2558–2569.

48 Aston KI, Punj V, Liu L, Carrell DT: Genome-wide sperm deoxyribonucleic acid methylation is altered in some men with abnormal chromatin packaging or poor in vitro fertilization embryogenesis. Fertil Steril 2012;97:285–292.

49 de Mateo S, Ramos L, de Boer P, Meistrich M, Oliva R: Protamine 2 precursors and processing. Rotein Pept Lett 2011; 18:778–785.

50 Carrell DT, Emery BR, Hammoud S: Altered protamine expression and diminished spermatogenesis: what is the link? Hum Reprod Update 2007;13:313–327.

51 Torregrosa N, Domínguez-Fandos D, Camejo MI, Shirley CR, Meistrich ML, Ballescà JL, Oliva R: Protamine 2 precursors, protamine 1/protamine 2 ratio, DNA integrity and other sperm parameters in infertile patients. Hum Reprod 2006;21:2084–2089.

52 Huser T, Orme CA, Hollars CW, Corzett MH, Balhorn R: Raman spectroscopy of DNA packaging in individual human sperm cells distinguishes normal from abnormal cells. J Biophotonics 2009;2: 322–332.

53 Aoki VW, Emery BR, Liu L, Carrell DT: Protamine levels vary between individual sperm cells of infertile human males and correlate with viability and DNA integrity. J Androl 2006;27:890–898.

54 Schagdarsurengin U, Paradowska A, Steger K: Analysing the sperm epigenome: roles in early embryogenesis and assisted reproduction. Nat Rev Urol 2012;9:609–619.

55 Ankolkar M, Patil A, Warke H, Salvi V, Kedia Mokashi N, Pathak S, Balasinor NH: Methylation analysis of idiopathic recurrent spontaneous miscarriage cases reveals aberrant imprinting at H19 ICR in normozoospermic individuals. Fertil Steril 2012;98:1186–1192.

56 El Hajj N, Zechner U, Schneider E, Tresch A, Gromoll J, Hahn T, Schorsch M, Haaf T: Methylation status of imprinted genes and repetitive elements in sperm DNA from infertile males. Sex Dev 2011;5:60–69.

57 Benchaib M, Braun V, Ressnikof D, Lornage J, Durand P, Niveleau A, Guérin JF: Influence of global sperm DNA methylation on IVF results. Hum Reprod 2005; 20:768–773.

58 Falls JG, Pulford DJ, Wylie AA, Jirtle RL: Genomic imprinting: implications for human disease. Am J Path 1999;154: 635–641.

59 Isles AR, Wilkinson LS: Imprinted genes, cognition and behaviour. Trends Cogn Sciences 2000;4:309–318.

Douglas T. Carrell, PhD
Department of Human Genetics, University of Utah
675 Arapeen Drive, Suite 201
Salt Lake City, UT 84108 (USA)
E-Mail douglas.carrell@hsc.utah.edu

Vogt PH (ed): Genetics of Human Infertility. Monogr Hum Genet.
Basel, Karger, 2017, vol 21, pp 128–142 (DOI: 10.1159/000477283)

Characteristic Features of Male Germline Development in Primates

Rüdiger Behr

Platform Degenerative Diseases, German Primate Center – Leibniz Institute for Primate Research, and DZHK (German Center for Cardiovascular Research), Göttingen, Germany

Abstract

The germline is constituted by all cells that have the potential to transmit their genetic information to the next generation. The germline can be considered as a defined sequence of genetic, cellular, and developmental processes recurring in each generation in order to ensure the continuity of a species-specific reproduction program. Although basic mechanisms of germline development in mammals are highly conserved, relatively slight yet relevant modifications of germline development evolved in different groups of mammals to adapt the entire process to the specific requirements of and conditions in each species. This review highlights selected aspects that illustrate germline adaptations and characteristics in primates mainly in comparison to the mouse, which is the best investigated mammalian model organism in reproductive biology.

The germline is constituted by all cells that have the potential to submit their genetic information to the next generation. The cycle of the germline in mammals is characterized by the recurring sequence of (1) fertilization, i.e., fusion of 2 haploid gametes, resulting in (2) a diploid phase of early embryonic development, which leads to (3) the specification and separation of germ cells (primordial germ cells; PGCs) from somatic cells, followed by (4) several rounds of mitotic divisions of the germ cells. Then (5) the germ cells enter meiosis, i.e., the genetic reduction division, resulting in (6) haploid cells forming gametes again. Fusion of the haploid male and the female gametes completes the cycle of the germline and begins the next generation (Fig. 1). This sequence of events occurs in all mammals. However, different species exhibit specific adaptations and characteristics of 1 or more phases of the cycle of the germline. Remarkably, the cycle of the germline is an extremely robust process that works “endlessly”. On the other hand, certain dynamics of the germline is essential for evolution since only modifications of the germline cells can lead to (genetically or epigenetically) inherited traits possibly resulting in better-adapted offspring and, hence, supporting species diversion. In light of these conflicting goals, namely germline stability and genome dynamics, some selected characteristic features of male germ cell development in pri-

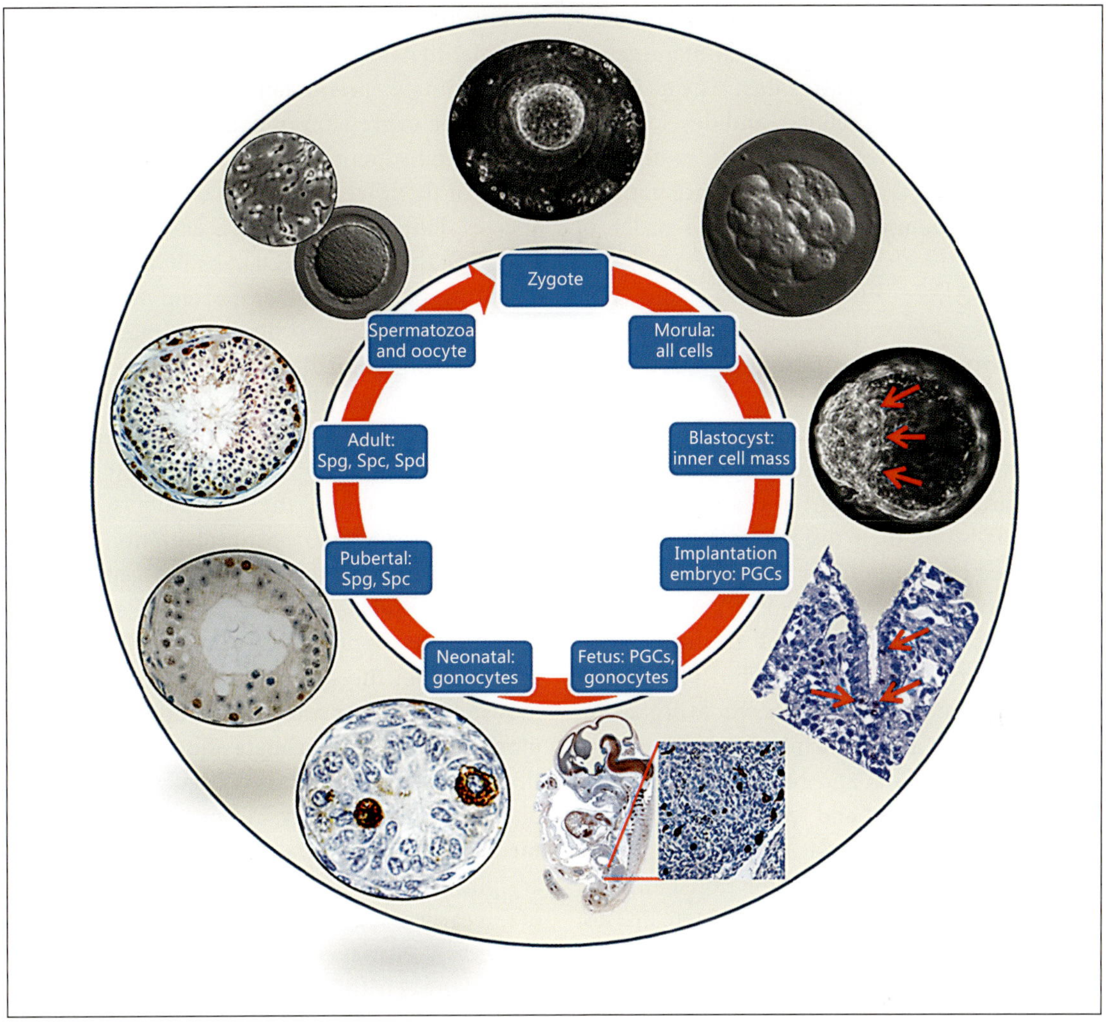

Fig. 1. Illustration of the cycle of the germline. All cells that have the potential to transmit their genetic information to the next generation belong to the germline. Germline cells are mentioned in the blue boxes. A new generation is initiated by the formation of a zygote, i.e., the fertilized oocyte. In the morula-stage embryo, the individual cells (blastomeres) are not yet specified. They are all potential progenitor cells of the prospective germ cells. The blastocyst consists of 2 clearly distinguishable cell populations: the inner cell mass cells (highlighted by red arrows) and the outer cell layer, i.e., the trophoblast. The germ cells develop from the inner cell mass cells. In the implantation embryo the first specified germ cells, called PGCs, occur. In the somite-stage embryos they are frequently located in the epithelium of the developing hind gut (red arrows). In the fetus, most PGCs have entered the forming gonad. The magnified area shows the distribution of germ cells in the gonadal primordium. In the neonatal testis the germ cells are mostly gonocytes, which are premeiotic germ cells located mostly in the center of the developing seminiferous tubule. At that stage, the tubule has no lumen. The gonocytes were stained using immunohistochemistry. In the pubertal testis, the seminiferous tubules form a lumen, and spermatogonia (Spg; stained brown) start to proliferate, giving rise to meiotic spermatocytes (Spc). In the adult testis, there are premeiotic Spg, meiotic Spc, and postmeiotic spermatids (Spd). Undifferentiated spermatogonia were stained by immunohistochemistry. Elongated spermatids are positioned on the apical (adluminal) surface of the germinal epithelium. Spermatozoa and oocytes are the gametes released from sexually mature male and female gonads, respectively. Fusion of the gametes initiates the next cycle of the germline. The different stages are illustrated using micro images (which are not shown to scale) of the Platform Degenerative Diseases of the DPZ.

mates will be discussed in this chapter in comparison with the best-characterized mammalian species, the mouse (*Mus musculus*). The major focus will be on genetic, cellular, and developmental aspects. The term primate includes non-human primates (NHP) and humans, since both belong to the taxonomical (biological) order of primates.

The Totipotent and Pluripotent Stages of the Germline

After fertilization in mammals, the cells of the embryo are first totipotent and after only very few cell divisions their differentiation potential is restricted to pluripotency. A cell is totipotent if it can form a whole organism. In contrast, pluripotency is the ability of a cell to differentiate into all cell types of the body, but pluripotent cells lack the potential to form a whole organism. Both totipotent as well as pluripotent cells belong to the germline, and both states require a finely tuned temporal and spatial control [1, 2]. Interestingly, the molecular regulation of pluripotency and the signal transduction pathways associated with this developmental state are not fully conserved in different mammalian species as has been shown for pluripotent cells of human and mouse origin [3, 4]. Recently, marmoset monkey and mouse pluripotent cells directly isolated from embryos were also compared [5]. Some factors that have important roles in the mouse system [6, 7], like *KLF2* and *NR0B1* (also known as *DAX-1*), were also highly expressed in the mouse preimplantation embryo [5] but were basically undetectable in the marmoset monkey (*Callithrix jacchus*) preimplantation embryo [5]. Also, the pluripotency-associated gene *FBX015*, although not essential for mouse development and fertility [8], shows dramatic differences in the expression levels in mouse and monkey preimplantation embryos. These selected examples highlight molecular differences in the regulation of pluripotency and, thereby, also differences in the maintenance of the germline at the mouse and primate preimplantation embryo stage. When the expression of components of specific signal transduction pathways was analyzed, many of them were found to be present in both species. However, transcripts encoding components of the TGF-β/NODAL, FGF, and WNT signaling pathways, all important for different early developmental processes in mammals [9–11], were differentially expressed [5], suggesting that the utilization of specific signal transduction pathways is different between mouse and primate preimplantation embryos. Recent groundbreaking studies on the cynomolgus monkey (*Macaca fascicularis*) postimplantation embryo also revealed clear differences between primate and mouse epiblast [12], which is the embryonic precursor tissue of the PGCs, and PGC specification between the cynomolgus monkey and the mouse [13]. These comparative approaches employing mouse and primate allowed differentiation between basic pathways involved in the regulation of pluripotency in mammals and those mechanisms that apparently exhibit evolutionary plasticity [14]. In summary, general features of the early phase of embryonic development are conserved. However, there are also clear differences between the mouse and the primate regarding the regulation of pluripotency in preimplantation and implantation embryos. At present, the phenotypic and particularly the functional consequences of these molecular findings can only be speculated on, since functional and gene deletion studies are very demanding and challenging in NHP.

Embryonic Specification of Primordial Germ Cells in Primates and the Mouse

In the mouse, about 45 PGCs can be detected around embryonic day (E) 7–7.25 by alkaline phosphatase staining [15, 16]. Lawson and Hage

[15] also showed through lineage tracing experiments that PGCs are not finally specified in the mouse before E6.5. However, around E6.25–6.5, marked expression of *fragilis*, a gene important for germ cell specification, was found in nascent PGCs, followed by expression of *stella* around E7 [17]; *stella* is germ cell specific. However, recent data may suggest that the activation of a germ cell-characteristic gene expression program may start before E7, possibly already around E3.5–4 [18]. Hence, in the mouse there is a period of currently unknown length during which cells of the implanted embryo have the competence to differentiate into germ cells. The final specification, however, apparently occurs only around or even shortly after E7. These early implantation stages are difficult to obtain from humans (for ethical and practical reasons) as well as from NHP. Nevertheless, very recent in vitro as well as in situ studies delineated this phase of primate germ cell specification. Instructive in vitro systems employing human pluripotent stem cells suggested significant differences between mouse and human germ cell specification [19–22]. In the mouse, it has been shown that the interplay of BLIMP1 (also known as PRDM1), PRDM14, and AP2γ (TFAP2C) initiates a unique cellular program resulting in the specification of PGCs [23]. These factors synergistically suppress the ongoing somatic differentiation and activate the reexpression of pluripotency- and germ cell-specific genes [23]. *PRDM14* is essential for PGC specification in mice [24]. Contrastingly, the role of *PRDM14* in human germ cell specification seems to be only minor since this gene was only minimally expressed in in vitro assays of germ cell development compared to the mouse [21]. Remarkably, Sasaki et al. [13] showed that cynomolgus monkey PCGs did express *PRDM14* in the context of natural embryos. This discrepancy between monkey and human *PRDM14* expression in PGCs may either represent a species-specific difference (human vs. cynomolgus monkey) or may reflect the different approaches of PGC investigation, i.e., pluripotent stem cell based for human PGC development and natural embryo based for monkey PGC investigation. A clear difference between primate and mouse PGC specification is the role of *SOX17*. This transcription factor is a key regulator of human PGC specification [19] and acts upstream of *BLIMP1*. In the absence of SOX17, no germ cell-like cells were obtained from pluripotent stem cells, highlighting the role of SOX17 in human germ line specification [19]. Importantly, *SOX17* has also been shown to be highly expressed, together with *TFAP2C*, in cynomolgus monkey PGCs [13]. In striking contrast, *SOX17* has no apparent role during germ cell specification in mice [19]. In general, the pluripotent stem cell-based system for the (functional) investigation of primate PGC development appears to be a very useful alternative for potential in vivo studies in NHP for the following reasons. First, Sasaki et al. [22] compared the gene expression signatures of their in vitro-derived PGC-like cells with those of PGCs isolated from monkey embryos and found significant matching of both gene signatures, nicely validating the in vitro data. Second, SOX2 is a core pluripotency transcription factor expressed by mouse PGCs, and it is essential for mouse PGC development in vivo [25]. In striking contrast to the mouse, human PGCs neither express SOX2 during in vivo development, nor upon in vitro culture [26], while OCT4 and Nanog as additional core pluripotency factors [27] are expressed [28]. This pattern was recently confirmed by Sasaki et al. [13] for cynomolgus monkey PGCs and in our lab for marmoset monkey PGCs [29; unpubl. data], suggesting that a lack of SOX2 expression is a common characteristic of primate PGCs. Importantly, *SOX2* was expressed in human pluripotent stem cells, but was undetectable or strongly repressed in human PGC-like cells derived from pluripotent stem cells [19, 30], which nicely recapitulates the dynamics of SOX2 expression during human and cynomolgus monkey PGC

development in vivo. In summary, molecular players essential for mouse PGC development like SOX2 appear to have only minor or even no role in primate PGC formation. In contrast, SOX17 is essential for human PGC formation, but not in the mouse. These examples highlight clear differences in the molecular regulation of PGC specification and development between primates and the mouse.

The Role of the Amnion and the Extraembryonic Ectoderm

The extraembryonic ectoderm (ExE) plays an important role during mouse PGC specification [23]. PGCs respond to BMP4, which is secreted from the ExE during embryonic days E6.5–7.5 [31]. Mouse embryos lacking BMP4 fail to develop PGCs; they do not contain any germ cells [32]. These data suggest that the ExE is essential for proper PGC specification and development in the mouse. However, since the anatomy and morphology of the mouse and the primate embryo are fundamentally different, with a flat germ disc in primates and an egg cylinder in the mouse [4, 33], there is no direct structural counterpart of the mouse ExE in the primate embryo [34]. Recently, it was shown that the nascent (pregastrulation) amnion is the origin of PGCs in the cynomolgus monkey [13]. Giving rise to PGCs appears to be a unique function of the amnion in primates [13]. Furthermore, this study also provided insights into (potential) inductive processes regulating PGC specification and determination in primates. The amnion itself as the PGC-generating tissue produces BMP4 and WNT3A, to which the PGCs may respond [13]. In summary, the significant anatomical differences between mouse and primate embryos at the time of PGC specification [4] and the amnion as the origin of primate PGCs [13] demonstrate significant species-specific adaptations in primates compared to the mouse.

Gonocytes and Spermatogonial Stem Cells

PGC specification and their initial development occur outside the gonads and even outside the embryo proper. In order to constitute a functional gonad, the PGCs have to be translocated from their extraembryonic position into the developing gonad, which is free of germ cells during the first steps of its differentiation. Only little is known about the primate (-specific aspects of) PGC migration and translocation [26, 29, 35–38]. Upon arrival in the male gonad, postmigratory PGCs are surrounded by cells forming the somatic parts of the developing testicular cords, which eventually become the seminiferous tubules in the adult testis. Upon inclusion in the testicular cords, the PGCs are called gonocytes. The gonocyte stage developmentally links the PGC stage with the spermatogonial stage and involves phases of relative quiescence, proliferation, migration from a central position within the testicular cord to the basement membrane of the developing germinal epithelium, and finally differentiation to a spermatogonial stem cell [39, 40]. However, in mice, a subpopulation of gonocytes directly initiates spermatogenesis in order to fuel the first wave of sperm production without passing through an undifferentiated spermatogonial stage [41]. Again, only little is known about the molecular regulation of the development of gonocytes in primates [40, 42–45]. However, one aspect is evident: in primates there is an extended phase of relative quiescence of the gonocytes between the beginning of the gonocyte stage and the initiation of puberty, i.e., spermatogonia start to proliferate in order to initiate spermatogenesis. Although it has been shown that there is some germ cell proliferation and differentiation during the prepubertal period in the monkey [46] and in the human [47, 48] testis, this prepubertal period of relative testicular quiescence has no direct counterpart in rodents. In fact, a comparative analysis of the germ cell population in the neo- and postnatal human, marmoset, and rat testis showed that GC differentiation and loss of pluripotency marker expression in marmosets is remarkably similar to that in the human but fundamentally different from the situation in rats [40]. Based on their findings, McKinnell et al. [40] concluded that researchers and clinicians need to be very cautious when extrapolating the results from rodent studies into humans. In mice, no gonocytes were found on postnatal day 11 [46], and all germ cells had developed to spermatogonia or spermatocytes. The first haploid round spermatids were seen in postnatal day 21 mouse testes, and spermatogenesis was already completed by postnatal day 35 in the mouse [49]. This is in sharp contrast to the marmoset, which first produces sperm cells around 12 months after birth [50], and to the human testis, where puberty is usually initiated around the age of 11–13 years. Although some signals involved in the initiation and regulation of puberty have also been identified in NHP [51], there are still major gaps of knowledge in this field [52]. In general, an extended period of relative testicular quiescence before the initiation of the first meiotic wave occurs in primates, but not in rodents. These are relevant adaptations to the different reproductive strategies of primates as K-selected species with few offspring, long periods of gestation, long and intensive parental care, and a long period until the reproductive age is reached. In contrast, as r-selected species, rodents have high numbers of offspring, short periods of gestation, little parental care, and reach adulthood and sexual maturity early [53].

According to the classical model, ongoing spermatogenesis in rodents is fueled by spermatogonial stem cells, which are called A single (A_s) spermatogonia [54]. These are individual cells that are believed to be the starting point of a new clone of differentiating germ cells. They are characterized by the expression of several marker proteins such as GFRα1 (the GDNF receptor), NGN3, PLZF [for a review, see 55], SALL4 [56], and LIN28 [57]. In primates, the different putative stem cell types were classified and named after their morphological appearance: A_{dark} are considered to represent reserve stem cells, and A_{pale} spermatogonia are considered to represent active stem cells in terms of sperm production [for a review, see 55]. However, 10 years ago Ehmcke and Schlatt [58] proposed a model of spermatogonial self-renewal and differentiation that was based on the assumption that the primate spermatogonial population is more plastic than previously thought. Moreover, the relatively simple mouse model was also recently profoundly revised [59]. In fact, these novel data suggest that an extended heterogeneous population of spermatogonia forms a flexible and to a certain extent reversible pool of cells with stem cell characteristics on the one hand, and on the other hand differentiating characteristics. These important findings may lead to a revised model of spermatogonial self-renewal, expansion, and differentiation in mammals. However, even if the unexpected finding of plasticity of the spermatogonia population in the mouse testis applies to all mammals, there are significant differences between the mouse and the primate spermatogonial stem cell pool. Regarding marker expression, this is very obvious for LIN28 [44] (Fig. 2). While many mouse spermatogonia strongly express this important developmental and pluripotency-associated factor [60], it could be detected only in an extremely minor subpopulation of primate spermatogonia [44]. Also, NGN3, an important lineage-specifying transcription factor in the pancreas [61], is already expressed in mouse spermatogonia from the A_s stage onwards, but is absent from rhesus monkey A_{dark} and A_{pale} stem spermatogonia [55]. Irrespective of the validity of the different models of spermatogonial self-renewal and differentiation, it appears that mouse spermatogonia are in a more primitive, gonocyte-like state compared to primate spermatogonia. Single cell transcriptome analysis in combination with functional assays will further clarify the mode of the spermatogonial system in different

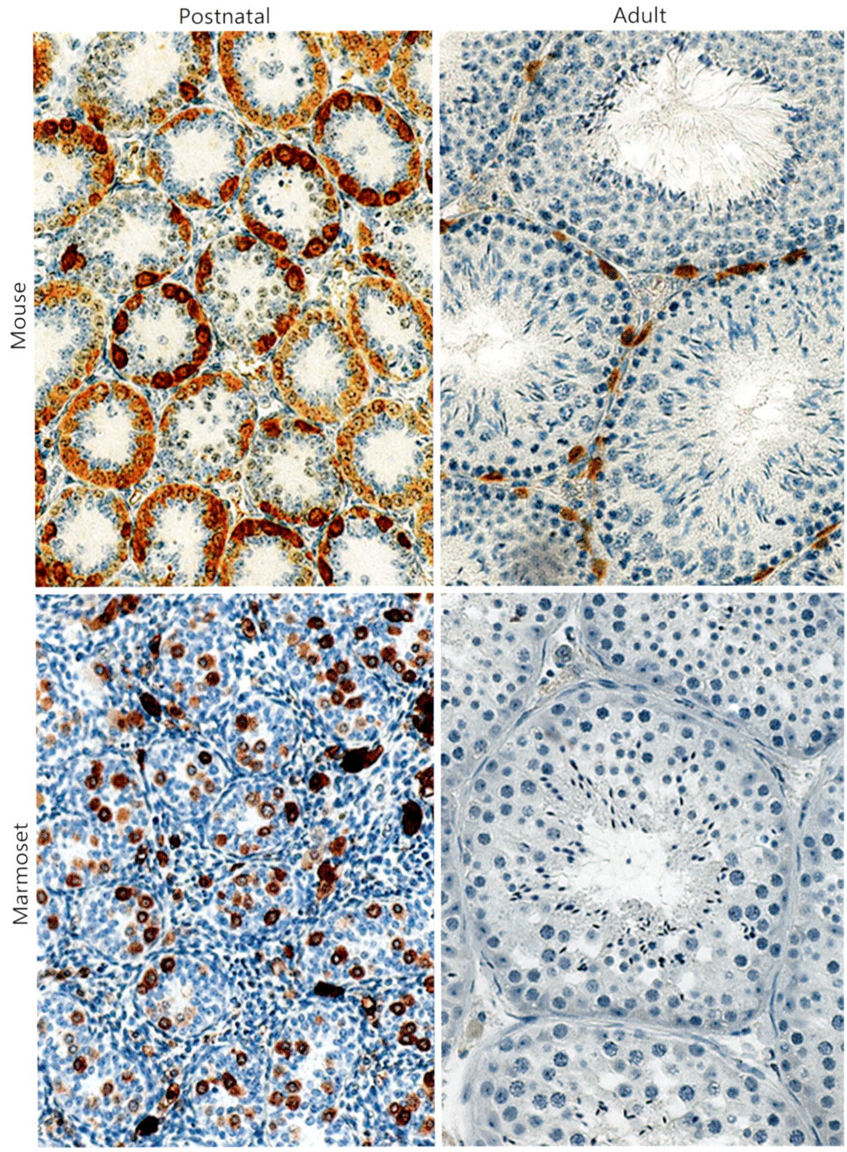

Fig. 2. Differential expression of the stem cell factor LIN28 in adult spermatogonia of marmoset monkey and mouse testes. In the immature postnatal testes, the gonocytes/spermatogonia are LIN28-positive in both species. In contrast, in the adult testes, only mouse spermatogonia are positive for LIN28, while the marmoset monkey spermatogonia (and those of all other NHP species tested so far) are generally negative for LIN28. Only very few primate spermatogonia express LIN28 [44].

mammals, including primates, within the next few years.

One highly significant and undoubted difference between premeiotic germ cell expansion in the mouse and primate testis, however, is the number of mitotic cell divisions before the spermatogonia eventually enter meiosis. While there are 10 or 11 mitotic divisions of spermatogonia in the mouse before they enter meiosis, in primates there are significantly fewer premeiotic cell divisions: 5 in Rhesus monkeys and only 2 in humans (for a review, see Ehmcke and Schlatt [58]). This means that the size of the clones emerging from 1 stem cell is much bigger in the mouse than in the human. The rhesus monkey clone size is between that of the mouse and the human. This difference in clone size in turn also implies that the density of stem cells in the primate testis is much higher than in the mouse testis. It was hypothesized that the germ cell clonal size (which is inversely correlated with the stem cell density) determines whether a primate species predominantly exhibits a single- or a multistage organization of the cross-section of the germinal epithelium [62]. The human testis shows a multistage system in around 80% of all seminiferous tubule cross-sections [62], which corresponds to the small germ cell clone size in the human testis [63]. Similarly, the marmoset monkey also predominantly shows a multistage organization, with up to 5 stages per cross-section [62, 64]. This high number of stages per cross-section suggests a very small clone size and very few premeiotic mitotic divisions of spermatogonia in this species. In contrast, the macaque species showed a multistage organization of the germinal epithelium cross-section in only 20–33% of all cross-sections [62], correlating well with the larger number of premeiotic spermatogonial cell divisions [63]. Hence, in primates, the species-specific histological organization of the seminiferous epithelium most likely evolved depending on the number of premeiotic spermatogonial cell divisions. The fact that both the human and the marmoset exhibit a multistage system makes the marmoset monkey a very good model for human spermatogenesis [64]. Finally, when NHP are used as experimental animals in reproductive biology, it must be considered that some primate species, including the rhesus monkey, have seasonal testicular activity with a transient block of spermatogonial proliferation [65], while seasonality has never been described for the human and the marmoset testis.

Spermatogonial Stem Cell Culture

For more than 20 years, it has been possible to culture mouse spermatogonia [66]. Nagano et al. [66] demonstrated the spermatogonial stem cell identity of the cultured cells by transplantation into a recipient testis, where the cells repopulated the seminiferous tubule and initiated complete spermatogenesis. Since then, mouse spermatogonia have been cultured in many laboratories around the world. They were genetically manipulated in vitro and transplanted into appropriate recipients in order to generate genetically modified mice [67], and were converted to a pluripotent state resembling embryonic stem cells [68]. Furthermore, rodent in vitro spermatogenesis was intensely investigated and finally successful [69–73] even when initiated from cultured spermatogonial stem cell lines [74]. Altogether, the culture of mouse spermatogonial stem cells is well established. In the primate, it is still a matter of debate whether long-term culture and the expansion of spermatogonial stem cells, i.e., the culture of functional stem cells, is possible. While some studies could detect human [75, 76] and marmoset monkey [77, 78] spermatogonia only for very limited periods in culture, other reports described the long-term culture of human spermatogonia [79–82] and even their differentiation into haploid germ cells [83]. However, since some markers used in human long-term spermatogonial culture studies are not unequivocal germ cell markers, it remains a matter of contention at present whether the cultured cells are really functional germ cells. The only functional test currently possible would be transplantation of long-term cultured NHP germ cells into a recipient testis of the same species and subsequent generation of offspring from the long-term cultured and transplanted germ cells. This is currently not possible in humans for ethical reasons due to the very limited knowledge about the safety of the procedure for the potential offspring. Nevertheless, in the long term, this procedure may be a promising strategy to preserve the prospective fertility of male prepubertal cancer survivors [84], and a very promising spermatogonial stem cell transplantation study has already been conducted in NHP with cryopreserved, but not long-term cultured spermatogonia [85]. In general, the long-term primate spermatogonial cell culture has to be improved. The robust spermatogonial stem cell culture in mice may reflect the more primitive developmental state of the mouse spermatogonial stem cells compared to the primate counterparts. In this context, it is tempting to speculate that the recently established concept of a naïve and a primed state of pluripotent stem cells [86] can also be translated to mouse (naïve) and primate (primed) spermatogonial stem cells.

Considering Potential Limitations of Mouse Models of Human Male Infertility

There exist excellent reviews on the genetic causes of male infertility [87, 88]. Hundreds of mouse mutants exhibiting spermatogenic defects leading to infertility have been generated, illuminating the roles of many conserved mammalian fertility genes. However, although many of the mouse genes investigated in the context of infertility were also analyzed in infertile patients, only few mouse fertility genes were also found to be mutated in patients, like TEX11 [89]. Even if all mouse genes were to be mutated soon [90], it remains questionable whether these mice represent appropriate models of the majority of human infertile patients. This may be due to the following facts: (1) male infertility is a multifactorial disease, and the interplay of several factors in primates may be different from that in mice, (2) there might be significant epigenetic differences between mouse and primate germ cells, and (3) there are primate-specific genes that have no counterpart in the mouse genome. Importantly, the primate-specific transcripts are highly enriched in the brain and in the testis [91] (see also below). Therefore, it is likely that some aspects of male primate germ cell development as well as some cases of human infertility cannot be modeled in mice due to the absence of the relevant genes. In general, the aspect of the evolution of novel genes, particularly in the testis, has probably been underestimated until recently [92], except for the sex chromosomes [93–95].

The Genome Perspective: Primate-Specific Genes and Mobile Elements

In terms of the evolutionary perspective, genomes are highly dynamic, and several mechanisms for the birth of new genes have been identified [96]. While new protein-coding genes usually evolve from preexisting protein-coding genes, recently even “motherless” new protein-coding genes, which probably developed de novo from ancestral noncoding DNAs, were described in the human and ape genome [97]. Hence, during evolution, genome dynamics resulted in highly diverse genomes. Importantly, it was recently estimated that the human genome encodes more than 300 human-specific genes and around 1,000 primate-specific genes [91]. Since the number of human genes is less than 20,000, more than 5% of all human genes are primate specific. These new genes are predominantly implicated in brain and testis development and function. Within the testis, most of the “male genes" appear to be expressed by germ cells [98], but not by the somatic compartment of the testis. Consequently, testicular transcriptomes are also different in different species [98], and, probably even more strikingly, gene expression levels evolve faster in primates than in rodents [99]. Furthermore, primates exhibit a faster accumulation of alternatively spliced transcripts than other mammalian orders [100]. On the molecular level, the global removal of repressive epigenetic marks and a permissive chromatin state during meiosis may boost gene expression in male germ cells. This molecular environment in germ cells most likely represents the delivery room for novel genes, and based on this, the "out-of-the-testis hypothesis" of gene/genome evolution was established [98]. To summarize: (1) testicular germ cells are most likely the hotbed of genomic evolution; (2) there are hundreds of primate-specific genes with enriched activity in the testis; (3) the testicular transcriptome is significantly different from those of other organs, and (4) interestingly, there is a primate-specific acceleration of transcriptome evolution.

Retrotransposons are mobile self-replicating genetic elements that can spread over the genome via an RNA intermediate [101] and can be considered to resemble retroviruses. However, viruses spread horizontally between organisms. In contrast, retrotransposons spread vertically through the germ line. Alu elements are a subclass of retrotransposons of about 300 base pairs in length. Since there is no specific defense or removal mechanism for Alu sequences, there is a steady accumulation of Alu sequences during evolution [101]. Importantly, Alu sequences are unique to primates, and they comprise around 11% of the human genome [102], while all transposable elements together constitute around 50% of the human genome [103]. Alu germline activity is the highest of all human retrotransposons and significantly contributes to genome instability and, hence, genetic population diversity [101]. Furthermore, another family of retrotransposons, the hominid-specific SINE-VNTR-Alus (called SVA), are the youngest of these elements, constituting 0.13% of the genome and originating approximately 25 million years ago [104]. The SVA are present in the human genome in about 3,000 copies. It has been shown that the elements of this family also contribute to the development of new genes in primates [104]. These examples highlight that significant parts of the primate genome are specific to primates and do not have any counterpart in the genomes of other mammalian taxa. Furthermore, these primate-specific portions of the genome are clearly not "junk DNA," but have functional relevance [105] – also in terms of primate-specific evolution [106].

The Haploid Phase of the Germline

Postmeiotic spermatids condense their chromatin in preparation for their release from the germinal epithelium and their subsequent passage through the female reproductive tract. Because of the block of transcription in spermatids [107] and the release of the residual body (a droplet of unnecessary cytoplasm also containing RNA), it was previously thought that sperm cells are free of RNA transcripts. Therefore, the transcriptome of the spermatids and sperm cells was not appreciated for a long time. This changed in recent years, and a very interesting study detected the highly surprising number of 16,900 different gene transcripts in spermatozoa [108]. This is more than in whole liver and in Sertoli cells, for instance [108]. Many spermatozoa transcripts may represent non- or incompletely destructed and retained transcripts from round and elongating spermatids. However, even if only a small fraction of the 16,900 transcripts encode functional RNAs, it becomes more and more evident that these transcripts (respectively, their corresponding genes) have evolutionary [109] and fertility-related [110] relevance. That species-specific differences also occur in the spermatozoa transcriptome is nicely reflected by the fact that protamine expression is different in man and rat. While 2 protamines (protamine 1 and protamine 2) are expressed in human spermatozoa at a specific ratio (0.98 P1/P2 in normozoospermic men) [111], in rat spermatozoa protamine 2 transcripts are barely present, and the corresponding protein was not detected in rat spermatozoa [112]. Deviation from the 0.98 P1/P2 ratio in humans is a useful parameter to estimate a reduction of the fertilizing potential of human spermatozoa [111]. The importance of the tightly controlled P1/P2 ratio in human sperm samples, on the one hand, and the evolutionary plasticity of the protamine system in mammals, on the other hand, suggest that fertility-relevant haploid expressed genes are regulated in a human-specific way. Unfortunately, only very limited data are available on protamines in NHP [113], and, to the best of my knowledge, P1/P2 ratios are yet to be determined in NHP.

Conclusion and Outlook

Primates and rodents differ in many relevant biological aspects, including neurobiology, life span, gestation period, and the number of progeny. This review highlights selected primate-specific features of germ line development, which are not as evident as other biological differences between primates and rodents, but which are probably not less significant with regard to reproduction, ontogenesis, and evolution. These include the differential regulation of developmental potency in the preimplantation embryo, the apparently different origins of PGCs in the primate and mouse postimplantation embryo, and the differential expression of some important (transcription) factors in primate and mouse premeiotic germ cells, namely SOX2, SOX17, and LIN28. Furthermore, the size and expansion of germ cell clones in the testis is regulated in a species-specific way – also within the order of primates – resulting in typical patterns of tubular cross-sections (preferentially single-stage organization in human and marmoset monkey vs. preferentially multistage organization in the macaques). Mouse spermatogonial stem cell culture is well established. In contrast, it remains controversial whether human and NHP long-term spermatogonial stem cell culture and expansion has thus far been successful. Regardless, the fact that the mouse spermatogonial stem cell culture protocols were not applicable to human and NHP spermatogonial stem cells may reflect biological differences between rodent and primate spermatogonial stem cells. Moreover, it must always be considered that the primate genome significantly differs from the rodent genome; there are up to 1,000 primate-specific genes, and there are also primate-specific mobile genetic elements. Taking into account that the primate-specific genes are particularly active in germ cells, this genomic difference between primates and rodents cannot be overestimated in germ cell biology. Furthermore, it appears reasonable to assume that upcoming research will uncover many additional primate-specific factors and characteristics of germline development, particularly in light of high-throughput transcriptome and epigenome analyses of single cells and the emergence of genetically modified monkeys. Finally, with regard to the investigation of infertility in humans, it is on the one hand important to realize potential limitations of non-primate animal models for primate (including human) germ cell biology and fertility. On the other hand, human geneticists, andrologists, and reproductive biologists may be well advised to consider and investigate specific aspects of the primate germline as causes of human infertility in more detail. It therefore appears to be essential to further investigate the primate – including the human – germline and germ cell biology in order to obtain better insights into human reproductive function and failure.

Acknowledgements

I highly appreciate the support by and fruitful discussions with many colleagues and friends. I would like to apologize to all colleagues whose great work could not be discussed in this review although so many excellent publications deserve acknowledgement. I thank Kerstin Zaft and Ellen Wiese for their great and patient support.

The work performed in the author's lab was supported by institutional resources of the German Primate Center and by grants from the Deutsche Forschungsgemeinschaft (DFG) and the Bundesministerium für Bildung und Forschung (BMBF).

References

1 Zernicka-Goetz M, Morris SA, Bruce AW: Making a firm decision: multifaceted regulation of cell fate in the early mouse embryo. Nat Rev Genet 2009;10: 467–477.
2 Goolam M, Scialdone A, Graham SJ, Macaulay IC, Jedrusik A, Hupalowska A, et al: Heterogeneity in Oct4 and Sox2 targets biases cell fate in 4-cell mouse embryos. Cell 2016;165:61–74.
3 Davidson KC, Mason EA, Pera MF: The pluripotent state in mouse and human. Development 2015;142:3090–3099.
4 Rossant J: Mouse and human blastocyst-derived stem cells: vive les differences. Development 2015;142:9–12.
5 Boroviak T, Loos R, Lombard P, Okahara J, Behr R, Sasaki E, et al: Lineage-specific profiling delineates the emergence and progression of naive pluripotency in mammalian embryogenesis. Dev Cell 2015;35:366–382.
6 Wani MA, Means RT Jr, Lingrel JB: Loss of LKLF function results in embryonic lethality in mice. Transgenic Res 1998;7: 229–238.
7 Khalfallah O, Rouleau M, Barbry P, Bardoni B, Lalli E: Dax-1 knockdown in mouse embryonic stem cells induces loss of pluripotency and multilineage differentiation. Stem Cells 2009;27: 1529–1537.
8 Tokuzawa Y, Kaiho E, Maruyama M, Takahashi K, Mitsui K, Maeda M, et al: Fbx15 is a novel target of Oct3/4 but is dispensable for embryonic stem cell self-renewal and mouse development. Mol Cell Biol 2003;23:2699–2708.
9 Papanayotou C, Collignon J: Activin/Nodal signalling before implantation: setting the stage for embryo patterning. Philos Trans R Soc Lond B Biol Sci 2014, DOI: 10.1098/rstb.2013.0539.
10 Kuijk EW, van Tol LT, van de Velde H, Wubbolts R, Welling M, Geijsen N, et al: The roles of FGF and MAP kinase signaling in the segregation of the epiblast and hypoblast cell lineages in bovine and human embryos. Development 2012;139:871–882.
11 Denicol AC, Dobbs KB, McLean KM, Carambula SF, Loureiro B, Hansen PJ: Canonical WNT signaling regulates development of bovine embryos to the blastocyst stage. Sci Rep 2013;3:1266.
12 Nakamura T, Okamoto I, Sasaki K, Yabuta Y, Iwatani C, Tsuchiya H, et al: A developmental coordinate of pluripotency among mice, monkeys and humans. Nature 2016;537:57–62.
13 Sasaki K, Nakamura T, Okamoto I, Yabuta Y, Iwatani C, Tsuchiya H, et al: The germ cell fate of cynomolgus monkeys is specified in the nascent amnion. Dev Cell 2016;39:169–185.
14 Frankenberg SR: Different species choose their own paths to pluripotency. Dev Cell 2015;35:267–268.
15 Lawson KA, Hage WJ: Clonal analysis of the origin of primordial germ cells in the mouse. Ciba Found Symp 1994;182: 68–84, discussion 84–91.
16 McLaren A: Primordial germ cells in the mouse. Dev Biol 2003;262:1–15.
17 Saitou M, Barton SC, Surani MA: A molecular programme for the specification of germ cell fate in mice. Nature 2002; 418:293–300.
18 Gerovska D, Arauzo-Bravo MJ: Does mouse embryo primordial germ cell activation start before implantation as suggested by single-cell transcriptomics dynamics? Mol Hum Reprod 2016;22: 208–225.
19 Irie N, Weinberger L, Tang WW, Kobayashi T, Viukov S, Manor YS, et al: SOX17 is a critical specifier of human primordial germ cell fate. Cell 2015;160: 253–268.
20 Tang WW, Dietmann S, Irie N, Leitch HG, Floros VI, Bradshaw CR, et al: A unique gene regulatory network resets the human germline epigenome for development. Cell 2015;161:1453–1467.
21 Sugawa F, Arauzo-Bravo MJ, Yoon J, Kim KP, Aramaki S, Wu G, et al: Human primordial germ cell commitment in vitro associates with a unique PRDM14 expression profile. EMBO J 2015;34: 1009–1024.
22 Sasaki K, Yokobayashi S, Nakamura T, Okamoto I, Yabuta Y, Kurimoto K, et al: Robust in vitro induction of human germ cell fate from pluripotent stem cells. Cell Stem Cell 2015;17:178–194.
23 Gunesdogan U, Magnusdottir E, Surani MA: Primordial germ cell specification: a context-dependent cellular differentiation event [corrected]. Philos Trans R Soc Lond B Biol Sci 2014, DOI: 10.1098/rstb.2013.0543.
24 Yamaji M, Seki Y, Kurimoto K, Yabuta Y, Yuasa M, Shigeta M, et al: Critical function of Prdm14 for the establishment of the germ cell lineage in mice. Nat Genet 2008;40:1016–1022.
25 Campolo F, Gori M, Favaro R, Nicolis S, Pellegrini M, Botti F, et al: Essential role of Sox2 for the establishment and maintenance of the germ cell line. Stem Cells 2013;31:1408–1421.
26 Perrett RM, Turnpenny L, Eckert JJ, O'Shea M, Sonne SB, Cameron IT, et al: The early human germ cell lineage does not express SOX2 during in vivo development or upon in vitro culture. Biol Reprod 2008;78:852–858.

27 Boyer LA, Lee TI, Cole MF, Johnstone SE, Levine SS, Zucker JP, et al: Core transcriptional regulatory circuitry in human embryonic stem cells. Cell 2005; 122:947–956.

28 Turnpenny L, Spalluto CM, Perrett RM, O'Shea M, Hanley KP, Cameron IT, et al: Evaluating human embryonic germ cells: concord and conflict as pluripotent stem cells. Stem Cells 2006;24:212–220.

29 Aeckerle N, Drummer C, Debowski K, Viebahn C, Behr R: Primordial germ cell development in the marmoset monkey as revealed by pluripotency factor expression: suggestion of a novel model of embryonic germ cell translocation. Mol Hum Reprod 2015;21:66–80.

30 Lin IY, Chiu FL, Yeang CH, Chen HF, Chuang CY, Yang SY, et al: Suppression of the SOX2 neural effector gene by PRDM1 promotes human germ cell fate in embryonic stem cells. Stem Cell Rep 2014;2:189–204.

31 Magnusdottir E, Surani MA: How to make a primordial germ cell. Development 2014;141:245–252.

32 Lawson KA, Dunn NR, Roelen BA, Zeinstra LM, Davis AM, Wright CV, et al: Bmp4 is required for the generation of primordial germ cells in the mouse embryo. Genes Dev 1999;13:424–436.

33 Skreb N, Solter D, Damjanov I: Developmental biology of the murine egg cylinder. Int J Dev Biol 1991;35:161–176.

34 De Felici M: Origin, migration, and proliferation of human primordial germ cells; in Coticchio G, Albertini DF, De Santis L (eds): Oogenesis. London, Springer, 2013, p 364.

35 Politzer G: Die Keimbahn des Menschen. Z Anat Entwicklungsgesch 1933; 100:331–361.

36 Witschi E: Migration of the germ cells of human embryo from the yolk sac to the primitive gonadal folds. Contrib Embryol 1948;32:67–97.

37 Kerr CL, Hill CM, Blumenthal PD, Gearhart JD: Expression of pluripotent stem cell markers in the human fetal testis. Stem Cells 2008;26:412–421.

38 Mamsen LS, Brochner CB, Byskov AG, Mollgard K: The migration and loss of human primordial germ stem cells from the hind gut epithelium towards the gonadal ridge. Int J Dev Biol 2012;56: 771–778.

39 Manku G, Culty M: Mammalian gonocyte and spermatogonia differentiation: recent advances and remaining challenges. Reproduction 2015;149:R139–R157.

40 McKinnell C, Mitchell RT, Walker M, Morris K, Kelnar CJ, Wallace WH, et al: Effect of fetal or neonatal exposure to monobutyl phthalate (MBP) on testicular development and function in the marmoset. Hum Reprod 2009;24:2244–2254.

41 Yoshida S, Sukeno M, Nakagawa T, Ohbo K, Nagamatsu G, Suda T, et al: The first round of mouse spermatogenesis is a distinctive program that lacks the self-renewing spermatogonia stage. Development 2006;133:1495–1505.

42 Su S, Szarek M, Vooght A, Hutson J, Li R: Gonocyte transformation to spermatogonial stem cells occurs earlier in patients with undervirilisation syndromes. J Pediatr Surg 2014;49:323–327.

43 Lin ZY, Hirano T, Shibata S, Seki NM, Kitajima R, Sedohara A, et al: Gene expression ontogeny of spermatogenesis in the marmoset uncovers primate characteristics during testicular development. Dev Biol 2015;400:43–58.

44 Aeckerle N, Eildermann K, Drummer C, Ehmcke J, Schweyer S, Lerchl A, et al: The pluripotency factor LIN28 in monkey and human testes: a marker for spermatogonial stem cells? Mol Hum Reprod 2012;18:477–488.

45 Eildermann K, Aeckerle N, Debowski K, Godmann M, Christiansen H, Heistermann M, et al: Developmental expression of the pluripotency factor sal-like protein 4 in the monkey, human and mouse testis: restriction to premeiotic germ cells. Cells Tissues Organs 2012; 196:206–220.

46 Kelnar CJ, McKinnell C, Walker M, Morris KD, Wallace WH, Saunders PT, et al: Testicular changes during infantile "quiescence" in the marmoset and their gonadotrophin dependence: a model for investigating susceptibility of the prepubertal human testis to cancer therapy? Hum Reprod 2002;17:1367–1378.

47 Hilscher B, Engemann A: Histological and morphometric studies on the kinetics of germ cells and immature Sertoli cells during human prespermatogenesis. Andrologia 1992;24:7–10.

48 Gueler B, Sonne SB, Zimmer J, Hilscher B, Hilscher W, Graem N, et al: AZFa protein DDX3Y is differentially expressed in human male germ cells during development and in testicular tumours: new evidence for phenotypic plasticity of germ cells. Hum Reprod 2012;27:1547–1555.

49 Vergouwen RP, Huiskamp R, Bas RJ, Roepers-Gajadien HL, Davids JA, de Rooij DG: Postnatal development of testicular cell populations in mice. J Reprod Fertil 1993;99:479–485.

50 Li LH, Donald JM, Golub MS: Review on testicular development, structure, function, and regulation in common marmoset. Birth Defects Res B Dev Reprod Toxicol 2005;74:450–569.

51 Wahab F, Drummer C, Schlatt S, Behr R: Dynamic regulation of hypothalamic DMXL2, KISS1, and RFRP expression during postnatal development in non-human primates. Mol Neurobiol 2017, DOI: 10.1007/s12035-016-0329-x.

52 Wahab F, Shahab M, Behr R: The involvement of gonadotropin inhibitory hormone and kisspeptin in the metabolic regulation of reproduction. J Endocrinol 2015;225:R49–R66.

53 Larke A, Crews DE: Parental investment, late reproduction, and increased reserve capacity are associated with longevity in humans. J Physiol Anthropol 2006;25:119–131.

54 De Rooij DG: Proliferation and differentiation of spermatogonial stem cells. Reproduction 2001;121:347–354.

55 Hermann BP, Sukhwani M, Hansel MC, Orwig KE: Spermatogonial stem cells in higher primates: are there differences from those in rodents? Reproduction 2010;139:479–493.

56 Hobbs RM, Fagoonee S, Papa A, Webster K, Altruda F, Nishinakamura R, et al: Functional antagonism between Sall4 and Plzf defines germline progenitors. Cell Stem Cell 2012;10:284–298.

57 Zheng K, Wu X, Kaestner KH, Wang PJ: The pluripotency factor LIN28 marks undifferentiated spermatogonia in mouse. BMC Dev Biol 2009;9:38.

58 Ehmcke J, Schlatt S: A revised model for spermatogonial expansion in man: lessons from non-human primates. Reproduction 2006;132:673–680.

59 Hara K, Nakagawa T, Enomoto H, Suzuki M, Yamamoto M, Simons BD, et al: Mouse spermatogenic stem cells continually interconvert between equipotent singly isolated and syncytial states. Cell Stem Cell 2014;14:658–672.
60 Tsialikas J, Romer-Seibert J: LIN28: roles and regulation in development and beyond. Development 2015;142:2397–2404.
61 Gradwohl G, Dierich A, LeMeur M, Guillemot F: *neurogenin3* is required for the development of the four endocrine cell lineages of the pancreas. Proc Natl Acad Sci USA 2000;97:1607–1611.
62 Wistuba J, Schrod A, Greve B, Hodges JK, Aslam H, Weinbauer GF, et al: Organization of seminiferous epithelium in primates: relationship to spermatogenic efficiency, phylogeny, and mating system. Biol Reprod 2003;69:582–591.
63 Ehmcke J, Wistuba J, Schlatt S: Spermatogonial stem cells: questions, models and perspectives. Hum Reprod Update 2006;12:275–282.
64 Millar MR, Sharpe RM, Weinbauer GF, Fraser HM, Saunders PT: Marmoset spermatogenesis: organizational similarities to the human. Int J Androl 2000; 23:266–277.
65 Herndon JG, Bein ML, Nordmeyer DL, Turner JJ: Seasonal testicular function in male rhesus monkeys. Horm Behav 1996;30:266–271.
66 Nagano M, Avarbock MR, Leonida EB, Brinster CJ, Brinster RL: Culture of mouse spermatogonial stem cells. Tissue Cell 1998;30:389–397.
67 Kanatsu-Shinohara M, Ikawa M, Takehashi M, Ogonuki N, Miki H, Inoue K, et al: Production of knockout mice by random or targeted mutagenesis in spermatogonial stem cells. Proc Natl Acad Sci USA 2006;103:8018–8023.
68 Guan K, Nayernia K, Maier LS, Wagner S, Dressel R, Lee JH, et al: Pluripotency of spermatogonial stem cells from adult mouse testis. Nature 2006;440:1199–1203.
69 Stukenborg JB, Wistuba J, Luetjens CM, Elhija MA, Huleihel M, Lunenfeld E, et al: Coculture of spermatogonia with somatic cells in a novel three-dimensional soft-agar-culture-system. J Androl 2008;29:312–329.
70 Reda A, Hou M, Landreh L, Kjartansdottir KR, Svechnikov K, Soder O, et al: In vitro spermatogenesis – optimal culture conditions for testicular cell survival, germ cell differentiation, and steroidogenesis in rats. Front Endocrinol (Lausanne) 2014;5:21.
71 Stukenborg JB, Schlatt S, Simoni M, Yeung CH, Elhija MA, Luetjens CM, et al: New horizons for in vitro spermatogenesis? An update on novel three-dimensional culture systems as tools for meiotic and post-meiotic differentiation of testicular germ cells. Mol Hum Reprod 2009;15:521–529.
72 Reda A, Hou M, Winton TR, Chapin RE, Soder O, Stukenborg JB: In vitro differentiation of rat spermatogonia into round spermatids in tissue culture. Molr Hum Reprod 2016;22:601–612.
73 Sato T, Katagiri K, Gohbara A, Inoue K, Ogonuki N, Ogura A, et al: In vitro production of functional sperm in cultured neonatal mouse testes. Nature 2011;471: 504–507.
74 Sato T, Katagiri K, Yokonishi T, Kubota Y, Inoue K, Ogonuki N, et al: In vitro production of fertile sperm from murine spermatogonial stem cell lines. Nat Commun 2011;2:472.
75 Kossack N, Terwort N, Wistuba J, Ehmcke J, Schlatt S, Scholer H, et al: A combined approach facilitates the reliable detection of human spermatogonia in vitro. Hum Reprod 2013;28:3012–3025.
76 Zheng Y, Thomas A, Schmidt CM, Dann CT: Quantitative detection of human spermatogonia for optimization of spermatogonial stem cell culture. Hum Reprod 2014;29:2497–2511.
77 Eildermann K, Gromoll J, Behr R: Misleading and reliable markers to differentiate between primate testis-derived multipotent stromal cells and spermatogonia in culture. Hum Reprod 2012;27: 1754–1767.
78 Langenstroth D, Kossack N, Westernstroer B, Wistuba J, Behr R, Gromoll J, et al: Separation of somatic and germ cells is required to establish primate spermatogonial cultures. Hum Reprod 2014;29:2018–2031.
79 Sadri-Ardekani H, Mizrak SC, van Daalen SK, Korver CM, Roepers-Gajadien HL, Koruji M, et al: Propagation of human spermatogonial stem cells in vitro. JAMA 2009;302:2127–2134.
80 Nickkholgh B, Mizrak SC, van Daalen SK, Korver CM, Sadri-Ardekani H, Repping S, et al: Genetic and epigenetic stability of human spermatogonial stem cells during long-term culture. Fertil Steril 2014;102:1700–1707.e1.
81 Smith JF, Yango P, Altman E, Choudhry S, Poelzl A, Zamah AM, et al: Testicular niche required for human spermatogonial stem cell expansion. Stem Cells Transl Med 2014;3:1043–1054.
82 Conrad S, Azizi H, Hatami M, Kubista M, Bonin M, Hennenlotter J, et al: Differential gene expression profiling of enriched human spermatogonia after short- and long-term culture. Biomed Res Int 2014;2014:138350.
83 Yang S, Ping P, Ma M, Li P, Tian R, Yang H, et al: Generation of haploid spermatids with fertilization and development capacity from human spermatogonial stem cells of cryptorchid patients. Stem Cell Reports 2014;3:663–675.
84 Jahnukainen K, Mitchell RT, Stukenborg JB: Testicular function and fertility preservation after treatment for haematological cancer. Curr Opin Endocrinol Diabetes Obes 2015;22:217–223.
85 Hermann BP, Sukhwani M, Winkler F, Pascarella JN, Peters KA, Sheng Y, et al: Spermatogonial stem cell transplantation into rhesus testes regenerates spermatogenesis producing functional sperm. Cell Stem Cell 2012;11:715–726.
86 Weinberger L, Ayyash M, Novershtern N, Hanna JH: Dynamic stem cell states: naive to primed pluripotency in rodents and humans. Nat Rev Mol Cell Biol 2016;17:155–169.
87 Massart A, Lissens W, Tournaye H, Stouffs K: Genetic causes of spermatogenic failure. Asian J Androl 2012;14: 40–48.
88 Yatsenko AN, Iwamori N, Iwamori T, Matzuk MM: The power of mouse genetics to study spermatogenesis. J Androl 2010;31:34–44.
89 Yatsenko AN, Georgiadis AP, Ropke A, Berman AJ, Jaffe T, Olszewska M, et al: X-linked TEX11 mutations, meiotic arrest, and azoospermia in infertile men. New Engl J Med 2015;372:2097–2107.
90 Archambeault DR, Matzuk MM: Disrupting the male germ line to find infertility and contraception targets. Ann Endocrinol 2014;75:101–108.
91 Zhang YE, Long M: New genes contribute to genetic and phenotypic novelties in human evolution. Curr Opin Genet Dev 2014;29C:90–96.

92 Carelli FN, Hayakawa T, Go Y, Imai H, Warnefors M, Kaessmann H: The life history of retrocopies illuminates the evolution of new mammalian genes. Genome Res 2016;26:301–314.

93 Gromoll J, Weinbauer GF, Skaletsky H, Schlatt S, Rocchietti-March M, Page DC, et al: The Old World monkey DAZ (deleted in azoospermia) gene yields insights into the evolution of the DAZ gene cluster on the human Y chromosome. Hum Mol Genet 1999;8:2017–2024.

94 Kuroda-Kawaguchi T, Skaletsky H, Brown LG, Minx PJ, Cordum HS, Waterston RH, et al: The AZFc region of the Y chromosome features massive palindromes and uniform recurrent deletions in infertile men. Nat Genet 2001;29:279–286.

95 Rozen SG, Marszalek JD, Irenze K, Skaletsky H, Brown LG, Oates RD, et al: AZFc deletions and spermatogenic failure: a population-based survey of 20,000 Y chromosomes. Am J Hum Genet 2012;91:890–896.

96 Kaessmann H: Origins, evolution, and phenotypic impact of new genes. Genome Res 2010;20:1313–1326.

97 Xie C, Zhang YE, Chen JY, Liu CJ, Zhou WZ, Li Y, et al: Hominoid-specific de novo protein-coding genes originating from long non-coding RNAs. PLoS Genet 2012;8:e1002942.

98 Necsulea A, Kaessmann H: Evolutionary dynamics of coding and non-coding transcriptomes. Nat Rev Genet 2014;15:734–748.

99 Brawand D, Soumillon M, Necsulea A, Julien P, Csardi G, Harrigan P, et al: The evolution of gene expression levels in mammalian organs. Nature 2011;478:343–348.

100 Merkin J, Russell C, Chen P, Burge CB: Evolutionary dynamics of gene and isoform regulation in Mammalian tissues. Science 2012;338:1593–1599.

101 Ade C, Roy-Engel AM, Deininger PL: Alu elements: an intrinsic source of human genome instability. Curr Opin Virol 2013;3:639–645.

102 Deininger P: Alu elements: know the SINEs. Genome Biol 2011;12:236.

103 Callinan PA, Batzer MA: Retrotransposable elements and human disease. Genome Dyn 2006;1:104–115.

104 Xing J, Wang H, Belancio VP, Cordaux R, Deininger PL, Batzer MA: Emergence of primate genes by retrotransposon-mediated sequence transduction. Proc Natl Acad Sci USA 2006;103:17608–17613.

105 Elbarbary RA, Lucas BA, Maquat LE: Retrotransposons as regulators of gene expression. Science 2016;351:aac7247.

106 Denli AM, Narvaiza I, Kerman BE, Pena M, Benner C, Marchetto MC, et al: Primate-specific ORF0 contributes to retrotransposon-mediated diversity. Cell 2015;163:583–593.

107 Steger K: Transcriptional and translational regulation of gene expression in haploid spermatids. Anat Embryol 1999;199:471–487.

108 Soumillon M, Necsulea A, Weier M, Brawand D, Zhang X, Gu H, et al: Cellular source and mechanisms of high transcriptome complexity in the mammalian testis. Cell Rep 2013;3:2179–2190.

109 Joseph SB, Kirkpatrick M: Haploid selection in animals. Trends Ecol Evol 2004;19:592–597.

110 Jodar M, Sendler E, Moskovtsev SI, Librach CL, Goodrich R, Swanson S, et al: Absence of sperm RNA elements correlates with idiopathic male infertility. Sci Transl Med 2015;7:295re6.

111 Rogenhofer N, Dansranjavin T, Schorsch M, Spiess A, Wang H, von Schonfeldt V, et al: The sperm protamine mRNA ratio as a clinical parameter to estimate the fertilizing potential of men taking part in an ART programme. Hum Reprod 2013;28:969–978.

112 Bunick D, Balhorn R, Stanker LH, Hecht NB: Expression of the rat protamine 2 gene is suppressed at the level of transcription and translation. Exp Cell Res 1990;188:147–152.

113 Hecht N, Behr R, Hild A, Bergmann M, Weidner W, Steger K: The common marmoset (*Callithrix jacchus*) as a model for histone and protamine expression during human spermatogenesis. Hum Reprod 2009;24:536–545.

Rüdiger Behr
German Primate Center, Platform Degenerative Diseases
Kellnerweg 4
DE-37077 Göttingen (Germany)
E-Mail rbehr@dpz.eu

Vogt PH (ed): Genetics of Human Infertility. Monogr Hum Genet.
Basel, Karger, 2017, vol 21, pp 143–161 (DOI: 10.1159/000477284)

Genetic and Epigenetic Mouse Models of Human Male Infertility

Maren Godmann · Sandra Zemter · Christian Kosan

Center for Molecular Biomedicine (CMB), Department of Biochemistry, Friedrich Schiller University Jena, Jena, Germany

Abstract

Spermatogenesis describes a complex multistep differentiation process to produce millions of mature spermatozoa daily. Spermatogenesis is fueled by spermatogonial stem cells. It comprises a variety of unique genetic and epigenetic mechanisms to eventually generate haploid sperm, which provides half of the genetic material and epigenetic information that is needed to create a new life upon fertilization. Due to its intricacy, germ cell differentiation is error prone and problems at all stages of spermatogenesis might contribute to human infertility. Male infertility accounts for half of all infertility cases and is considered a multifactorial disease with highly heterogeneous phenotype manifestation. The molecular mechanisms causing fertility problems are largely unknown in many cases. At present, epigenetics take center stage in male reproduction since there is increasing evidence that an intact epigenome is required for reproductive health and prevention of paternal disease transmission. Transgenic mouse models represent a valuable tool with which to study the significance of single genes or epimutations for proper germ cell development, though there are some limitations when translating this information from mice to humans. Nevertheless, mouse models greatly enhance our understanding of fertility pathways, which is critical in order to identify genes and epigenetic signatures involved in the pathophysiology of male reproductive disorders and offspring health. This review will provide prominent examples of mouse models with single gene mutations directly affecting spermatogenesis, thereby mimicking primary human infertility. The main focus though will be on mouse models with defects in genes encoding for epigenetic regulators, such as histone-modifying enzymes and DNA methyltransferases, and the consequences for spermatogenesis and offspring health.

According to the World Health Organization (WHO), human infertility describes "a disease of the reproductive system by the failure to achieve a clinical pregnancy after 12 months of regular unprotected sexual intercourse" [1]. It affects 10–15% of couples worldwide with an equal contribution from both partners [2].

Infertility is a heterogeneous disorder with a complex etiology resulting from various genetic aberrations and critical environmental influences, or a combination of both. In men with semen defects, known genetic causes account for approximately 20% of infertility conditions. Here, clinical genetic screenings are applied to analyze numerical and structural chromosomal aberrations, Y chromosome microdeletions, and single gene alterations, e.g., in the gene encoding for the cystic fibrosis transmembrane conductance regulator (*CFTR*), among others [3–5]. However, the remaining 80% of primary male infertility causes are unknown and classified as "idiopathic."

In humans, more than 2,300 genes are expressed in the testis and their function is mostly not fully understood yet [3, 6]. Each of these genes – individually or in combinations with others – may have an influence on a man's reproductive potential, and their aberrations most likely account for some fertility problems that are so far unexplained. Additionally, alterations of epigenetic signatures in germ cells – e.g., changes in patterns of posttranslational histone modifications and/or alterations in the DNA methylation profile – have been associated with some idiopathic infertility cases [7–10]. However, studying male infertility in humans is limited by the fact that patients have different genetic predispositions, lead unique lifestyles, and are exposed to diverse environments. All of these factors might lead to the heterogeneous nature of sperm quality and a male's reproductive potential. A thorough phenotyping of large patient cohorts as well as large screening approaches are required to detect genetic and epigenetic alterations, in order to eventually understand the multifaceted etiology of male infertility. Mouse models represent a precious tool with which to mimic human disease conditions and may essentially contribute to unraveling of the intricate molecular networks controlling spermatogenesis.

In this review, we will describe powerful mechanisms of targeted mutagenesis in the mouse to study primary defects in candidate genes important for male fertility. Moreover, we will discuss key genetic factors in spermatogenesis that have been identified and characterized in mouse models, and will eventually be correlated with human male infertility conditions. The main focus of this review will be on the impact of epigenetic modifiers on spermatogenesis and offspring health. We will discuss the ablation or overexpression of epigenetic modifiers in mice – and consequently changes in the murine sperm epigenome – in a possible context with impaired human male reproductive health.

Genetic Engineering of Mouse Models to Study Spermatogenesis

Spermatogenesis describes the development of a diploid spermatogonial stem cell (SSC) into a haploid mature spermatozoa capable of fertilizing an oocyte. It is a highly complex process that is controlled by the endocrine system and a coordinated interplay of testicular somatic cells and gametes of different developmental stages [11–14]. Given the endocrine and paracrine signaling mechanisms and complex cellular interactions, it is not possible to entirely copy spermatogenesis *in vitro*, although germ cell maturation beyond meiosis has been accomplished in a cell culture dish [15, 16]. Since mouse spermatogenesis is generally comparable to human spermatogenesis and well defined in developmental and histological terms [17], mice provide an attractive model for studying the function of candidate genes during germ cell development.

Conventional or systemic knockout mice and conditional knockout mice are indispensable tools with which to study the functionality of individual genes in the entire organism or specific cell types at a given developmental time point, respectively. Since the production of mature sperm occurs stepwise with distinct intermediate stages, a conditional system depicts the preferable option of properly evaluating the function of a candidate gene in a specific germ cell subpopulation. Today, many Cre deleter lines and inducible Cre systems are available that enable a germ cell-type and de-

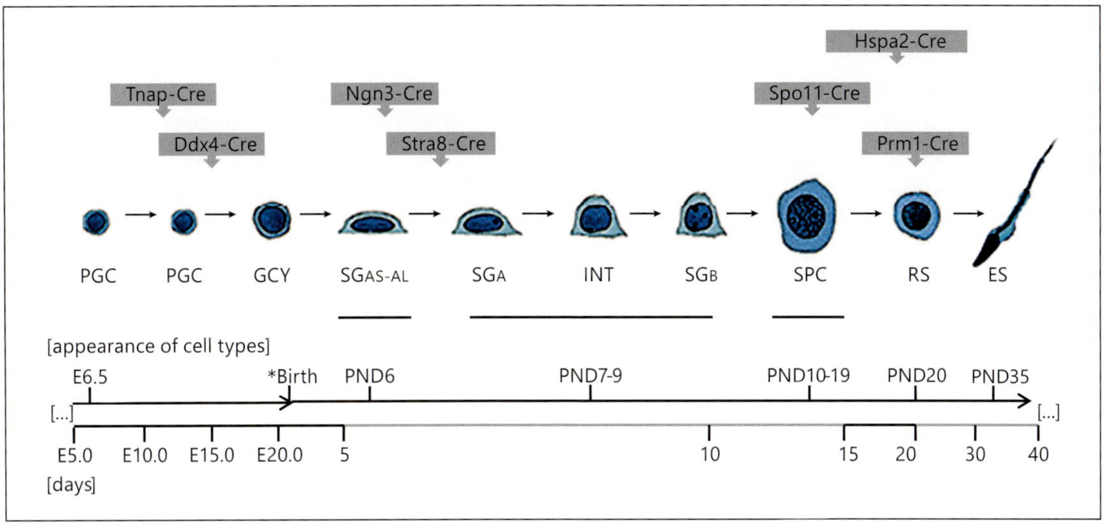

Fig. 1. Common Cre-deleter lines in developing male germ cells. A schematic depiction of developmental germ cell stages from the determination of PGCs in the embryo to elongated spermatids (ES) in the postnatal testis. Tnap-Cre recombinase expression starts on E13.5 in PGCs [148], whereas Ddx4-Cre is specifically expressed in PGCs from E15.0 [147]. Stra8-Cre expression is male germ cell specific and limited to spermatogonia (mainly from PND7 on) and preleptotene SPC [149]. Neurogenin 3 (Ngn3) expression starts on PND3/4 and increases through PND5–7 [150]. Ngn3-Cre activity is also detectable in defined cell types of the pancreas, small intestine, and stomach [151]. Spo11-Cre activity is found in early meiotic stages [152], whereas the Hspa2-Cre transgene is expressed in SPCs from the leptotene/zygotene stage onwards to spermatids until PND30 [153]. E, embryonic day; PND, postnatal day; GCY, gonocytes; SGAS-AL, Asingle + Apaired + Aaligned spermatogonia; SGA, type A spermatogonia; Int, intermediate spermatogonia; SGB, type B spermatogonia; SPC, meiotic spermatocytes; RS, round spermatids; Tnap, tissue nonspecific alkaline phosphatase; Ddx4, dead box polypeptide 4; Stra8, stimulated by retinoic acid gene 8; Spo11, SPO11 meiotic protein covalently bound to double-strand breaks; Hspa2, heat-shock protein 2; Prm1, protamin 1.

velopmental-specific deletion of a gene-of-interest in combination with the corresponding floxed allele [18, 19] (Fig. 1). An inappropriate time point of gene deletion – not only during gametogenesis – might result in a milder or delayed manifestation of the phenotype, or even no phenotype at all [20, 21].

However, homologous gene targeting strategies are very time consuming and costly [22]. As of late, more attractive gene targeting strategies are rapidly evolving – one very interesting system is the type II CRISPR/Cas9-mediated genome editing approach. Here, depicted in a simplified way, the CRISPR (clustered regularly interspaced short palindromic repeats)-associated endonuclease Cas9 is guided by a short RNA to its target sequence, where it introduces sequence-specific double-strand breaks. This leads to the activation of NHEJ (nonhomologous end joining) or HDR (homology directed repair). Repair of the cleaved DNA by NHEJ introduces random mutations into the cleaved site, while HDR employs a homologous DNA template to introduce specific "knock-in" sequences, as in traditional homologous recombination [23]. This principle enables a fast and efficient genome engineering, e.g., in embryonic stem cells [24, 25] or 1-cell mouse embryos in the pronuclear stage [26] to generate transgenic mice. Interestingly, the CRISPR/Cas9 technology has recently been used to correct a disease-causing mutation in mouse SSCs, resulting in healthy offspring after in vitro fertilization [27]. Originally, this RNA-guided DNA endonuclease activity was first observed in bacteria as protective mechanisms against viruses [28, 29].

Thus, CRISPR/Cas9-mediated genomic targeting and genome editing is a fascinating new approach to the study of gene function, which allows the targeting of any genomic region in a very fast and specific way. Important details on CRISPR/Cas genome editing can be found elsewhere [24, 25, 30, 31].

It is worth mentioning that there are other techniques, such as TALENs (transcription activator-like effector nucleases) or ZFNs (zinc-finger nucleases) that allow precise genome editing, which are discussed in other excellent reviews [32, 33].

Genetic Aberrations in Primary Male Infertility – Benefits and Limitations of Mouse Models

Selected Autosomal Single-Gene Mutations Causing Male Fertility Problems in Mice and Humans

Primary male infertility is caused by defects in germ cell maturation and function, and is often associated with an abnormal sperm count, sperm morphology, and/or sperm motility, whereas secondary infertility comprises systemic or syndromic effects, including developmental, endocrine, and metabolic defects [34]. Mouse models play an important role not only in identifying individual genes critical for spermatogenesis, but also in understanding their functions in multifaceted molecular pathways. Here, we will present some important examples of single-gene mutations affecting murine spermatogenesis that might explain the causes of primary human infertility (summarized in Table 1).

Aurora kinases are serine-threonine kinases that are involved in cell cycle regulation, cytokinesis, and chromosome dynamics. Aurora kinase C (AURKC) is highly expressed in the testis, following a stage-specific pattern. *Aurkc* null mice are viable, though males show compromised fertility. *Aurkc* mutant sperm display abnormalities that include heterogeneous chromatin condensation, loose acrosomes, and blunted heads [35]. In humans, *AURKC* mutations are frequently found in infertile men of the North African populations. Interestingly, these patients often have polyploidy large-headed spermatozoa, indicating that meiosis cannot be completed [36–38]. Both *Aurkc* knockout mice as well as infertile human patients with a nonfunctional AURKC protein show sperm head abnormalities due to erroneous meiosis.

Heat-shock transcription factors transactivate genes encoding for heat-shock proteins in response to stress stimuli, but are also involved in developmental processes [39, 40]. Heat-shock transcription factor 2 (*Hsf2*)-deficient mice that survive to adulthood exhibit a reduction in testis size and in sperm count due to impaired meiosis. Fertility is only slightly affected in young adult mice [41]. However, genetic ablation of both transcription factors, *Hsf1* and *Hsf2*, results in a more severe phenotype with a complete block in meiosis and eventually infertility [41]. Mutations that cause a loss of HSF2 function have also been found in humans suffering from azoospermia, a complete loss of mature sperm, indicating that an intact HSF2 might be essential for successful human spermatogenesis [42].

Kelch-like 10 (KLHL10) is a testis-specific BTB/POZ domain-containing protein with 6 kelch repeats that is exclusively expressed in elongating and elongated spermatids. Ablation of only 1 *Klhl10* allele in mice leads to male infertility. Disrupted spermiogenesis in heterozygous mice is characterized by asynchronous spermatid maturation and the degeneration of late spermatids. Thus, *Klhl10* haploinsufficiency results in a global failure of spermiogenesis in mice [43]. Interestingly, a screening of oligozoospermic patients (men with a low semen sperm concentration) revealed

Table 1. Examples of autosomal single gene mutations associated with primary human infertility compared to the corresponding mouse model

Gene name	Human gene symbol (localization)	Human phenotype (mutations found to be associated with ...)	References	Mouse homologue (localization)	Mouse model	Mouse phenotype	References
Aurora kinase C	*AURKC* (19q13.43)	abnormal sperm morpho-logy, sperm polyploidy, teratozoospermia	36–38, 154	*Aurkc* (chr.7, 4.06 cM, A2-A3)	conventional knockout	compromised fertility, heterogeneous chromatin condensation, sperm head defects	35
Heat-shock transcription factor 2	*HSF2* (6q22)	azoospermia	42	*Hsf2* (chr. 10, 29.19 cM, B3–B4)	conventional single knockout; conventional double knockout	*Hsf2* knockout: slightly impaired fertility, reduced testis size and sperm count; *Hsf1* and *Hsf2* knockout: meiotic arrest at pachytene stage	41, 155
Kelch-like 10	*KLHL10* (17q21.2)	oligozoospermia	44	*Klhl10* (chr.11, 63.47 cM, D)	conventional knockout	haploinsufficiency causes infertility, disrupted spermiogenesis, asynchronous spermatid maturation, spermatid degeneration	43
Solute carrier family 26 member 8	*SLC26A8* (6p21)	asthenozoospermia	47	*Slc26a8* (chr.17, 14.82 cM)	conventional knockout	infertile, impaired sperm motility, reduced sperm fertilization potential	46
Spermatogenesis- and oogenesis-specific basic helix-loop-helix 1	*SOHLH1* (9q34.3)	nonobstructive azoospermia	52	*Sohlh1* (chr.2, 18.21 cM)	conventional knockout	gradual loss of fertility, due defective spermatogonial differentiation	49
Spermatogenesis- and oogenesis-specific basic helix-loop-helix 2	*SOHLH2* (13q13.3)	nonobstructive azoospermia	53	*Sohlh2* (chr.3, 26.53 cM)	conventional knockout	Infertile, impaired spermatogonial differentiation, defective synaptonemal complex formation	50, 51
Zona pellucida binding protein	*ZPBP* (7p14.3)	teratozoospermia	55	*Zpbp* (chr.11, 6.76 cM, A2)	conventional knockout	infertile, abnormal sperm head morphology, impaired sperm motility	156

missense and splicing mutations in the *KLHL10* gene that were absent in corresponding controls, suggesting a critical, dose-dependent function for KHLH10 also in human spermatogenesis [44].

The solute carrier family 26 member 8 (*Slc26a8/TAT1*) gene encodes for a testis-specific sulfate transporter with restricted expression to spermatocytes and spermatids in humans and rodents [45]. In mature spermatozoa, Slc26a8 is found at the annulus, a ring-shaped region located at the junction of a sperm's midpiece and principal piece of the tail. Targeted disruption of both *Slc26a8* alleles in mice results in infertility due to structural defects of sperm flagella and sperm immobility [46]. A recent study in humans identified various missense mutations in the *SLC26A8* locus in men suffering from asthenozoospermia, a form of spermatogenic failure due to structural abnormalities of sperm flagella and impaired sperm motility [47]. Thus, SLC26A8 is another example for a single autosomal gene that has the same severe phenotypic effects in mouse and human spermatogenesis in case the protein is nonfunctional.

The spermatogenesis and oogenesis specific basic helix-loop-helix transcription factors 1 and 2 (*Sohlh1* and *Sohlh2*) are exclusively expressed in spermatogonia [48, 49]. Targeted ablation of *Sohlh1* in mice causes infertility by disrupting spermatogonial differentiation into spermatocytes. Interestingly, Sohlh2 was upregulated in spermatogonia lacking Sohlh1 [49]. *Sohlh2*-null mice are also sterile due to strong impairment of type A spermatogonia differentiation [50]. Further analyses demonstrated that Sohlh2 is critical for the formation of synaptonemal complexes by regulation of the expression of meiotic factors [51]. However, in humans, mutations in the *SOHLH1* gene could be observed in a subset of Korean patients suffering from nonobstructive azoospermia (complete spermatogenic failure resulting in semen without any sperm) [52]. Another study supported the importance of functional SOHLH proteins in spermatogenesis and demonstrated a correlation of genetic variants in the *SOHLH2* gene and an increased risk of nonobstructive azoospermia in Chinese men [53].

The zona pellucida-binding protein 1 (Zpbp1) is a spermatid- and spermatozoon-specific protein that localizes to the acrosome. Male mice with a genetic ablation of *Zpbp1* were sterile due to disrupted acrosome development and impaired sperm morphogenesis. Spermatozoa lacking *Zpbp1* exhibit morphological defects with a round-headed appearance and the absence of an acrosome [54]. Globozoospermia in humans is characterized by a round-headed sperm morphology and absence of the acrosome. Interestingly, Yatsenko et al. [55] identified missense and splicing mutations in the *ZPBP1* gene in 4% of patients with abnormal sperm head morphology.

These examples emphasize the assumption that single-gene defects might be a cause of most severe primary infertility conditions in humans. However, today, only a few single-gene aberrations have been strongly associated with primary human infertility. One should consider that in knockout mice a defined genomic sequence is usually ablated to completely disrupt the function of the corresponding gene product. Consequences of small in-frame genetic alterations or few amino acid exchanges might result in a less severe phenotype in humans than predicted from mouse models. Restrictions may also arise if there are no orthologous genes or if there is a functional redundancy. Mouse models may not recapitulate the phenotype manifestation of a human disease if alternative pathways exist that can compensate for the loss of a given protein.

A well-known example for such a compensatory effect is found in mice mimicking cystic fibrosis. In *CFTR* knockout mice fertility is only little affected, since secretory functions of the epididymis, which are usually ensured by a functional CFTR protein, are maintained by an alternative mechanism. However, in humans, mutations in the *CFTR* gene result in azoospermia due to a congenital bilateral aplasia of the vas deferens

(CBAVD) considered as secondary infertility [34, 56, 57]. CBAVD accounts for approximately 2% of infertility cases and *CFTR* mutations are responsible in about 95% of men with CBAVD [58, 59].

The most prominent and important example where mouse models face their limitations are Y-chromosomal (micro)deletions. They are among the most frequent genetic aberrations that contribute to human male infertility [60–62]. The human Y chromosome essentially contains sex-determining genetic material and triggers testis development. Unlike autosomes, there is only 1 copy of the Y chromosome, which does not undergo meiotic recombination, but evolved a mechanism called "gene conversion" to maintain the fidelity of its genetic information [63]. The human Y chromosome harbors massive palindromes that undergo intrapalindromic arm-to-arm recombination and any perturbation of this delicate process might cause deletions of (critical) genetic material and spermatogenic failure [64–66]. However, defined genomic microdeletions of the long arm of the human Y chromosome have not been associated with human male infertility due to abnormal semen parameters [67, 68], whereas others do not affect the fertility status [61, 69]. Moreover, there are candidate genes located on the human Y chromosome that have X chromosome-linked or autosomal homologues in the mouse. [70]. Due to this genetic heterogeneity and Y-chromosomal structural variations, it is difficult to directly model these defects in the mouse.

Epimutations as Causes of Primary Male Infertility? What Mouse Models Teach Us about Abnormal Epigenetic Profiles in Male Germ Cells

What is Epigenetics?

Nearly all cells of an organism – including somatic cell and premeiotic germ cells – share per se the same genome, although they have different phenotypes and carry out a multitude of diverse processes to eventually ensure proper body function [71, 72]. What finally puts a face on cells and evolves them into true specialists to fulfill different body functions is an additional layer of so-called epigenetic information that is superimposed on the DNA or histones, the fundamental proteins that enable DNA packaging into an organized chromatin structure. Today, the best-studied epigenetic modifications are probably the methylation of the fifth carbon of the cytosine base (5mC) in the DNA itself, and posttranslational modifications (PTMs) of histones, e.g., methylation, acetylation, and phosphorylation, among others [73]. However, epigenetic mechanisms are by definition the sum of biochemical information that induces heritable changes in gene expression without changing the genetic information itself. This includes phenomena such as higher-order chromatin structures, ATP-dependent chromatin remodeling processes, the incorporation of histone variants, as well as non-coding RNA-mediated pathways, while the epigenetic lexicon is still expanding [74]. Epigenetic marks are controlled by chromatin regulators, like DNA-modifying enzymes (e.g., DNA methyltransferases) or histone modifiers. The latter are classified as "writers," enzymes that transfer PTMs to histones, "erasers," enzymes that remove PTMs, and "readers," proteins that recognize and interpret either a specific modification or combination of PTMs [75, 76]. Chromatin regulators function mostly in multisubunit protein complexes: (a) to create and maintain the epigenetic landscape of a cell, or (b) to read and translate the given epigenetic information. The malfunctioning of chromatin regulators might result in the introduction of epigenetic errors (so-called epimutations), the disturbance of a cell's epigenetic profile, and pathogenic cellular states [77–79].

Spermatogenesis involves unique epigenetic mechanisms starting with the erasure of parental epigenetic signatures in embryonic primordial germ cells (PGC) and the resetting of sex-specific epigenetic profiles prior to implantation [80, 81]. Postnatally, epigenetic mechanisms enable the progression from a diploid SCC to a haploid mature spermatozoon, regulating mitotic and meiotic cell divisions, testis-specific gene transcription, and histone-to-protamine transitions, though the latter process is not complete. Approximately 2% of histones are retained in murine spermatozoa, whereas as much as 15% of the DNA in human sperm remain packaged by histones [82–85].

Intriguingly, retained histones are loaded with specific PTMs and found at genes important for embryo development [85–87]. Epimutations can occur at any step of spermatogenesis – naturally with different consequences. Epigenetic aberrations that are introduced during SSC self-renewal or premeiotic mitotic divisions might reduce the stem cell pool or impair spermatogonial differentiation. Alterations of epigenetic profiles specifically found during meiosis might result in erroneous chromosome paring, inaccurate homologues recombination, or even chromosomal nondisjunction. Postmeiotically, during spermiogenesis, disruption of epigenetic signatures might influence histone-to-protamine transition, histone retention, or higher DNA packing [88–90]. For a long time, a father's germ cell epigenome was considered insignificant, since: (a) PGCs undergo massive waves of epigenetic reprogramming with an almost complete erasure of the parental epigenome [80], (b) sperm become transcriptionally inactive during spermiogenesis [91], and (c) existing mRNA molecules are predominantly fragmented [92]. However, there is increasing evidence that the maintenance of epigenome integrity is absolutely critical for embryo development and offspring health [77]. Understanding of the molecular mechanisms remains at an early stage.

Again, critical knowledge of epigenetic molecular pathways, the function of chromatin regulators and DNA methyltransferases, and, consequently, the integrity of a defined epigenetic profile in gametogenesis and reproduction has been gained by the generation of transgenic mouse models [93] (Table 2). The translation of this information to human counterparts though is highly complicated due to the dynamic nature of an epigenome and its subjection to environmental influences [94, 95].

Aberrant Epigenetic Profiles Are Found in Infertile Men

Mammalian DNA is predominantly methylated within CpG dinucleotides found in transposable elements, satellite sequences, and differentially methylated regions (DMR) of imprinted genes, among others. Methylation of CpG nucleotides within promoter regions typically results in gene silencing [96–98]. Establishing specific DNA methylation patterns and inheriting them to daughter cells is absolutely critical for normal embryo development and disease susceptibility in the course of life [99].

Importantly, methylation defects have been found in human sperm at imprinted loci, e.g., *MEST* and *IGF2/H19* [10], and developmental genes [100], and are often associated with impaired fertility and also abnormal embryo development [101, 102]. The group of Douglas Carrell discusses this topic in detail [this vol., pp. 116–127]. However, to date there are only few examples where human infertility is associated with erroneous DNA methylation at nonimprinted loci. For instance, in patients with abnormal protamine ratios or oligozoospermia, DNA hypermethylation at CpG islands of the *CREM* promoter could be observed [103, 104]. The *Crem* gene encodes for the Crem (cAMP-responsive element modulator) transcription factor that is specifically expressed in postmeitotic spermatids and its genetic ablation in mice results in a complete absence of spermatozoa [105, 106].

The epigenome is highly dynamic and influenced by an interplay of multiple factors, such as lifestyle, nutrition, or environmental stress [93, 107, 108]. A phenomenon called "epigenetic drift" that is naturally associated with aging (e.g., DNA hypermethylation of distinct genomic regions) also contributes to individual alterations of the epigenetic landscape [109]. This and the fact that the patients in most studies are not well phenotyped and patient groups are often small, makes it challenging to identify epimutations in humans and might be an explanation for why only little is known about the contribution of disturbed epigenetic profiles and human infertility to date.

Importantly, erroneous DNA methylation patterns or epimutations in germ cells might emerge from malfunctioning DNA methyltransferases or epigenetic modifiers, which has been proven in mice (see below), but also in humans. Intriguingly, a large screening approach revealed a significant excess of nonsilent variants in genes encoding for key epigenetic regulators, like the DNA methyltransferases DNMT1, DNMT3B, or the bromo- and WD-containing protein 1 (BRWD1) in patients with nonobstructive azoospermia [110]. Thus, it is very likely that genetic defects in genes encoding for epigenetic modifiers also contribute to epigenetically caused human infertility.

Mouse Models to Study Epigenetic Modifiers

Today there are increasing numbers of mouse models, in which genes encoding for epigenetic modifiers have been manipulated to unravel their function. A significant number of studies describe the effect of perturbed function on epigenetic profiles and the consequences of altered histone PTMs and DNA methylation patterns on gametogenesis and, consequently, embryogenesis (Table 2).

Using genetic mouse models to understand the impact of epigenetic mechanisms on fertility conditions is of special interest, since mice have a defined genetic background, are kept under controlled conditions, and allow phenotype analysis of age-matched littermates at defined developmental time points. These "artificial" conditions, which are in striking contrast to human lifestyle, make it easier to bring out epimutations and meaningful epigenetic signatures in the dynamic epigenetic landscape of defined cell populations, which is fundamental for further mechanistic analyses.

DNA Modifying Enzymes

DNA methyltransferases, DNMTs, are enzymes that catalyze de novo DNA methylation or maintain existing patterns during cell divisions. DNA methyl marks are either lost after cell divisions, when no maintenance DNA methyltransferase is present (passive dilution), or actively removed by yet unknown enzymes or a combinatorial action of DNA repair enzymes, namely members of the ten-eleven translocation (TET) family and the thymine DNA glycosylase [111].

DNA methylation in male germ cells is unique and differs from that found in somatic cells [112]. The expression of the maintenance DNA methyltransferases *Dnmt1* and the de novo methyltransferases *Dnmt3a* and *Dnmt3b*, as well as the catalytically inactive though regulatory important *Dnmt3l*, correlate with the precisely coordinated appearance of stage-specific DNA methylation patterns in PGCs of the embryo and in postnatal germ cells [81, 110, 113, 114]. Genetic ablation experiments in mice provide significant information on the functional role of DNA methyltransferases in gametogenesis. Dnmt3a deficiency in germ cells results in infertility due to meiotic defects and failure to establish paternal methylation imprints at defined loci, e.g., *H19* and *Dlk1/Gtl2* [115]. In contrast, conditional ablation of *Dnmt3b* does not impair spermatogenesis, though Dnmt3b targets *Rasgrf1* DMR and satellite repeats [115]. However, mice with a germ cell-specific ablation of *Dnmt3l* – a catalytically inactive cofactor of Dnmt3a and Dnmt3b – are infertile due to azoospermia and display almost the same spermatogenic phenotype as conditional *Dnmt3a*

Table 2. Selected mouse models to functionally explain the role of important epigenetic-modifying enzymes in spermatogenesis

Epigenetic modifier	Gene symbol (localization)	Function	Target(s)/ formation of …	Mouse models	Male reproductive phenotype	References
DNA methyl-transferase 1	*Dnmt1* (chr.9, 7.66 cM)	maintenance DNA methyltransferase	CpG	(1) heterozygous for a Dnmt1 loss-of-function mutation; (2) heterozygous for Dnmt1 null allele (conventional knock-out); $Dnmt1^{+/-}$/Sca1 mice	(1) impaired imprinting in spermatozoa (partial hypermethylation of Snrpn DMR); (2) Dnmt1 haploinsufficiency causes genome instability and germline-specific intergenerational expansion of CAG repeats at the spinocerebellar ataxia type 1 locus	120, 121
DNA methyl-transferase 3A	*Dnmt3a* (chr.12, 1.99 cM, A2-A3)	de novo DNA methyltransferase	CpG	conditional knockout	meiotic defects, reactivation of retrotransposons, imprinting defects (hypomethylation of e.g. H19), progressive loss of germ cells followed by azoospermia (similar to Dnmt3l)	115
DNA methyl-transferase 3B	*Dnmt3b* (chr.2, 75.79 cM, A2-A3)	de novo DNA methyltransferase	CpG	conditional knockout	dispensable for spermatogenesis	115
DNA methyl-transferase 3L	*Dnmt3l*(chr.10, 39.72 cM)	no catalytic activity	CpG	conditional knockout	meiotic defects, reactivation of retrotransposons, imprinting defects (hypomethylation of e.g., H19), progressive loss of germ cells followed by azoospermia (similar to Dnmt3a)	116–119
Tet methyl-cytosine dioxygenase 1	*Tet1* (chr.10, 32.48 cM)	methylcytosine dioxygenase	5mC (5-methylcytosine)	conventional knockout	knockout testes are morphologically and functionally normal; imprinting defects (hypermethylation at DMR of imprinted alleles) result in impaired offspring health	123
Lysine-specific methyl-transferase 2E	*Kmt2e, Mll5* (chr.5, 10.33 cM, A3)	histone methyltransferase	H3K4me1,2	conventional knockout	infertile due to disturbed spermiogenesis, abnormal head morphology, packaging defects in maturing sperm, impaired sperm motility	136
PR domain containing 9	*Prdm9, Meisetz* (chr.17, 8.95 cM)	histone methyltransferase	H3K4me3	conventional knockout	infertile due to impaired double-stranded break repair pathway, deficient homologues chromosome pairing, impaired sex body formation, reduced H3K4me3 levels, altered gene expression	157

Table 2. Continued

Epigenetic modifier	Gene symbol (localization)	Function	Target(s)/ formation of …	Mouse models	Male reproductive phenotype	References
Euchromatic histone lysine N-methyl-transferase 2	*Ehmt2, Kmt1c, G9a* (chr.17, 18.45 cM)	Histone methyltransferase	H3K9me1,2	conditional knockout	infertile due to meiotic disruption at early pachytene stage, incomplete synaptonemal complex formation, global reduction of H3K9me1,2 at meiotic prophase	132
Suppressor of variegation 3–9 homolog 1 and 2	*Suv39h1, Kmt1a* (chr.X, 3.64 cM, A1-A2) *Suv39h2, Kmt1b* (chr.2, 1.95 cM, A)	histone methyltransferase histone methyltransferase	H3K9me3 H3K9me3	conventional double knockout	double knockout infertile, complete spermatogenic failure; impaired H3K9 methylation in type B spermatogonia and preleptotene spermatocytes, defective pairing of homologues chromosomes during meiosis, delayed chromosome synapsis, missegregation of bivalents (aneuploidy), genomic instability. Single knockouts of either *Suv39h1* or *Suv39h2* do not affect fertility	124
SET domain, bifurcated 1	*Setdb1, Kmt1e, Eset* (chr.3, 40.74 cM, F2)	histone methyltransferase	H3K9me3	ENU mutagenesis: *Setdb1* allele has a splice site mutation → introduction of a premature stop codon → null allele	haploinsufficiency causes DNA hypomethylation at specific classes of transposable elements → altered epigenetic profiles are transgenerationally inherited	127
Lysine-specific demethylase 1	*Lsd1, Kdm1a, Aof2* (chr.4, 68.80 cM)	histone demethylase	H3K4me1,2 and H3K9me1,2	(1) conditional knockout (2) transgene overexpression	(1) infertility due to reduced self-renewal capacity of SSC, impaired spermatogonial differentiation, meiotic failure (2) testes of transgenic mice are morphologically and functionally normal; histone methylation defects (H3K4me2 hypomethylation) and altered RNA content in sperm result in severely impaired offspring health; altered epigenetic profiles are transgenerationally inherited	77, 141

Table 2. Continued

Epigenetic modifier	Gene symbol (localization)	Function	Target(s)/ formation of …	Mouse models	Male reproductive phenotype	References
Lysine-specific demethylase 3a	*Kdm3a, Jmjd1a, Jhdm2a* (chr.6, 32.18 cM)	histone demethylase	H3K9me1,2	(1) null allele through gene trap approach (2) conditional knockout: ablation of JmjC catalytic domain	(1) infertile due to postmeiotic chromatin condensation defects, impaired Tnp1 and Prmt1 expression, altered heterochromatin distribution, abnormal sperm head morphology, sperm are immotile (2) see above; cytoplasmic defects preceding histone replacement and chromatin compaction: deformed acrosomes, incomplete manchettes, and detached centrosomes	88, 142, 158
Jumonji domain containing 1C	*Jmjd1c, Trip8* (10, 34.85 cM)	histone demethylase – *controversially discussed*	H3K9me1,2 – *controversially discussed*	conventional knock-out	Infertile with increasing age due to progressive germ cell loss; impaired meiotic prophase progression; no effect on global H3K9 methylation	143, 144

knockout mice [115]. *Dnmt3l* null spermatocytes are not able to progress through meiosis and some imprinted loci, such as *H19*, are found to be hypomethylated. Moreover, retrotransposons regain activity due to failed de novo methylation of both long terminal repeat (LTR) and non-LTR retrotransposons [116–119]. Thus, de novo methylation during postnatal sperm development is critical for meiotic progression, the establishment of genomic imprinting, germ cell-specific methylation of non-imprinted genes, and genome stability [112].

Recent studies demonstrated an essential function of the maintenance DNA methyltransferases Dnmt1 in spermatogenesis and offspring health, since *Dnmt1* haploinsufficiency causes imprinting defects (e.g., *Snrpn* DMR) [120]. Importantly, *Dnmt1* haploinsufficiency in a spinocerebellar ataxia type 1 mouse model causes the expansion of CAG repeats in offspring, indicating a transgenerational inheritance of genomic instability due to impaired Dnmt1 availability [121].

Tet1 is a member of the TET family of proteins, which have the capacity to oxidize 5-methylcytosine (5mC) to 5-hydroxymethylcytosine (5mhC) and are supposed to play a key role in active DNA demethylation [111]. Tet1 has an important function during PGC reprogramming [122]. Genome-wide DNA methylation analysis of embryonic day 13.5 PGCs and sperm of *Tet1* knockout mice revealed hypermethylation of DMRs of imprinted genes in sperm, which can be traced back to PGCs [123]. Although *Tet1* knockout testes appear to be normal, offspring sired by a *Tet1*-deficient father show growth defects, underlining the importance of a correct establishment and maintenance of DNA methylation profiles during pre- and postnatal gametogenesis [123].

Histone Modifiers

DNA methylation and histone modifications act in concert to establish and maintain an epigenetic profile that controls chromatin structure and gene expression, and eventually determines a cell's phenotype [96–98]. Thus, besides DNA-modifying enzymes, histone modifiers take center stage in epigenetic reprogramming events during gametogenesis (Tables 2).

Peters et al. [124] were the first to demonstrate a key role for histone methyltransferases (HMTs) in spermatogenesis. The HMT suppressor of variegation 3–9 homolog 1 and 2 (Suv39h1/Kmt1a, Suv39h2/Kmt1b) are encoded by 2 different loci and show a distinct expression pattern in adult tissues: Suv39h1 is broadly abundant, whereas *Suv39h2* is predominantly expressed in the testis. Here, Suv39h2 is found at heterochromatic regions in meiotic and early postmeiotic cells. Moreover, Suv39h2 specifically accumulates at sex bodies, specific regions on sex chromosomes that undergo transcriptional silencing during the first meiotic prophase [125]. Both HMTs catalyze trimethylation of histone H3 lysine 9 (H3K9me3), which is usually associated with heterochromatin formation and gene silencing [126]. The single knockout of either *Suv39h1* or *Suv39h2* does not affect spermatogenesis, implying a functional redundancy. However, double knockout of *Suv39h1* and *Suv39h2* H3K9 trimethyltransferases leads to complete spermatogenic failure due to severely disturbed meiosis. Homologous chromosomes fail to associate correctly, chromosome synapsis is delayed, and segregation of bivalents is defective, which results in aneuploidy. Importantly, the authors demonstrate a perturbation of H3K9 methylation patterns in type B spermatogonia and preleptotene spermatocytes, probably leading to chromosomal instability and altered gene expression [124].

Another histone-modifying enzyme that forms H3K9me3 in germ cells is the SET domain bifurcated 1 (Setdb1/Kmt1e/Eset) methyltransferase. Mice haploinsufficient for *Setdb1* are fertile. However, *Setdb1* haploinsufficiency causes DNA hypomethylation at specific classes of transposable elements [127]. Interestingly, Setdb1 haploinsufficiency in a mouse model with a metastable epiallele (A^{vy} locus) demonstrates the transfer of altered epigenetic signatures in sperm to the offspring, strongly supporting the hypothesis that the paternal sperm epigenome matters to offspring health [127].

The formation of H3K9 mono- and dimethylation is catalyzed by the euchromatic histone lysine N-methyltransferase 2 (Ehmt2/Kmt1c/G9a). In contrast to Suv39h1 and Suv39h2, which are found at heterochromatin, Ehmt2 localizes to euchromatin and is involved in transcriptional silencing [128–131]. In the testis, *Ehmt2* expression takes place in a specific developmental window and is found in spermatogonia to early leptotene spermatocytes [132]. Conditional knockout studies revealed a critical function for Ehmt2 in meiotic progression. Spermatocytes lacking *Emht2* show a block at early meiotic stages due to impaired chromosome synapsis. Lack of Ehmt2 results in a strong reduction of global H3K9me1,2 levels during the meiotic prophase, whereas H3K9me3 is not affected. Interestingly, *Ehmt2* haploinsufficiency also causes mono- and dihypomethylation, though to a lesser extent than observed in *Ehmt2* null germ cells. Concomitant with the loss of H3K9 methylation, *Ehmt2* null germ cells show aberrant transcription profiles, which might explain the erroneous meiotic prophase progression [132].

Meisetz, also known as PR domain containing 9 (Prdm9), is another well-studied HMT important for proper meiotic progression, which specifically trimethylates lysine 4 of histone H3 (H3K4me3). Genetic ablation of *Meisetz* leads to infertility in both sexes due to meiotic failure at the pachytene stage. Germ cells lacking *Meisetz* have a severely impaired double-strand break repair, defective homologues chromosome pairing, and sex body formation [133]. *Meisetz* null germ cells show reduced H3K4 trimethylation, a mark that associates with active gene transcription [126]. Thus, the authors assume that meiotic failure results from inappropriate activation of critical meiotic genes due to H3K4 hypomethylation

[133]. It is noteworthy that 2 independent studies describe a possible association of single nucleotide polymorphisms in the *MEISETZ/PRDM9* gene and primary human infertility due to azoospermia [134, 135].

Taken together, the abovementioned HMTs are responsible for creating a unique epigenetic profile in distinct postnatal germ cell populations that is indispensable for successful spermatogenesis. Thereby, Suv39h1,2, Ehmt2, and Meisetz act independently on distinct genomic loci to ensure progression through specific critical steps of meiosis.

The correct positioning of histone methylation marks is not only critical for meiosis, but also for the terminal differentiation of germ cells during spermiogenesis. The lysine-specific methyltransferase 2E (Kmt2e/Mll5) catalyzes the formation of H3K4 mono- and dimethylation [136]. In the adult testis, Mll5 is mainly detected in developing spermatocytes and early spermatids. Genetic ablation of *Mll5* results in infertility due to disturbed spermiogenesis. Maturing sperm show an abnormal head morphology and packaging defects. Sperm motility is also impaired. However, changes in H3K4 methylation levels have not been reported [136].

To confer the postulated dynamic uniquely characterizing the epigenome, HMTs need antagonists. A decade ago, histone methylation was still believed to be a nonreversible PTM of histones. Importantly, in 2004, Shi et al. [137] identified the first lysine-specific demethylase 1 (Lsd1/Kdm1a/Aof2), which is highly evolutionarily conserved. Depending on cofactor availability, Kdm1a might promote gene activation through the removal of silencing H3K9me1,2 marks, or gene silencing through the removal of activating H3K4me1,2 marks. In cooperation with the androgen receptor, for example, Kdm1a specifically removes repressive H3K9me1 and H3K9me2 marks in normal and pathogenic prostate tissue, which results in the initiation of androgen receptor-dependent transcription [138]. As a component of the nucleosome and remodeling (NuRD) complex, Kdm1a removes activating H3K4 dimethyl marks in breast cancer cells [139].

During postnatal testis development, *Kdm1a* is specifically expressed according to cell type and stage [140]. Conditional knockout studies reveal a critical role for *Kdm1a* in spermatogenesis, since germ cells harboring 2 *Kdm1a* null alleles display a reduced self-renewal capacity of SSC, impaired spermatogonial differentiation, and meiotic failure. Thus, *Kdm1a* knockout males are infertile. *Kdm1a* loss is associated with an increase of H3K4me2 global methylation levels in spermatogonia and consequently altered gene expression, whereas global H3K4me1 levels are not altered [141]. Strikingly, overexpression of *Kdm1a* does not impair the spermatogenesis and fertility of transgenic mice, though H3K4me2 levels at specific loci are significantly reduced in sperm. Instead, offspring health and survivability is severely impaired, when sired by a *Kdm1a* transgenic father. An altered paternal epigenome due to *Kdm1a* overexpression results in increased pregnancy loss and embryo malformations, such as skeletal abnormalities and limb deformation, among others. Intriguingly, the observed defects persist transgenerationally in the absence of KDM1A transgene germline expression and are also associated with altered RNA profiles in sperm and offspring at the 2-cell stage [77].

Kdm3a/Jmjd1a/Jhdm2a is another lysine-specific demethylase (KDM) that targets mono- and dimethylation of H3K9. Today, 2 mouse models exist to analyze the function of Kdm3a in spermatogenesis. *Kdm3a* expression is absent in spermatogonia and early meiotic cells, but culminates in round spermatids [88]. Chromatin condensation during spermiogenesis is defective in germ cells lacking a functional *Kdm3a*. Sperm display an altered heterochromatin distribution, abnormal heads, and are unable to move. Interestingly, Kdm3a controls the expression of transition protein 1 (*Tnp1*) and protamine 1 (*Prm*), which are key factors in spermiogenesis, enabling chromatin compaction. Impaired *Tnp1* and *Prtm1* expression might explain the observed phenotype, which resembles azoospermia or globozoospermia in humans [88]. A continuative study used a different mouse model, in which the catalytic domain of *Kdm3a* has been deleted. Mice lacking a functional Kdm3a display the same phenotype as observed in *Kdm3a* null germ cells. Deeper structural analyses revealed cytoplasmic defects preceding histone replacement and chromatin compaction due to deformed acrosomes, incomplete manchettes, and detached centrosomes [142].

The histone demethylase activity of jumonji domain containing 1C (*Jmjd1c/Trip8*) is controversially discussed and it remains a matter of debate whether it targets H3K9me1,2 methylation or functions as a nonhistone protein demethylase [33, 143]. Knockout studies revealed that mice with a *Jmjd1c* null allele are infertile, displaying an age-dependent, progressive loss of germ cells, at least partially due to increased apoptosis in premeiotic cells. Interestingly, H3K9me1,2 levels are not changed in sperm of Jmjd1c knockout mice [144], probably pointing towards a role as a nonhistone protein demethylase.

In contrast, the lysine (K)-specific demethylase 4D (Kdm4d/Jmjd2), which removes H3K9 di- and trimethylation marks, is dispensable for spermatogenesis, although H3K9me3 accumulates significantly in round spermatids and methylated H3K9 is aberrantly distributed in distinct germ cell subpopulations. The authors suggest that possible defects in spermatozoa might be rescued by another histone demethylase, namely *Kdm4d*, which is predominantly expressed in elongating spermatids [145].

H3K27me2,3 which is associated with paused or silenced gene transcription [85, 98], is targeted by the histone demethylase Kdm6b/Jmjd3. Germ cell-specific ablation of *Kdm6b* does not negatively affect postnatal spermatogenesis. However, *Kdm6b* conditional knockout males have larger testes, prolonged fertility (the litter size after 1 year is not reduced, as it typically is in ageing wildtype controls), and an enhanced SSC self-renewal capacity due to frequent fragmentation of spermatogonial cysts [146].

In summary, all of the studies described in this chapter clearly indicate that genetically induced alterations in germ cell histone methylation profiles – either through knockout or overexpression of a specific epigenetic modifier – most likely affect postnatal gametogenesis or the development of offspring sired by a transgenic father (summarized in Table 2). Translating these findings to human fertility implicates critical requirements for establishing and maintaining specific epigenetic profiles during spermatogenesis. Disruption of proper HMT or HDM function through genetic mutations might not only impair spermatogenesis, but also links pregnancy loss or birth defects to a malformed sperm epigenome of the father.

Conclusions

The broad spectrum of male infertility and subfertility conditions is, without much doubt, a result of cumulative genetic and epigenetic alterations in multiple genes and gene regulatory elements. Of course, it is difficult to mimic such a complex disease with all its facets in a mouse model. Joint efforts have to be made in order to better understand the primary causes of male infertility and eventually to develop new fertility treatments and to improve the outcome of assisted reproductive techniques. Data of genome-wide association studies and profound epigenetic screening in humans should be combined with sound knowledge of the molecular mechanisms underlying fertility pathways gained through the creation and analysis of transgenic mouse models.

References

1 Zegers-Hochschild F, et al: International Committee for Monitoring Assisted Reproductive Technology (ICMART) and the World Health Organization (WHO) revised glossary of ART terminology, 2009. Fertil Steril 2009;92:1520–1524.
2 De Kretser DM, Baker HW: Infertility in men: recent advances and continuing controversies. J Clin Endocrinol Metab 1999;84:3443–3450.
3 Hotaling J, Carrell DT: Clinical genetic testing for male factor infertility: current applications and future directions. Andrology 2014;2:339–350.
4 Esteves SC: A clinical appraisal of the genetic basis in unexplained male infertility. J Hum Reprod Sci 2013;6:176–182.
5 Crosignani PG, Rubin BL: Optimal use of infertility diagnostic tests and treatments. The ESHRE Capri Workshop Group. Hum Reprod 2000;15:723–732.
6 Gibson G: Hints of hidden heritability in GWAS. Nat Genet 2010;42:558–560.
7 Carrell DT: Epigenetics of the male gamete. Fertil Steril 2012;97:267–274.
8 Carrell DT, Hammoud SS: The human sperm epigenome and its potential role in embryonic development. Mol Hum Reprod 2010;16:37–47.
9 Hammoud SS, et al: Genome-wide analysis identifies changes in histone retention and epigenetic modifications at developmental and imprinted gene loci in the sperm of infertile men. Hum Reprod 2011;26:2558–2569.
10 Poplinski A, Tuttelmann F, Kanber D, Horsthemke B, Gromoll J: Idiopathic male infertility is strongly associated with aberrant methylation of MEST and IGF2/H19 ICR1. Int J Androl 2010;33:642–649.
11 Clermont Y: The cycle of the seminiferous epithelium in man. Am J Anat 1963;112:35–51.
12 De Rooij DG: Proliferation and differentiation of spermatogonial stem cells. Reproduction 2001;121:347–354.
13 McLachlan RI, et al: Identification of specific sites of hormonal regulation in spermatogenesis in rats, monkeys, and man. Recent Prog Horm Res 2002;57:149–179.
14 Plant T, Zeleznik A: Knobil and Neill's Physiology of Reproduction, ed 4. Cambridge, Academic Press, 2015.
15 Geijsen N, et al: Derivation of embryonic germ cells and male gametes from embryonic stem cells. Nature 2004;427:148–154.
16 Hunter D, Anand-Ivell R, Danner S, Ivell R: Models of in vitro spermatogenesis. Spermatogenesis 2012;2:32–43.
17 Russell LD, Ettlin RA, Sinha Hikim AP, Clegg ED: Histological and Histopathological Evaluation of the Testis. St. Louis, Cache River Press, 1990.
18 Smith L: Good planning and serendipity: exploiting the Cre/Lox system in the testis. Reproduction 2011;141:151–161.
19 Metzger D, Chambon P: Site- and time-specific gene targeting in the mouse. Methods 2001;24:71–80.
20 Hobbs RM, et al: Functional antagonism between Sall4 and Plzf defines germline progenitors. Cell Stem Cell 2012;10:284–298.
21 Kosan C, et al: Transcription factor miz-1 is required to regulate interleukin-7 receptor signaling at early commitment stages of B cell differentiation. Immunity 2010;33:917–928.
22 Friedel RH, Wurst W, Wefers B, Kuhn R: Generating conditional knockout mice. Methods Mol Biol 2011;693:205–231.
23 Tschaharganeh DF, Lowe SW, Garippa RJ, Livshits G: Using CRISPR/Cas to study gene function and model disease in vivo. FEBS J 2016;283:3194–3203.
24 Cong L, et al: Multiplex genome engineering using CRISPR/Cas systems. Science 2013;339:819–823.
25 Mali P, et al: RNA-guided human genome engineering via Cas9. Science 2013;339:823–826.
26 Wang H, et al: One-step generation of mice carrying mutations in multiple genes by CRISPR/Cas-mediated genome engineering. Cell 2013;153:910–918.
27 Wu Y, et al: Correction of a genetic disease by CRISPR-Cas9-mediated gene editing in mouse spermatogonial stem cells. Cell Res 2015;25:67–79.
28 Barrangou R, et al: CRISPR provides acquired resistance against viruses in prokaryotes. Science 2007;315:1709–1712.
29 Hale CR, et al: RNA-guided RNA cleavage by a CRISPR RNA-Cas protein complex. Cell 2009;139:945–956.
30 Deltcheva E, et al: CRISPR RNA maturation by trans-encoded small RNA and host factor RNase III. Nature 2011;471:602–607.
31 Jinek M, et al: A programmable dual-RNA-guided DNA endonuclease in adaptive bacterial immunity. Science 2012;337:816–821.
32 Gaj T, Gersbach CA, Barbas CF 3rd: ZFN, TALEN, and CRISPR/Cas-based methods for genome engineering. Trends Biotechnol 2013;31:397–405.
33 Kim H, Kim JS: A guide to genome engineering with programmable nucleases. Nat Rev Genet 2014;15:321–334.
34 Zorrilla M, Yatsenko AN: The genetics of infertility: current status of the field. Curr Genet Med Rep 2013, DOI: 10.1007/s40142-013-0027-1.
35 Kimmins S, et al: Differential functions of the Aurora-B and Aurora-C kinases in mammalian spermatogenesis. Mol Endocrinol 2007;21:726–739.
36 Ounis L, et al: Mutations of the aurora kinase C gene causing macrozoospermia are the most frequent genetic cause of male infertility in Algerian men. Asian J Androl 2015;17:68–73.
37 Dieterich K, et al: Homozygous mutation of AURKC yields large-headed polyploid spermatozoa and causes male infertility. Nat Genet 2007;39:661–665.
38 Dieterich K, et al: The Aurora Kinase C c.144delC mutation causes meiosis I arrest in men and is frequent in the North African population. Hum Mol Genet 2009;18:1301–1309.
39 Kingston RE, Schuetz TJ, Larin Z: Heat-inducible human factor that binds to a human hsp70 promoter. Mol Cell Biol 1987;7:1530–1534.
40 Wu C, et al: Purification and properties of *Drosophila* heat shock activator protein. Science 1987;238:1247–1253.
41 Wang G, Zhang J, Moskophidis D, Mivechi NF: Targeted disruption of the heat shock transcription factor (*hsf*)-2 gene results in increased embryonic lethality, neuronal defects, and reduced spermatogenesis. Genesis 2003;36:48–61.
42 Mou L, et al: A dominant-negative mutation of HSF2 associated with idiopathic azoospermia. Hum Genet 2013;132:159–165.
43 Yan W, Ma L, Burns KH, Matzuk MM: Haploinsufficiency of kelch-like protein homolog 10 causes infertility in male mice. Proc Natl Acad Sci USA 2004;101:7793–7798.

44 Yatsenko AN, et al: Non-invasive genetic diagnosis of male infertility using spermatozoal RNA: KLHL10 mutations in oligozoospermic patients impair homodimerization. Hum Mol Genet 2006; 15:3411–3419.
45 Toure A, et al: Tat1, a novel sulfate transporter specifically expressed in human male germ cells and potentially linked to RhoGTPase signaling. J Biol Chem 2001;276:20309–20315.
46 Toure A, et al: The testis anion transporter 1 (Slc26a8) is required for sperm terminal differentiation and male fertility in the mouse. Hum Mol Genet 2007; 16:1783–1793.
47 Dirami T, et al: Missense mutations in SLC26A8, encoding a sperm-specific activator of CFTR, are associated with human asthenozoospermia. Am J Hum Genet 2013;92:760–766.
48 Ballow DJ, Xin Y, Choi Y, Pangas SA, Rajkovic A: *Sohlh2* is a germ cell-specific bHLH transcription factor. Gene Expr Patterns 2006;6:1014–1018.
49 Ballow D, Meistrich ML, Matzuk M, Rajkovic A: *Sohlh1* is essential for spermatogonial differentiation. Dev Biol 2006;294:161–167.
50 Hao J, et al: *Sohlh2* knockout mice are male-sterile because of degeneration of differentiating type A spermatogonia. Stem Cells 2008;26:1587–1597.
51 Park YH, et al: Prostate-specific extracellular vesicles as a novel biomarker in human prostate cancer. Sci Rep 2016;6: 30386.
52 Choi Y, et al: Mutations in *SOHLH1* gene associate with nonobstructive azoospermia. Hum Mutat 2010;31:788–793.
53 Song B, et al: Association of genetic variants in *SOHLH1* and *SOHLH2* with non-obstructive azoospermia risk in the Chinese population. Eur J Obstet Gynecol Reprod Biol 2015;184:48–52.
54 Li Q, et al: Redundant roles of SMAD2 and SMAD3 in ovarian granulosa cells in vivo. Mol Cell Biol 2008;28:7001–7011.
55 Yatsenko AN, et al: Association of mutations in the zona pellucida binding protein 1 (*ZPBP1*) gene with abnormal sperm head morphology in infertile men. Mol Hum Reprod 2012;18:14–21.
56 Costes B, et al: Frequent occurrence of the CFTR intron 8 (TG)n 5T allele in men with congenital bilateral absence of the vas deferens. Eur J Hum Genet 1995; 3:285–293.
57 Riordan JR, et al: Identification of the cystic fibrosis gene: cloning and characterization of complementary DNA. Science 1989;245:1066–1073.
58 Carrell DT, De Jonge C, Lamb DJ: The genetics of male infertility: a field of study whose time is now. Arch Androl 2006;52:269–274.
59 Shah K, Sivapalan G, Gibbons N, Tempest H, Griffin DK: The genetic basis of infertility. Reproduction 2003;126:13–25.
60 Krausz C, et al: The Y chromosome-linked copy number variations and male fertility. J Endocrinol Invest 2011;34: 376–382.
61 Vogt PH, Falcao CL, Hanstein R, Zimmer J: The AZF proteins. Int J Androl 2008;31:383–394.
62 Simoni M, Tuttelmann F, Gromoll J, Nieschlag E: Clinical consequences of microdeletions of the Y chromosome: the extended Munster experience. Reprod Biomed Online 2008;16:289–303.
63 Rozen S, et al: Abundant gene conversion between arms of palindromes in human and ape Y chromosomes. Nature 2003;423:873–876.
64 Lange J, et al: Isodicentric Y chromosomes and sex disorders as byproducts of homologous recombination that maintains palindromes. Cell 2009;138:855–869.
65 Skaletsky H, et al: The male-specific region of the human Y chromosome is a mosaic of discrete sequence classes. Nature 2003;423:825–837.
66 Repping S, et al: Recombination between palindromes P5 and P1 on the human Y chromosome causes massive deletions and spermatogenic failure. Am J Hum Genet 2002;71:906–922.
67 Reijo R, et al: Diverse spermatogenic defects in humans caused by Y chromosome deletions encompassing a novel RNA-binding protein gene. Nat Genet 1995;10:383–393.
68 Vogt P, et al: Microdeletions in interval 6 of the Y chromosome of males with idiopathic sterility point to disruption of AZF, a human spermatogenesis gene. Hum Genet 1992;89:491–496.
69 Krausz C: Y chromosome and male infertility. Andrologia 2005;37:219–223.
70 Cooke HJ, Saunders PT: Mouse models of male infertility. Nat Rev Genet 2002; 3:790–801.
71 Bedzhov I, Graham SJ, Leung CY, Zernicka-Goetz M: Developmental plasticity, cell fate specification and morphogenesis in the early mouse embryo. Philos Trans R Soc Lond B Biol Sci 2014, DOI: 10.1098/rstb.2013.0538.
72 Zernicka-Goetz M, Morris SA, Bruce AW: Making a firm decision: multifaceted regulation of cell fate in the early mouse embryo. Nat Rev Genet 2009;10: 467–477.
73 Kouzarides T: Chromatin modifications and their function. Cell 2007;128:693–705.
74 Tan MK, Lim HJ, Harper JW: SCF(FBXO22) regulates histone H3 lysine 9 and 36 methylation levels by targeting histone demethylase KDM4A for ubiquitin-mediated proteasomal degradation. Mol Cell Biol 2011;31:3687–3699.
75 Musselman CA, et al: Molecular basis for H3K36me3 recognition by the Tudor domain of PHF1. Nat Struct Mol Biol 2012;19:1266–1272.
76 Musselman CA, Lalonde ME, Cote J, Kutateladze TG: Perceiving the epigenetic landscape through histone readers. Nat Struct Mol Biol 2012;19:1218–1227.
77 Siklenka K, et al: Disruption of histone methylation in developing sperm impairs offspring health transgenerationally. Science 2015;350:aab2006.
78 Oakes CC, et al: DNA methylation dynamics during B cell maturation underlie a continuum of disease phenotypes in chronic lymphocytic leukemia. Nat Genet 2016;48:253–264.
79 Hamidi T, Singh AK, Chen T: Genetic alterations of DNA methylation machinery in human diseases. Epigenomics 2015;7:247–265.
80 Hajkova P, et al: Chromatin dynamics during epigenetic reprogramming in the mouse germ line. Nature 2008;452:877–881.
81 Hajkova P, et al: Epigenetic reprogramming in mouse primordial germ cells. Mech Dev 2002;117:15–23.
82 Bench GS, Friz AM, Corzett MH, Morse DH, Balhorn R: DNA and total protamine masses in individual sperm from fertile mammalian subjects. Cytometry 1996;23:263–271.
83 Brykczynska U, et al: Repressive and active histone methylation mark distinct promoters in human and mouse spermatozoa. Nat Struct Mol Biol 2010;17: 679–687.

84 Gatewood JM, Cook GR, Balhorn R, Schmid CW, Bradbury EM: Isolation of four core histones from human sperm chromatin representing a minor subset of somatic histones. J Biol Chem 1990; 265:20662–20666.
85 Hammoud SS, et al: Distinctive chromatin in human sperm packages genes for embryo development. Nature 2009;460: 473–478.
86 Erkek S, et al: Molecular determinants of nucleosome retention at CpG-rich sequences in mouse spermatozoa. Nat Struct Mol Biol 2013;20:868–875.
87 Hammoud SS, et al: Chromatin and transcription transitions of mammalian adult germline stem cells and spermatogenesis. Cell Stem Cell 2014;15:239–253.
88 Okada Y, Scott G, Ray MK, Mishina Y, Zhang Y: Histone demethylase JHDM2A is critical for Tnp1 and Prm1 transcription and spermatogenesis. Nature 2007; 450:119–123.
89 Montellier E, et al: Chromatin-to-nucleoprotamine transition is controlled by the histone H2B variant TH2B. Genes Dev 2013;27:1680–1692.
90 Bao J, Bedford MT: Epigenetic regulation of the histone-to-protamine transition during spermiogenesis. Reproduction 2016;151:R55–R70.
91 Grunewald S, Paasch U, Glander HJ, Anderegg U: Mature human spermatozoa do not transcribe novel RNA. Andrologia 2005;37:69–71.
92 Johnson GD, et al: Cleavage of rRNA ensures translational cessation in sperm at fertilization. Mol Hum Reprod 2011; 17:721–726.
93 Godmann M, Lambrot R, Kimmins S: The dynamic epigenetic program in male germ cells: its role in spermatogenesis, testis cancer, and its response to the environment. Microsc Res Tech 2009;72:603–619.
94 Jirtle RL, Skinner MK: Environmental epigenomics and disease susceptibility. Nat Rev Genet 2007;8:253–262.
95 Furrow RE, Christiansen FB, Feldman MW: Environment-sensitive epigenetics and the heritability of complex diseases. Genetics 2011;189:1377–1387.
96 Meissner A, et al: Genome-scale DNA methylation maps of pluripotent and differentiated cells. Nature 2008;454: 766–770.
97 Lister R, et al: Human DNA methylomes at base resolution show widespread epigenomic differences. Nature 2009; 462:315–322.
98 Azuara V, et al: Chromatin signatures of pluripotent cell lines. Nat Cell Biol 2006;8:532–538.
99 Peters J: The role of genomic imprinting in biology and disease: an expanding view. Nat Rev Genet 2014;15:517–530.
100 Aston KI, Punj V, Liu L, Carrell DT: Genome-wide sperm deoxyribonucleic acid methylation is altered in some men with abnormal chromatin packaging or poor in vitro fertilization embryogenesis. Fertil Steril 2012;97:285–292.
101 Schagdarsurengin U, Paradowska A, Steger K: Analysing the sperm epigenome: roles in early embryogenesis and assisted reproduction. Nat Rev Urol 2012;9:609–619.
102 Aston KI, et al: Aberrant sperm DNA methylation predicts male fertility status and embryo quality. Fertil Steril 2015;104:1388–1397.e15.
103 Nanassy L, Carrell DT: Analysis of the methylation pattern of six gene promoters in sperm of men with abnormal protamination. Asian J Androl 2011;13:342–346.
104 Nanassy L, Carrell DT: Abnormal methylation of the promoter of CREM is broadly associated with male factor infertility and poor sperm quality but is improved in sperm selected by density gradient centrifugation. Fertil Steril 2011;95:2310–2314.
105 Nantel F, et al: Spermiogenesis deficiency and germ-cell apoptosis in CREM-mutant mice. Nature 1996;380: 159–162.
106 Blendy JA, Kaestner KH, Weinbauer GF, Nieschlag E, Schutz G: Severe impairment of spermatogenesis in mice lacking the CREM gene. Nature 1996; 380:162–165.
107 Lambrot R, et al: Low paternal dietary folate alters the mouse sperm epigenome and is associated with negative pregnancy outcomes. Nat Commun 2013;4:2889.
108 Terashima M, et al: Effect of high fat diet on paternal sperm histone distribution and male offspring liver gene expression. Epigenetics 2015;10:861–871.
109 Yuan T, et al: An integrative multiscale analysis of the dynamic DNA methylation landscape in aging. PLoS Genet 2015;11:e1004996.
110 Schaefer CB, Ooi SK, Bestor TH, Bourc'his D: Epigenetic decisions in mammalian germ cells. Science 2007; 316:398–399.
111 Kohli RM, Zhang Y: TET enzymes, TDG and the dynamics of DNA demethylation. Nature 2013;502:472–479.
112 Trasler JM: Epigenetics in spermatogenesis. Mol Cell Endocrinol 2009;306: 33–36.
113 La Salle S, Trasler JM: Dynamic expression of DNMT3a and DNMT3b isoforms during male germ cell development in the mouse. Dev Biol 2006; 296:71–82.
114 La Salle S, et al: Windows for sex-specific methylation marked by DNA methyltransferase expression profiles in mouse germ cells. Dev Biol 2004; 268:403–415.
115 Kaneda M, et al: Essential role for de novo DNA methyltransferase Dnmt3a in paternal and maternal imprinting. Nature 2004;429:900–903.
116 Bourc'his D, Xu GL, Lin CS, Bollman B, Bestor TH: Dnmt3L and the establishment of maternal genomic imprints. Science 2001;294:2536–2539.
117 La Salle S, et al: Loss of spermatogonia and wide-spread DNA methylation defects in newborn male mice deficient in DNMT3L. BMC Dev Biol 2007;7:104.
118 Webster KE, et al: Meiotic and epigenetic defects in Dnmt3L-knockout mouse spermatogenesis. Proc Natl Acad Sci USA 2005;102:4068–4073.
119 Bourc'his D, Bestor TH: Meiotic catastrophe and retrotransposon reactivation in male germ cells lacking Dnmt3L. Nature 2004;431:96–99.
120 Saferali A, et al: DNA methyltransferase 1 (*Dnmt1*) mutation affects *Snrpn* imprinting in the mouse male germ line. Genome 2012;55:673–682.
121 Dion V, Lin Y, Hubert L Jr, Waterland RA, Wilson JH: Dnmt1 deficiency promotes CAG repeat expansion in the mouse germline. Hum Mol Genet 2008;17:1306–1317.
122 Yamaguchi S, et al: Tet1 controls meiosis by regulating meiotic gene expression. Nature 2012;492:443–447.
123 Yamaguchi S, Shen L, Liu Y, Sendler D, Zhang Y: Role of Tet1 in erasure of genomic imprinting. Nature 2013;504: 460–464.
124 Peters AH, et al: Loss of the *Suv39h* histone methyltransferases impairs mammalian heterochromatin and genome stability. Cell 2001;107:323–337.

125 O'Carroll D, et al: Isolation and characterization of Suv39h2, a second histone H3 methyltransferase gene that displays testis-specific expression. Mol Cell Biol 2000;20:9423–9433.
126 Jenuwein T, Allis CD: Translating the histone code. Science 2001;293:1074–1080.
127 Daxinger L, et al: Hypomethylation of ERVs in the sperm of mice haploinsufficient for the histone methyltransferase Setdb1 correlates with a paternal effect on phenotype. Sci Rep 2016;6:25004.
128 Tachibana M, et al: G9a histone methyltransferase plays a dominant role in euchromatic histone H3 lysine 9 methylation and is essential for early embryogenesis. Genes Dev 2002;16:1779–1791.
129 Rice JC, et al: Histone methyltransferases direct different degrees of methylation to define distinct chromatin domains. Mol Cell 2003;12:1591–1598.
130 Gyory I, Wu J, Fejer G, Seto E, Wright KL: PRDI-BF1 recruits the histone H3 methyltransferase G9a in transcriptional silencing. Nat Immunol 2004;5:299–308.
131 Roopra A, Qazi R, Schoenike B, Daley TJ, Morrison JF: Localized domains of G9a-mediated histone methylation are required for silencing of neuronal genes. Mol Cell 2004;14:727–738.
132 Tachibana M, Nozaki M, Takeda N, Shinkai Y: Functional dynamics of H3K9 methylation during meiotic prophase progression. EMBO J 2007;26:3346–3359.
133 Hayashi K, Yoshida K, Matsui Y: A histone H3 methyltransferase controls epigenetic events required for meiotic prophase. Nature 2005;438:374–378.
134 Irie S, et al: Single-nucleotide polymorphisms of the *PRDM9* (*MEISETZ*) gene in patients with nonobstructive azoospermia. J Androl 2009;30:426–431.
135 Miyamoto T, et al: Two single nucleotide polymorphisms in *PRDM9* (*MEISETZ*) gene may be a genetic risk factor for Japanese patients with azoospermia by meiotic arrest. J Assist Reprod Genet 2008;25:553–557.
136 Yap DB, et al: Mll5 is required for normal spermatogenesis. PLoS One 2011;6:e27127.
137 Shi Y, et al: Histone demethylation mediated by the nuclear amine oxidase homolog LSD1. Cell 2004;119:941–953.
138 Metzger E, et al: LSD1 demethylates repressive histone marks to promote androgen-receptor-dependent transcription. Nature 2005;437:436–439.
139 Wang Y, et al: LSD1 is a subunit of the NuRD complex and targets the metastasis programs in breast cancer. Cell 2009;138:660–672.
140 Godmann M, et al: Dynamic regulation of histone H3 methylation at lysine 4 in mammalian spermatogenesis. Biol Reprod 2007;77:754–764.
141 Lambrot R, Lafleur C, Kimmins S: The histone demethylase KDM1A is essential for the maintenance and differentiation of spermatogonial stem cells and progenitors. FASEB J 2015;29:4402–4416.
142 Kasioulis I, et al: Kdm3a lysine demethylase is an Hsp90 client required for cytoskeletal rearrangements during spermatogenesis. Mol Biol Cell 2014;25:1216–1233.
143 Brauchle M, et al: Protein complex interactor analysis and differential activity of KDM3 subfamily members towards H3K9 methylation. PLoS One 2013;8:e60549.
144 Kuroki S, et al: JMJD1C, a JmjC domain-containing protein, is required for long-term maintenance of male germ cells in mice. Biol Reprod 2013;89:93.
145 Iwamori N, Zhao M, Meistrich ML, Matzuk MM: The testis-enriched histone demethylase, KDM4D, regulates methylation of histone H3 lysine 9 during spermatogenesis in the mouse but is dispensable for fertility. Biol Reprod 2011;84:1225–1234.
146 Iwamori N, Iwamori T, Matzuk MM: H3K27 demethylase, JMJD3, regulates fragmentation of spermatogonial cysts. PLoS One 2013;8:e72689.
147 Gallardo T, Shirley L, John GB, Castrillon DH: Generation of a germ cell-specific mouse transgenic Cre line, *Vasa-Cre*. Genesis 2007;45:413–417.
148 Lomeli H, Ramos-Mejia V, Gertsenstein M, Lobe CG, Nagy A: Targeted insertion of Cre recombinase into the TNAP gene: excision in primordial germ cells. Genesis 2000;26:116–117.
149 Sadate-Ngatchou PI, Payne CJ, Dearth AT, Braun RE: Cre recombinase activity specific to postnatal, premeiotic male germ cells in transgenic mice. Genesis 2008;46:738–742.
150 Yoshida S, et al: The first round of mouse spermatogenesis is a distinctive program that lacks the self-renewing spermatogonia stage. Development 2006;133:1495–1505.
151 Schonhoff SE, Giel-Moloney M, Leiter AB: Neurogenin 3-expressing progenitor cells in the gastrointestinal tract differentiate into both endocrine and non-endocrine cell types. Dev Biol 2004;270:443–454.
152 Pellegrini M, et al: Targeted JAM-C deletion in germ cells by Spo11-controlled Cre recombinase. J Cell Sci 2011;124:91–99.
153 Inselman AL, et al: Heat shock protein 2 promoter drives Cre expression in spermatocytes of transgenic mice. Genesis 2010;48:114–120.
154 Ben Khelifa M, et al: Identification of a new recurrent aurora kinase C mutation in both European and African men with macrozoospermia. Hum Reprod 2012;27:3337–3346.
155 Wang G, et al: Essential requirement for both *hsf1* and *hsf2* transcriptional activity in spermatogenesis and male fertility. Genesis 2004;38:66–80.
156 Lin YN, Roy A, Yan W, Burns KH, Matzuk MM: Loss of zona pellucida binding proteins in the acrosomal matrix disrupts acrosome biogenesis and sperm morphogenesis. Mol Cell Biol 2007;27:6794–6805.
157 Hayashi T, Carthew RW: Surface mechanics mediate pattern formation in the developing retina. Nature 2004;431:647–652.
158 Okada Y, Tateishi K, Zhang Y: Histone demethylase JHDM2A is involved in male infertility and obesity. J Androl 2010;31:75–78.

Maren Godmann
Center for Molecular Biomedicine (CMB), Department of Biochemistry
Friedrich Schiller University Jena, Hans-Knöll-Strasse 2
DE–07745 Jena (Germany)
E-Mail maren.godmann@uni-jena.de

Vogt PH (ed): Genetics of Human Infertility. Monogr Hum Genet.
Basel, Karger, 2017, vol 21, pp 162–172 (DOI: 10.1159/000477285)

In vitro Spermatogenesis and Its Potential Clinical Implication for Patients

Jan-Bernd Stukenborg[a] · Kirsi Jahnukainen[a, b]

[a]Department of Women's and Children's Health, Paediatric Endocrinology Unit, NORDFERTIL Research Lab Stockholm; Q2:08, Karolinska Institute and University Hospital, Stockholm, Sweden; [b]Division of Haematology-Oncology and Stem Cell Transplantation, Children's Hospital, University of Helsinki, Helsinki University Central Hospital, Helsinki, Finland

Abstract

The establishment of a robust and reliable culture system to study the differentiation of male germ cells in vitro has been a topic in developmental biology and reproductive medicine for over 100 years. Although successful approaches resulting in full mammalian spermatogenesis have been developed for mice, development of a system to elucidate details of the complex process of spermatogenesis in humans is still needed. A huge variety of strategies employing different types of cells, cultured in different conditions, have been investigated so far. However, mostly because of limited access to human gonadal material from healthy donors, crucial information necessary to establish a functioning system remains missing. To picture the current status of information on human spermatogenesis in vitro, this short review mainly focuses on articles published over the last decade. However, important articles published before 2006 have also been included in the absence of more recent studies. A literature search was conducted, including articles written in English and German, cited in PubMed, and references identified in articles, with the focus on in vitro spermatogenesis and its clinical implication for paediatric oncology and haematology patients subjected to gonadotoxic anticancer treatments.

The transmission of genetic information from one generation to another highlights the important role of germ cells. In men, fertility is dependent on the spermatogenic process leading to the production of fertile male gametes. This process includes the proliferation and differentiation of spermatogonial stem cells (SSCs), meiotic divisions, and differentiation and maturation of spermatids during the process of spermiogenesis [1].

Spermatogenesis is a constant process that relies on SSCs. In contrast to the situation in women, where the oocyte pool decreases constantly, sperm production can be maintained until late in life, as long as the SSC pool is not lost. In humans, 2 types of undifferentiated spermatogonia have been described: A_{dark} and A_{pale} spermatogonia. These undifferentiated spermatogonia develop from gonocytes within the first months after birth [1]. While A_{dark} spermatogonia represent the reserve stem cell pool, and do not divide when spermatogenesis is active unless severe testicular damage occurs, type A_{pale} spermatogonia constantly divide during every spermatogenic cycle [2]. They self-renew and differentiate further into B-spermatogonia.

After the last mitotic division, primary spermatocytes, which originate from B-spermatogonia, enter meiosis and convert into round haploid spermatids. During the following process of spermiogenesis, elongated spermatids are formed. The time taken for SSCs to differentiate into elongated spermatids, including the proliferation of spermatogonia, is around 74 days in humans [3].

Although what is known about spermatogenesis has dramatically increased in recent decades, details of the highly complex process of human spermatogenesis are still inadequate. Limited access to human testicular material, often connected to ethical concerns, as well as the lack of functional in vitro models are the main reasons behind this. The use of animal models to elucidate the process of human spermatogenesis is limited as a result of species-dependent differences, e.g., the number of spermatogonial subtypes are 9 in mice and 3 in humans [4, 5].

In recent decades, many strategies, including animal studies with a focus on germ cell or tissue transplantation [6–10], as well as different types of in vitro culture [11–17], including pluripotent stem cells [18, 19] and the recently described very small embryonic-like stem cells [20, 21], have been considered to explore the spermatogenic progress in detail. Among these strategies, approaches employing germ cell or testicular tissue transplantation have provided options for maturing SSCs and more advanced germ cells in milieus similar to those that are present naturally. However, the advantages of these in vivo settings are limited, especially with a view to their future potential as clinical tools for fertility preservation techniques, e.g., for prepubertal boys with malignant haematological diseases subjected to highly gonadotoxic anticancer treatments. Therefore, experiments focusing on human male germ cell maturation in vitro are so far the most promising strategies. To summarise current knowledge of human in vitro spermatogenesis, the following sections are focused on strategies to monitor/evaluate mechanisms of proliferation and differentiation of human and rodent male germ cells ex vivo using germ cell or testicular tissue culture (Fig. 1), as well as the needs of fertility preservation techniques, with a focus on the situation for paediatric oncology and haematology patients, who might be the first real benefiters of these techniques.

A Century of Search for the Right Setting: A Historical View of Cell Culture Approaches Designed for the Differentiation of Male Germ Cells

Literature research concerning articles related to in vitro spermatogenesis dates back to the year 1915. At the beginning of the last century, organ culture conditions were developed for testicular tissue from a variety of different species, mainly from rodents in mammals. These revealed the supportive effects of in vitro maintenance of the microenvironment provided by the seminiferous epithelium and thereby the intact cell-to-cell communication pathways of somatic and germ cells [16]. These first experiments, followed by many others between the 1930s and 1990s, revealed many import aspects related to male germ cell differentiation, e.g., the positive effects of temperature below that of the body [22–26], the need for cell-cell contacts [27–29], the supportive effect on the viability of media components including pyruvate, glutamine, vitamins A, C, and E, the non-supportive effect of gonadotrophins for the success of germ cell cultures [22], and the fact that high oxygen levels can be toxic to cells in vitro.

In the late 1990s, Tesarik et al. [14, 30] reported the first successful differentiation of human male germ cells with completion of meiosis and the spermiogenic process in vitro via the use of seminiferous tubule cultures at 30°C. Fluorescence in situ hybridisation (FISH), morphologic analysis employing the Papanicolaou method, and immunocytochemical detection of

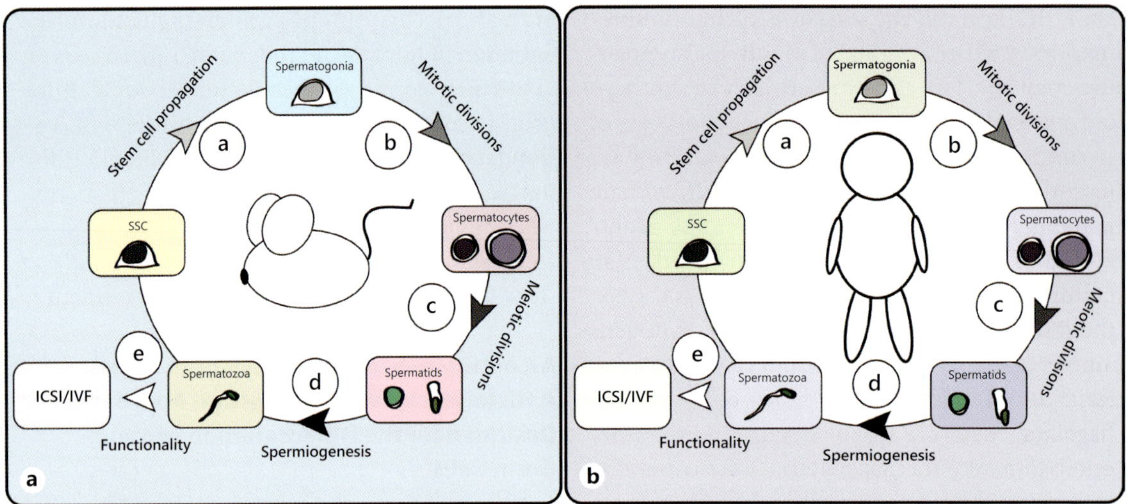

Rodents		Humans	
Maturation steps	References	Maturation steps	References
a/b - c	[15, 27, 40, 41]	a/b - c	[25, 26]
a/b - d	[16, 35, 39, 46]	a/b - d	[36, 44]
a/b - e	[11, 12, 37]	a/b - e	[---]
		c - d	[14, 30, 31, 32]
		c - e	[14]
		d - e	[33]

c

Fig. 1. Schematic overview of experimental conditions used for in vitro spermatogenesis in rodents (**a**) and humans (**b**). Different steps of the spermatogenic process are highlighted – (1) stem cell propagation; (2) mitotic divisions; (3) meiotic divisions; (4) spermiogenesis; (5) functionality – and selected articles describing the differentiation of murine or human spermatogonia, spermatocytes, or round spermatids into more advanced stages are mentioned (**c**). ICSI, intracytoplasmic sperm injection; IVF, in vitro fertilisation.

proacrosin 4D4 were used to identify haploid cells generated in vitro. Unfortunately, measurements of DNA contents supporting the haploid nature of the round spermatids are unavailable and the ploidy of the spermatids cannot be checked when injected into an oocyte due to the risk of abnormalities. These potential abnormalities could be related to the increased speed of maturation, as mentioned below. Although huge limitations concerning the quality control of the produced sperm and therefore on the safety of the procedure itself existed, ongoing experiments on the functionality of the sperm were performed. As a result of these experiments, the group reported the birth of healthy infants after intracytoplasmic sperm injection using in vitro-differentiated sperm from patients with azoospermia due to a meiotic block [14].

In addition, the differentiation of primary spermatocytes into haploid spermatids, which in vivo takes up to 32 days [3, 30], was reported to occur within 48 h [30]. However, the reason behind the increased differentiation speed remains unknown and was not addressed in these studies. Although earlier investigators reported a similar speed for germ cell differentiation in vivo and in vitro, another group observed a similar feature of in vitro maturation into round spermatids when culturing meiotic germ cells on Vero cells [31]. The haploid characteristic of the in vitro-matured round spermatids in this study was examined by FISH analysis and Giemsa staining after injecting the round spermatids into mouse oocytes. Both methods confirmed the haploid nature of the investigated round spermatids.

In 1999, Cremades et al. [32] reported the differentiation of round spermatids, obtained from patients with azoospermia due to a postmeiotic block, into mature elongated spermatids using culture conditions with Vero cells. In that study, the round spermatids, described as 6–8 μm in diameter with a round nucleus, used as starting material as well as the matured sperm, exhibiting a flagellum, were identified solely on morphologic criteria. In subsequent studies, in vitro-matured spermatids revealed low fertilisation potential. However, in the cases of successful fertilisation, a normal blastocyst formation potential was reported [33].

Although the results reported during the late 1990s and the follow-up studies were in the spotlight of the scientific community, the culture conditions resulted in low efficiency rates and could not be reproduced in a robust way. Therefore, these techniques have never been used as a standard procedure in clinical practice. The appearance of round spermatids after 48 h and the limited numbers of haploid cells reported raised questions of whether the postmeiotic cells were already present at the beginning of the cultures, since the reason behind the fast differentiation process (48 h in vitro vs. 32 days in vivo) could not be identified in detail. In addition, these studies exclusively used testicular tissue from adult patients with meiotic arrest (Fig. 2). Therefore, it is possible that parts from the testis tissue contained postmeiotic cells at the beginning of the experiments.

In search of a reproducible method, further studies focusing on the in vitro differentiation of murine or human male germ cells combined with somatic cells, as well as studies involving enriched germ cell types such as spermatogonia and spermatocytes, clearly demonstrated that a microenvironment resembling the 3-dimensional organisation of the seminiferous epithelium in situ (thereby providing cell-cell contact) should be provided [11, 16, 34–36]. So far, the differentiation of rodent spermatogonia to postmeiotic germ cells has been reported in connection with organ culture and 3-dimensional cell culture methodologies [11, 12, 16, 37–41] (Fig. 1).

The establishment of novel 3-dimensional culture systems in parallel with the establishment of organ cultures has recently provided novel insights into the process of mammalian male germ cell differentiation and proliferation, as well as formation of testicular microenvironments in vitro [15, 16, 35, 36, 42, 43] (Fig. 1). Three-dimensional culture systems, using agar, methylcellulose, or extracellular matrixes, were first established as clonogenic assays for multipotent haematopoietic cells [44]. These assays were subsequently further developed and adapted to the needs required for the clonal expansion of germ cells [15, 16, 35, 39, 40]. Regardless of the matrix used to generate the 3-dimensional environment, the differentiation of male germ cells through meiosis could be demonstrated, pointing out the important effect of physical contact between the cells, in accordance with results from previous organ culture experiments [16].

However, further studies are needed, including the characterisation of SSC niche formation and regulation in humans, to address the needs necessary for establishing a system for fertility preservation in humans. In this respect, another study using testicular material from 16 patients with cryptorchidism and 9 patients with obstructive azoospermia (mean age 29 ± 2 years) revealed the differentiation of human SSCs up to functional haploid spermatids [45]. This could be achieved by using DMEM/F12 cell culture medium, 10% foetal bovine serum, retinoic acid, and stem cell factor in a conventional single cell culture for 7–10 days [45]. The studies discussed above, using testicular tissue of adult patients, represent a step towards the goal of establishing a clinical tool for fertility preservation, by providing a new

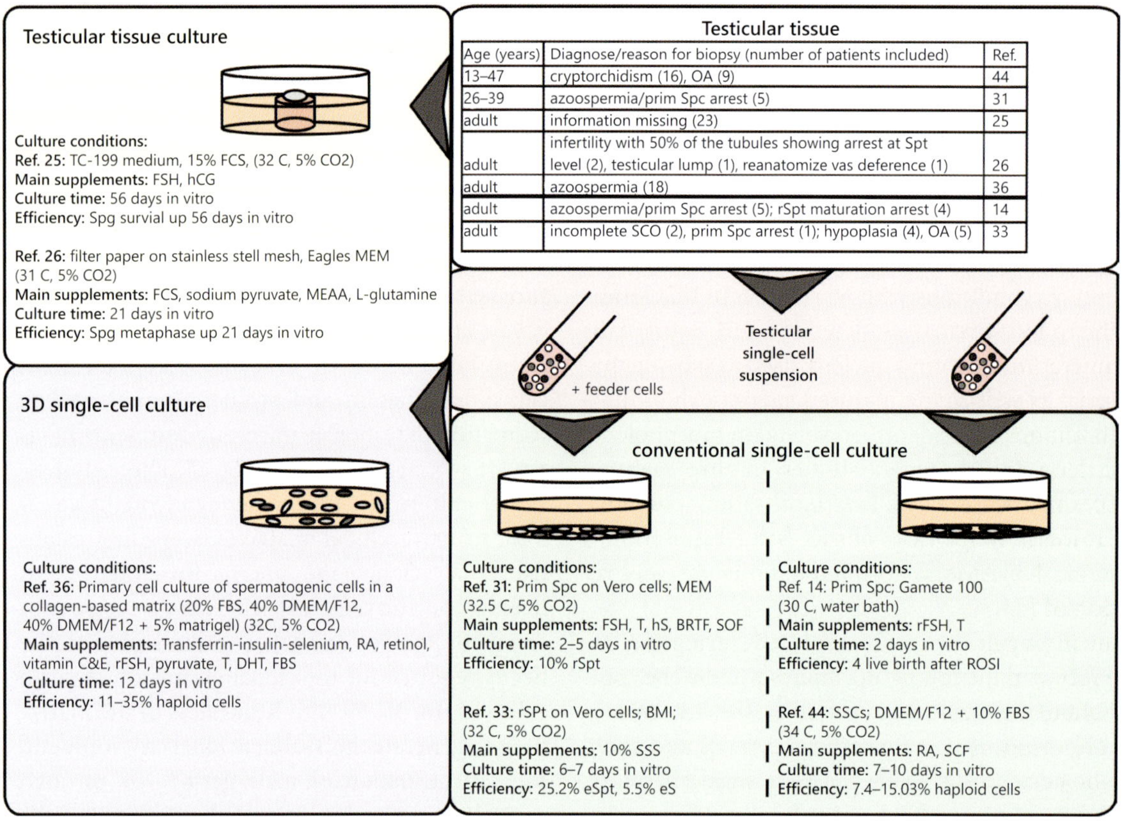

Fig. 2. Schematic overview of experimental conditions used for in vitro spermatogenesis in humans. Selected articles are mentioned describing the culture conditions and main factors employed, as well as culture periods and efficiency rates of haploid cell production of each study. The age, diagnosis, and number of patients that participated in the studies on male germ cell differentiation in vitro are provided. Detailed information regarding the limitations of each study are given in the text. Spg, spermatogonia; prim Spc, primary spermatocyte; rSpt, round spermatid; eSpt, elongating spermatid; eS, elongated spermatid; OA, obstructive azoospermia; SCO, Sertoli cell-only syndrome; ROSI, round spermatid injection; rFSH, recombinant follicle-stimulating hormone; hCG, human chorionic gonadotropin; T, testosterone; DHT, dihydrotestosterone; RA, retinoic acid; SCF, stem cell factor; FBS, foetal bovine serum; FCS, foetal calf serum; SSS, synthetic serum substitute; MEAA, minimal essential amino acids; hS, human serum; SOF, synthetic oviduct fluid; BRTF, bovine rete testicular fluid.

aspect to the in vitro behaviour of human testicular tissue. Thus, they are important for future fertility preservation strategies, especially for prepubertal boys suffering haematological diseases, who need a fertility preservation technique without the risk of reintroducing malignant cells, as discussed below.

Unfortunately, they do not automatically offer a working concept for male germ cell differentiation obtained from prepubertal boys, who are not able to produce sperm as their testes have not passed the maturation phase of the supporting somatic cell types (e.g., Sertoli and Leydig cells) that occurs during puberty. A very recent study by de Michele et al. [46] reported preserved seminiferous tubule structures, along with survival of spermatogonia and Sertoli and Leydig cell maturation in prepubertal testis tissue cultured after cryopreservation for up to 139 days in vitro. In that study, the organ culture condition was supplemented with transferrin, L-glutamine, vitamin A and C, and human serum albumin. Leydig cells produced testosterone, with a peak at 10 days in vitro, while anti-Müllerian hormone expression decreases after 16 days in vitro, suggesting a Sertoli cell maturation [46]. Although the results were negative in terms of germ cell differentiation, the study provides important insights into the features of maturation and functionality of somatic cells, cultured in testicular organ culture conditions.

However, only an organ culture setting with 10% knockout serum replacement or AlbuMAX (40 mg/mL) instead of conventional foetal bovine serum has been successfully used in the generation of functional murine sperm capable of producing fertile offspring [13, 37]. Interestingly, the effect of age on germ cell capacity to differentiate beyond meiosis, as reported in earlier studies [47], could also be observed in organ culture when using material from adult mice [48].

Lately, the concept of using a cytocompatible decellularised testicular matrix (DTM) for male germ cell differentiation has been reported [17, 49]. A study by Baert et al. [17], in addition to showing the impact of structural support provided by human DTM, revealed important insights into the components inside the basal membrane. Interestingly, proteomic analysis of the DTM used revealed (in addition to well-known components such as laminin, collagens I and IV, glycosaminoglycans, and fibronectin) more than 100 unique proteins belonging to or associated with the testicular extracellular matrix. These new and interesting findings offer insights needed for further experiments to elucidate the role and potential use of scaffolds made of human DTM in in vitro systems for fertility preservation and their future use in clinics.

In addition to the experimental definition of appropriate culture conditions, current studies, focusing on the available cryopreservation techniques, their effects on SSCs, and their future potential to differentiate further into functional sperm, have recently been performed with murine and human cells/tissue. These studies do not show a particularly negative effect of the cryopreservation process on germ cell survival or the differentiation potential of these cells [13, 50–53]. Nevertheless, additional studies are mandatory to address efficiency/safety concerns, and to avoid potential abnormalities such as genetic/epigenetic instabilities of in vitro-generated gametes, which have been described in connection with bone marrow or human embryonic and foetal mesenchymal stem cells, for example [54, 55]. However, initial experiments focusing on the effects of long-term culture of SSCs are encouraging, demonstrating the genomic stability of these cells [56].

In summary, experiments demonstrating a complete spermatogenesis in vitro, including differentiating SSCs up to postmeiotic cells from immature testicular tissue in humans, have not been reported so far. Studies employing testicular tissue from prepubertal boys for in vitro differentiation protocols are crucial in order to explore the aspects needed to set up a robust technique for fertility preservation in humans. Although the results of in vitro differentiation of rodent SSCs into functional sperm was recently reported, it is difficult to estimate how long it will take to create systems allowing the ex vivo maturation of human male germ cells. However, new research consortia, such as Growsperm (www.growsperm.eu), Androprotect (http://repro.klinikum.uni-muenster.de), Edinburgh Fertility Preservation (http://www.ed.ac.uk/integrative-physiology/edinburgh-fertility-preservation), or NORDFERTIL (www.nordfertil.org), have been initiated to coordinate research and educate young researchers with a special focus on fertility preservation in boys. Examples of the clinical implications for in vitro spermatogenesis will be discussed in the next chapter.

Clinical Implications for in vitro Spermatogenesis

Male infertility is a multifactorial and complex condition affecting around 10–15% of all couples worldwide [57]. The fact that only 1 in 8 infertile men has a treatable condition, and can subsequently father children naturally, highlights its impact on society. The reasons for subfertility and infertility are varied and relate to a wide number of different factors. The known causes of infertility can be grouped into sperm production problems, blockage of sperm transport, and sexual problems [57]. Therefore, the issue of subfertility or infertility in men has increased over the last 2 decades, leading to the "andrologist" subspecialisation in medicine. This has seen an increasing number of public and private medical-assisted reproduction clinics, new guidelines for toxicology tests in the pharmaceutical industry focusing on the reproductive organs, as well as discussions about the effects of environmental pollutions on fertility in animals and humans.

The problem of impaired sperm production, which accounts for the majority of all cases of fertility problems, especially needs to be the focus of new research approaches. This group includes chromosomal or genetic diseases (e.g., Klinefelter syndrome), Y-chromosome deletions, trisomy 21, undescended testis, infections, torsions, varicocele, medicines and chemicals, radiation damages (e.g., anticancer treatments), but also unknown causes.

However, as mentioned above, detailed knowledge about the biology of male human fertility is still inadequate and remains to be elucidated in order to create novel treatment options for patients. Considering the results of experiments on in vitro spermatogenesis mentioned above, the establishment of a robust technique for human in vitro spermatogenesis is more likely to be successful with healthy testicular tissue of prepubertal boys showing no genetic impairment or other diseases directly affecting the spermatogenic process. Therefore, prepubertal boys with childhood cancer, whose spermatogenesis is not affected by the anticancer treatment or the disease itself, might be among those first to really benefit. The following section discusses aspects of fertility preservation in this group in detail.

Fertility Preservation and Childhood Cancer: An Example of the Need for in vitro Spermatogenesis in Clinics

Treatments That Affect Male Fertility

Testicular cells, especially rapidly dividing germ cells, are highly sensitive to cytotoxic treatment and irradiation (Table 1). Low doses of these treatments deplete the differentiating spermatogonia pool, while less sensitive SSCs survive, and spermatocytes and spermatids continue their maturation to sperm [58]. The impact of combination chemotherapy on the spermatogenic epithelium is dependent on the drugs used and their dosage [59–61] (Table 1). Acute leukaemia, the most common cancer type in children, involves treatment with antimetabolites and vinca alkaloids. Treatment with these cell cycle-specific cytotoxic drugs, without a high dose of the alkylating agent cyclophosphamide, does not totally deplete SSCs and spermatogenesis recovers from the surviving reserve stem cell population [62, 63].

The germinal epithelium is very sensitive to irradiation damage and cytotoxic treatment with alkylating agents [64, 65]. Many investigators have described threshold doses of alkylating agents such as cyclophosphamide in relation to long-term subfertility [66]. However, a recent large study of non-irradiated childhood cancer survivors failed to reveal any threshold dose of alkylating agent exposure that could predict impaired spermatogenesis or azoospermia after a median follow-up period of 21 years [65]. There may be other factors, such as genetic variation in

Table 1. Gonadotoxic therapies used in the treatment of childhood cancers

Gonadotoxic therapy	Indications in paediatric oncology	Risk of infertility
Radiotherapy		
Radiotherapy of a field including the testes	Solid tumours and leukaemia	Very high
Total body irradiation	HSCT conditioning	Very high
Chemotherapy with alkylating agents		
Cyclophosphamide	Solid tumours and haematological cancers	High
Ifosfamide	Solid tumours	High
Nitrosoureas	Solid tumours	High
Chlorambucil	Solid tumours	High
Melphalan	HSCT conditioning	Very high
Busulfan	HSCT conditioning	Very high
Dacarbazine	Solid tumours and haematological cancers	High
Procarbazine	Solid tumours and lymphoma	High

HSCT, haematopoietic stem cell transplantation.

drug-metabolising pathways, which modulate the impact of alkylating agent exposure on spermatogenesis or its recovery [65]. Irradiation doses of 2–3 Gy, which also affect SSCs, cause long-term azoospermia [67]. Doses of more than 6 Gy are able to deplete the SSC pool and lead to permanent infertility [68].

Total body irradiation (TBI), as conditioning for haematological stem cell transplantation (HSCT), is associated with significant germ cell failure [69]. The probability of recovery of spermatogenesis after HSCT is associated with the type of conditioning therapy, age of the patient, time interval since transplantation, and absence of chronic graft-versus-host disease [70, 71]. Following TBI at doses of 10–14 Gy, recovery of spermatogenesis has been reported to never occur before the 4th year after transplantation [70]. Similar findings have recently been reported in the paediatric population. HSCT conditioning with chemotherapy-based regimens is associated with a larger adult testicular volume, lower serum levels of FISH, and the more frequent presence of spermatozoa compared with those conditioned with TBI at doses of 10–12 Gy [72].

Who Are the Patients that Need Artificially Generated Sperm?

Pubertal boys and men who are at risk of infertility should be offered the possibility to cryopreserve their sperm at the time of diagnosis of a malignant disease. Unfortunately, this is not an option for prepubertal boys before spermarche. Instead, cryopreservation of testicular tissue could be offered. Testicular biopsy is invasive, and can carry an operative risk among immunocompromised and pancytopenic cancer patients. These uncertainties, and the unknown effectiveness of the procedure for the restoration of fertility, dictate that it should only be offered to boys who are at high risk of permanent testicular damage and subsequent infertility [73].

A very high risk of infertility is associated with conditioning therapy for allogeneic or autologous HSCT and radiotherapy with testis in the field [71, 72]. Boys undergoing orchidectomy could also be offered cryopreservation of the removed tissue. Patients with leukaemia and lymphoma facing allogeneic HSCT represent a significant group of patients who would benefit from prepubertal testicular cryopreservation. However, leukaemia, lymphoma, and other haematological malignancies carry a high risk of testicular contamination [74]. The situation is similar to fertility preservation among females, where currently only patients with immune deficiency, bone marrow failure, benign haematological diseases, and cancers associated with a low risk of reproductive tract metastasis are considered for autotransplantation [75–77]. For the time being, it cannot be regarded as safe to perform testicular tissue or SSC transplantation among patients with haematological cancers because of the possibility of reseeding malignant cells into cured patients. The maturation of testicular tissue and spermatogonia in vitro, as discussed above, may be a promising strategy to overcome the problems of leukemic cell contamination [78]. In summary, patients that urgently need artificially generated sperm are those with haematological malignancies treated by means of HSCT or radiotherapy.

Conclusion

Male germ cells are among the most essential cells in male life. Although knowledge of the processes involved in the survival, proliferation, and differentiation of these cells has dramatically increased in recent decades, the detailed information needed for success in establishing an in vitro system for human germ cells is still unavailable. Owing to successful approaches in animal studies, techniques are now emerging to propagate and mature germ cells in vitro. Although there are still ethical, safety, and efficiency concerns, we expect that in the near future such methods, combined with advanced assisted reproductive techniques, will be introduced for personalised medicine in highly specialised medical centres all over the world.

References

1 Stukenborg JB, Kjartansdottir KR, Reda A, Colon E, Albersmeier JP, Soder O: Male germ cell development in humans. Horm Res Paediatr 2014;81:2–12.

2 Ehmcke J, Schlatt S: Identification and characterization of spermatogonial subtypes and their expansion in whole mounts and tissue sections from primate testes. Methods Mol Biol 2008;450: 109–118.

3 Amann RP: The cycle of the seminiferous epithelium in humans: a need to revisit? J Androl 2008;29:469–487.

4 Ehmcke J, Wistuba J, Schlatt S: Spermatogonial stem cells: questions, models and perspectives. Hum Reprod Update 2006;12:275–282.

5 Jahnukainen K, Stukenborg JB: Clinical review: present and future prospects of male fertility preservation for children and adolescents. J Clin Endocrinol Metab 2012;97:4341–4351.

6 Jahnukainen K, Ehmcke J, Nurmio M, Schlatt S: Fertility preservation after sterilizing therapy through autologous ectopic grafting of cryopreserved testicular tissue in prepubertal monkeys. Cancer Res, in press.

7 Brinster RL, Zimmermann JW: Spermatogenesis following male germ-cell transplantation. Proc Natl Acad Sci USA 1994;91:11298–11302.

8 Honaramooz A, Snedaker A, Boiani M, Schöler H, Dobrinski I, Schlatt S: Sperm from neonatal mammalian testes grafted in mice. Nature 2002;418:778–781.

9 Schlatt S, Honaramooz A, Ehmcke J, Goebell PJ, Rubben H, Dhir R, et al: Limited survival of adult human testicular tissue as ectopic xenograft. Hum Reprod 2006;21:384–389.

10 Galuppo AG: Spermatogonial stem cells as a therapeutic alternative for fertility preservation of prepubertal boys. Einstein (Sao Paulo) 2015;13:637–639.

11 Sato T, Katagiri K, Gohbara A, Inoue K, Ogonuki N, Ogura A, et al: In vitro production of functional sperm in cultured neonatal mouse testes. Nature 2011;471: 504–507.

12 Sato T, Yokonishi T, Komeya M, Katagiri K, Kubota Y, Matoba S, et al: Testis tissue explantation cures spermatogenic failure in c-Kit ligand mutant mice. Proc Natl Acad Sci USA 2012;109:16934–16938.

13 Yokonishi T, Sato T, Komeya M, Katagiri K, Kubota Y, Nakabayashi K, et al: Offspring production with sperm grown in vitro from cryopreserved testis tissues. Nat Commun 2014;5:4320.

14 Tesarik J, Bahceci M, Ozcan C, Greco E, Mendoza C: Restoration of fertility by in-vitro spermatogenesis. Lancet 1999; 353:555–556.

15 Reda A, Hou M, Landreh L, Kjartansdottir KR, Svechnikov K, Soder O, et al: In vitro spermatogenesis – optimal culture conditions for testicular cell survival, germ cell differentiation, and steroidogenesis in rats. Front Endocrinol 2014;5:21.

16 Stukenborg JB, Schlatt S, Simoni M, Yeung CH, Elhija MA, Luetjens CM, et al: New horizons for in vitro spermatogenesis? An update on novel three-dimensional culture systems as tools for meiotic and post-meiotic differentiation of testicular germ cells. Mol Hum Reprod 2009;15:521–529.

17 Baert Y, Stukenborg JB, Landreh M, De Kock J, Jornvall H, Soder O, et al: Derivation and characterization of a cytocompatible scaffold from human testis. Hum Reprod 2015;30:256–267.

18 Kurimoto K, Saitou M: Mechanism and reconstitution in vitro of germ cell development in mammals. Cold Spring Harb Symp Quant Biol 2015;80:147–154.
19 Kjartansdottir KR, Reda A, Panula S, Day K, Hultenby K, Soder O, et al: A combination of culture conditions and gene expression analysis can be used to investigate and predict hES cell differentiation potential towards male gonadal cells. PLoS One 2015;10:e0144029.
20 Kurkure P, Prasad M, Dhamankar V, Bakshi G: Very small embryonic-like stem cells (VSELs) detected in azoospermic testicular biopsies of adult survivors of childhood cancer. Reprod Biol Endocrinol 2015;13:122.
21 Anand S, Patel H, Bhartiya D: Chemoablated mouse seminiferous tubular cells enriched for very small embryonic-like stem cells undergo spontaneous spermatogenesis in vitro. Reprod Biol Endocrinol 2015;13:33.
22 Steinberger A: In vitro techniques for the study of spermatogenesis. Methods Enzymol 1975;39:283–296.
23 Mieusset R, Bujan L: Testicular heating and its possible contributions to male infertility: a review. Int J Androl 1995; 18:169–184.
24 Nakamura M, Romrell LJ, Hall PF: The effects of temperature and glucose on protein biosynthesis by immature (round) spermatids from rat testes. J Cell Biol 1978;79:1–9.
25 Kato S: Studies on human testicular organ culture (in Japanese). Nihon Hinyokika Gakkai Zasshi 1972;63:519–538.
26 Curtis D: In vitro differentiation of diakinesis figures in human testis. Hum Genet 1981;59:406–411.
27 Steinberger A, Steinberger E: In vitro culture of rat testicular cells. Exp Cell Res 1966;44:443–452.
28 Steinberger A, Steinberger E: Tissue culture of male mammalian gonads. In Vitro 1970;5:17–27.
29 Steinberger A, Steinberger E, Perloff WH: Mammalian testes in organ culture. Exp Cell Res 1964;36:19–27.
30 Tesarik J: Overcoming maturation arrest by in vitro spermatogenesis: search for the optimal culture system. Fertil Steril 2004;81:1417–1419.
31 Tanaka A, Nagayoshi M, Awata S, Mawatari Y, Tanaka I, Kusunoki H: Completion of meiosis in human primary spermatocytes through in vitro coculture with Vero cells. Fertil Steril 2003; 79(suppl 1):795–801.
32 Cremades N, Bernabeu R, Barros A, Sousa M: In vitro maturation of round spermatids using co-culture on Vero cells. Hum Reprod 1999;14:1287–1293.
33 Cremades N, Sousa M, Bernabeu R, Barros A: Developmental potential of elongating and elongated spermatids obtained after in vitro maturation of isolated round spermatids. Hum Reprod 2001;16:1938–1944.
34 Hofmann MC, Narisawa S, Hess RA, Millán JL: Immortalization of germ cells and somatic testicular cells using the SV40 large T antigen. Exp Cell Res 1992; 201:417–435.
35 Lee JH, Kim HJ, Kim H, Lee SJ, Gye MC: In vitro spermatogenesis by three-dimensional culture of rat testicular cells in collagen gel matrix. Biomaterials 2006;27:2845–2853.
36 Lee JH, Gye MC, Choi KW, Hong JY, Lee YB, Park DW, et al: In vitro differentiation of germ cells from nonobstructive azoospermic patients using three-dimensional culture in a collagen gel matrix. Fertil Steril 2007;87:824–833.
37 Sato T, Katagiri K, Yokonishi T, Kubota Y, Inoue K, Ogonuki N, et al: In vitro production of fertile sperm from murine spermatogonial stem cell lines. Nat Commun 2011;2:472.
38 Yokonishi T, Sato T, Katagiri K, Ogawa T: In vitro spermatogenesis using an organ culture technique. Methods Mol Biol 2013;927:479–488.
39 Abu Elhija M, Lunenfeld E, Schlatt S, Huleihel M: Differentiation of murine male germ cells to spermatozoa in a soft agar culture system. Asian J Androl 2012;14:285–293.
40 Stukenborg JB, Wistuba J, Luetjens CM, Elhija MA, Huleihel M, Lunenfeld E, et al: Coculture of spermatogonia with somatic cells in a novel three-dimensional soft-agar-culture-system. J Androl 2008;29:312–329.
41 Reda A, Hou M, Winton TR, Chapin RE, Soder O, Stukenborg JB: In vitro differentiation of rat spermatogonia into round spermatids in tissue culture. Mol Hum Reprod 2016;22:601–612.
42 Dores C, Alpaugh W, Dobrinski I: From in vitro culture to in vivo models to study testis development and spermatogenesis. Cell Tissue Res 2012;349:691–702.
43 Chapin RE, Winton T, Nowland W, Danis N, Kumpf S, Johnson K, Coburn A, Stukenborg JB: Lost in translation: the search for an in vitro screen for spermatogenic toxicity. Birth Defects Res B Dev Reprod Toxicol 2016;107:225–242.
44 Parent-Massin D: Relevance of clonogenic assays in hematotoxicology. Cell Biol Toxicol 2001;17:87–94.
45 Yang S, Ping P, Ma M, Li P, Tian R, Yang H, et al: Generation of haploid spermatids with fertilization and development capacity from human spermatogonial stem cells of cryptorchid patients. Stem Cell Rep 2014;3:663–675.
46 de Michele F, Poels J, Weerens L, Petit C, Evrard Z, Ambroise J, et al: Preserved seminiferous tubule integrity with spermatogonial survival and induction of Sertoli and Leydig cell maturation after long-term organotypic culture of prepubertal human testicular tissue. Hum Reprod 2017;32:32–45.
47 Creemers LB, den Ouden K, van Pelt AMM, de Rooij DG: Maintenance of adult mouse type A spermatogonia in vitro influence of serum and growth factors and comparison with prepubertal spermatogonial cell culture. Reproduction 2002;124:791–799.
48 Sato T, Katagiri K, Kojima K, Komeya M, Yao M, Ogawa T: In vitro spermatogenesis in explanted adult mouse testis tissues. PLoS One 2015;10:e0130171.
49 Baert Y DKJ, Alves-Lopes JP, Söder O, Stukenborg JB, Goossens E: Primary human testicular cells self-organize into organoids with testicular properties. Stem Cell Rep 2017;8:30–38.
50 Arkoun B, Dumont L, Milazzo JP, Rondanino C, Bironneau A, Wils J, et al: Does soaking temperature during controlled slow freezing of pre-pubertal mouse testes influence course of in vitro spermatogenesis? Cell Tissue Res 2016; 364:661–674.
51 Yokonishi T, Ogawa T: Cryopreservation of testis tissues and in vitro spermatogenesis. Reprod Med Biol 2016;15: 21–28.
52 Baert Y, Braye A, Struijk RB, van Pelt AM, Goossens E: Cryopreservation of testicular tissue before long-term testicular cell culture does not alter in vitro cell dynamics. Fertil Steril 2015;104: 1244–1252.e4.

53 Yango P, Altman E, Smith JF, Klatsky PC, Tran ND: Optimizing cryopreservation of human spermatogonial stem cells: comparing the effectiveness of testicular tissue and single cell suspension cryopreservation. Fertil Steril 2014;102: 1491–1498.e1.
54 Redaelli S, Bentivegna A, Foudah D, Miloso M, Redondo J, Riva G, et al: From cytogenomic to epigenomic profiles: monitoring the biologic behavior of in vitro cultured human bone marrow mesenchymal stem cells. Stem Cell Res Ther 2012;3:47.
55 Frost J, Monk D, Moschidou D, Guillot PV, Stanier P, Minger SL, et al: The effects of culture on genomic imprinting profiles in human embryonic and fetal mesenchymal stem cells. Epigenetics 2011;6:52–62.
56 Nickkholgh B, Mizrak SC, van Daalen SK, Korver CM, Sadri-Ardekani H, Repping S, et al: Genetic and epigenetic stability of human spermatogonial stem cells during long-term culture. Fertil Steril 2014;102:1700–1707.e1.
57 Tahmasbpour E, Balasubramanian D, Agarwal A: A multi-faceted approach to understanding male infertility: gene mutations, molecular defects and assisted reproductive techniques (ART). J Assist Reprod Genet 2014;31:1115–1137.
58 van Alphen MM, van de Kant HJ, de Rooij DG: Depletion of the spermatogonia from the seminiferous epithelium of the rhesus monkey after X irradiation. Radiat Res 1988;113:473–486.
59 Wallace WH, Anderson RA, Irvine DS: Fertility preservation for young patients with cancer: who is at risk and what can be offered? Lancet Oncol 2005;6:209–218.
60 Wyns C, Curaba M, Vanabelle B, van Langendonckt A, Donnez J: Options for fertility preservation in prepubertal boys. Hum Reprod Update 2010;16: 312–328.
61 Aubier F, Flamant F, Brauner R, Caillaud JM, Chaussain JM, Lemerle J: Male gonadal function after chemotherapy for solid tumors in childhood. J Clin Oncol 1989;7:304–309.
62 Jahnukainen K, Heikkinen R, Henriksson M, Cooper TG, Puukko-Viertomies LR, Makitie O: Semen quality and fertility in adult long-term survivors of childhood acute lymphoblastic leukemia. Fertil Steril 2011;96:837–842.
63 Nurmio M, Keros V, Lahteenmaki P, Salmi T, Kallajoki M, Jahnukainen K: Effect of childhood acute lymphoblastic leukemia therapy on spermatogonia populations and future fertility. J Clin Endocrinol Metab 2009;94:2119–2122.
64 Sklar CA, Robison LL, Nesbit ME, Sather HN, Meadows AT, Ortega JA, et al: Effects of radiation on testicular function in long-term survivors of childhood acute lymphoblastic leukemia: a report from the Children Cancer Study Group. J Clin Oncol 1990;8:1981–1987.
65 Green DM, Liu W, Kutteh WH, Ke RW, Shelton KC, Sklar CA, et al: Cumulative alkylating agent exposure and semen parameters in adult survivors of childhood cancer: a report from the St Jude Lifetime Cohort Study. Lancet Oncol 2014;15:1215–1223.
66 Rivkees SA, Crawford JD: The relationship of gonadal activity and chemotherapy-induced gonadal damage. JAMA 1988;259:2123–2125.
67 Rowley MJ, Leach DR, Warner GA, Heller CG: Effect of graded doses of ionizing radiation on the human testis. Radiat Res 1974;59:665–678.
68 Centola GM, Keller JW, Henzler M, Rubin P: Effect of low-dose testicular irradiation on sperm count and fertility in patients with testicular seminoma. J Androl 1994;15:608–613.
69 Sarafoglou K, Boulad F, Gillio A, Sklar C: Gonadal function after bone marrow transplantation for acute leukemia during childhood. J Pediatr 1997;130:210–216.
70 Anserini P, Chiodi S, Spinelli S, Costa M, Conte N, Copello F, et al: Semen analysis following allogeneic bone marrow transplantation: additional data for evidence-based counselling. Bone Marrow Transplant 2002;30:447–451.
71 Rovo A, Tichelli A, Passweg JR, Heim D, Meyer-Monard S, Holzgreve W, et al: Spermatogenesis in long-term survivors after allogeneic hematopoietic stem cell transplantation is associated with age, time interval since transplantation, and apparently absence of chronic GvHD. Blood 2006;108:1100–1105.
72 Wilhelmsson M, Vatanen A, Borgstrom B, Gustafsson B, Taskinen M, Saarinen-Pihkala UM, et al: Adult testicular volume predicts spermatogenetic recovery after allogeneic HSCT in childhood and adolescence. Pediatr Blood Cancer 2014; 61:1094–1100.
73 Jahnukainen K, Mitchell RT, Stukenborg JB: Testicular function and fertility preservation after treatment for haematological cancer. Curr Opin Endocrinol Diabetes Obes 2015;22:217–223.
74 Jahnukainen K, Hou M, Petersen C, Setchell B, Söder O: Intratesticular transplantation of testicular cells from leukemic rats causes transmission of leukemia. Cancer Res 2001;61:706–710.
75 Committee IP, Kim SS, Donnez J, Barri P, Pellicer A, Patrizio P, et al: Recommendations for fertility preservation in patients with lymphoma, leukemia, and breast cancer. J Assist Reprod Genet 2012;29:465–468.
76 Rosendahl M, Greve T, Andersen CY: The safety of transplanting cryopreserved ovarian tissue in cancer patients: a review of the literature. J Assist Reprod Genet 2013;30:11–24.
77 Bastings L, Beerendonk CC, Westphal JR, Massuger LF, Kaal SE, van Leeuwen FE, et al: Autotransplantation of cryopreserved ovarian tissue in cancer survivors and the risk of reintroducing malignancy: a systematic review. Hum Reprod Update 2013;19:483–506.
78 Sadri-Ardekani H, Homburg CH, van Capel TM, van den Berg H, van der Veen F, van der Schoot CE, et al: Eliminating acute lymphoblastic leukemia cells from human testicular cell cultures: a pilot study. Fertil Steril 2014;101: 1072–1078.e1.

Jan-Bernd Stukenborg
Department of Women's and Children's Health, Paediatric Endocrinology Unit
NORDFERTIL Research Lab Stockholm; Q2:08, Karolinska Institute and University Hospital
SE–171 76 Stockholm (Sweden)
E-Mail jan-bernd.stukenborg@ki.se

Author Index

Subject Index